Plastic Reason

Plastic Reason

AN ANTHROPOLOGY OF BRAIN SCIENCE
IN EMBRYOGENETIC TERMS

Tobias Rees

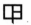

UNIVERSITY OF CALIFORNIA PRESS

University of California Press, one of the most distinguished university presses in the United States, enriches lives around the world by advancing scholarship in the humanities, social sciences, and natural sciences. Its activities are supported by the UC Press Foundation and by philanthropic contributions from individuals and institutions. For more information, visit www.ucpress.edu.

University of California Press
Oakland, California

Library of Congress Cataloging-in-Publication Data

Rees, Tobias, author.
    Plastic reason : an anthropology of brain science in embryogenetic terms / Tobias Rees.
        pages cm
    Includes bibliographical references and index.
    ISBN 978-0-520-28812-6 (cloth : alk. paper)
    ISBN 978-0-520-28813-3 (pbk. : alk. paper)
    ISBN 978-0-520-96317-7 (ebook)
    1. Developmental neurobiology.   2. Brain—Research—History.
3. Neuroplasticity.   4. Subject—Subsubject.   I. Title.
    QP363.5.R44   2016
    612.6'4018—dc23   2015032358

Manufactured in the United States of America

24   23   22   21   20   19   18   17   16
10   9   8   7   6   5   4   3   2   1

In keeping with a commitment to support environmentally responsible and sustainable printing practices, UC Press has printed this book on Natures Natural, a fiber that contains 30% post-consumer waste and meets the minimum requirements of ANSI/NISO Z39.48-1992 (R 1997) (*Permanence of Paper*).

For K.
whom I love so dearly.
without whom nothing would be.
to whom I owe so much.
take this.
it is for you.

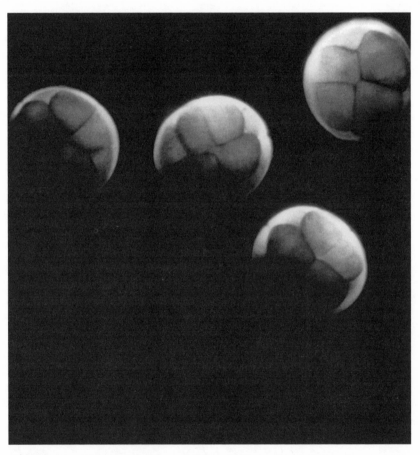

"7." © Ariel Ruiz i Altaba. Selenium-toned gelatin silver print, 15 × 15 inches, from the series *Embryonic Landscapes*. www.ruizialtaba.com. Frog embryos at the blastula stage.

CONTENTS

ILLUSTRATIONS

THE GROUND OF THE ARGUMENT

For most of the twentieth century, neuronal researchers took it for granted that the adult human brain is a thoroughly fixed and immutable cellular structure.

This book is an anthropological study of the intense turbulences provoked by the observation that some basic embryogenetic processes—most spectacularly the emergence of new cellular tissue in the form of new neurons, axons, dendrites, and synapses—continue to occur in the mature brain; that these new nervous tissues are still unspecified and hence literally plastic; and that this cellular plasticity is constitutive of the very possibility of being human.

Clandestine claims about the plasticity of the adult human brain first began to circulate in the margins of the neuronal sciences as early as the 1960s. However, it was only around the year 2000 that these claims consolidated enough to challenge fixity—just when I was arriving in Paris to begin my fieldwork in the laboratory of Alain Prochiantz, a critical site of this consolidation.

Could it be, Prochiantz and colleagues had been wondering since the early 1990s, that a "silent embryogenesis" continues to unfold in the adult brain and thereby renders it plastic and thus adaptable and hence open toward the future?

For the majority of neuronal scientists, such claims of plasticity were scandalous, for the very possibility of a continuity of embryogenetic processes in the mature nervous system threatened to undermine the one anatomical observation that had, tacitly, organized neuronal knowledge production since the late nineteenth century: adult cerebral fixity.

As early as the 1880s it had been determined that the birth of new nerve cells is an event of embryogenesis exclusively. And already by the late 1890s it had been firmly established that the spectacular growth of the brain's fine structure—the branches through which nerve cells connect to one another—ceases once adulthood is reached. "In fully grown animals," the Spanish histologist Santiago Ramón y Cajal put it in 1897, "the nervous system is essentially fixed."

Together these two observations defined a predicament that quietly structured the whole of twentieth-century neuroscience: How can an immutable brain allow for learning? For memory? For behavioral changes?

Conceptually and experimentally, the answers that emerged to these questions over the following century varied significantly. The brain, and with it the human, was successively known as a forest composed of neuronal trees (since the 1880s), as organized in closed (reticular) neuronal circuits (since the 1890s), as an electrical information-processing telegraph (since 1900), as a cybernetic machine (since the 1950s), and as a neurochemical organ composed of neurotransmitter-producing neurons connected to one another through synapses (1950s to 1990s). And yet, no matter how the conceptions of the brain changed over the course of the twentieth century, from the perspective of the nascent conception of the plastic brain they all had one thing in common: they were all grounded in the presupposition that the adult human brain is a fixed and immutable cellular structure.

What if this presupposition would prove to be wrong? What if thousands of new neurons were born in the adult human brain every day? If axons and dendrites continuously sprouted and connected neurons in new ways? If synapses were to ceaselessly appear and disappear?

When, while conducting fieldwork in Prochiantz's lab, I first began to understand that plasticity escapes the conceptual presuppositions that had organized twentieth-century brain research, I began to wonder if I could be the anthropologist of this escape—of the new, unanticipated space of possibility it opened up? The moment seemed opportune, as Prochiantz's lab was one of the key sites of the articulation of what I gradually came to call *plastic reason*—the effort to think of the adult human brain in terms of its retained embryogenetic plasticity.

Could I study the labor that goes into coming up with a whole new way of knowing the brain, by following the work of Prochiantz? By mapping the turbulences that surrounded his lab's project to make experimental embryology the science adequate to understanding the adult human brain? Could I use Prochiantz's lab as a lens for bringing into view the breaking open of the conceptual horizon that had organized, like a scaffold, the neuronal sciences for most of the twentieth century?

When I set out to address these questions in the fall of 2002, the old truth of fixity had already been undermined. But no new, coherent conception of the central nervous system had yet emerged to take its place. No one knew yet whether the brain actually was plastic or not. No one knew what plasticity would mean. Shortly after the turn of the millennium, the plastic brain did not yet exist, or only tentatively, in different, not always commensurate forms that flared up in expected and unexpected openings—in lab meetings, in conversations late at night, while conducting experiments, or while overhearing a conversation in the corridor or the elevator.

The challenge of my fieldwork has been to capture these openings, these unruly, untamed possibilities for conceptualizing the brain—the human as constituted by the brain—differently. The fact that they often didn't add up, that they went off in very different, partly mutually exclusive directions, only increased my excitement.

Plastic Reason is a study of knowledge in motion. It is about the breaking open of an established truth and the turbulence such a breaking open creates. It is about the emergences—in the plural—of efforts to work toward a new way of thinking and knowing the brain, its diseases, and its humans. *Plastic Reason* is about the emergence of possibilities where before there were none.

It has been said that the aim of an anthropology of reason is "to determine what can reasonably be said." *Plastic Reason* is a study of a situation in which what can reasonably be said (about the brain and the human) has been mutating.

NOTE ON TECHNICAL TERMS

Five independent but not unrelated technical vocabularies are of critical importance to this study.

The first one concerns the term *neuron*. Since the first appearance of the term in 1891, neurons have been known as the main functional building blocks of the nervous system. In humans, they make up—there is much current debate about this—between 10 and 50 percent of the total brain mass. The other 50 to 90 percent are *glia* cells, from the Greek *gloia,* meaning "glue." The assumption is that glia cells protect and nourish neurons. Each neuron is composed of a *soma,* or cell body, of one long projection called an *axon* and several shorter projections called *dendrites.* At their ends, axons and dendrites branch out. On dendrites grow tiny boughs called *dendritic spines.* Neurons communicate with one another through *synapses,* which release and take up chemical molecules referred to as *neurotransmitters.* The term *neurogenesis* refers to the generation and growth of new neurons. Until 1998, it was assumed that in humans all neurons are generated before or soon after birth. In that year, scientist discovered *adult neurogenesis*—the birth of new neurons in adult human brains.

The second technical vocabulary revolves around the term *plasticity,* which in this study refers to the continuity of some basic embryogenetic processes in the adult brain. *Embryogenesis* refers to the growth processes that lead from a fertilized egg through the multiplication of cells—termed *mitosis*—to the differentiation and migration of embryonic cells into all tissues and organs of a living organism. Because the early cells of the embryo are *pluripotent*—they can become a whole set of different kinds of cells, constitutive of different kinds of tissue—and because they still undergo growth processes through which they change their form, embryologists speak of *embryonic plasticity.* A plastic cell is thus either a cell that can still multiply and give rise to new, not yet differentiated cells, or a cell that can continue to change its form. Thus, to say that a *silent embryogenesis* continues to unfold in adult brains is to suggest that new, yet undifferentiated, and in that sense plastic, neurons still appear in the brain—adult neurogenesis—and that existing neurons maintain a basic level of plasticity so that they can continue to change their form, for example, in response to experience. Until the late 1990s, adult cerebral plasticity was deemed impossible. It was thought that once adulthood is reached, the brain is, on the level of neurons, axons, and dendrites or dendritic spines, devoid of any growth processes and hence of any plastic—embryonic—potential.

The third set of technical terms comes from genetics and is centered on *homeotic genes* and the proteins they give rise to, *homeoproteins.* Since the 1890s, biologists have used the term *homoiosis*—from the Greek word for "similar"—to refer to mutations in which one body part is replaced by another structurally similar one—say, an antenna by a leg. In the 1940s, genes were first identified that, when mutated, cause a homoiosis, and by the early 1980s it had been established that homeotic genes control the embryo-genetic formation of the basic anatomical structure in a large variety of animals. In 1985, after genetic sequencing had become widely available, it was discovered that all known animals have homeotic genes and that what all homeotic genes share, across the animal kingdom, is a 180 base pair long nucleotide sequence, called the *homeobox.* These discoveries led many to speculate that all homeotic genes are derived from a single ancestor and that all body plans are a variation of a single, original form. Homeotic genes became known as master control genes of embryogenesis. And homeoproteins? Each homeobox-containing gene encodes one particular kind of protein. Through a process of translation (from DNA to RNA) and transcription (from RNA to protein), the nucleotide sequence of a homeotic gene is changed into a set of amino acids. In that process the 180 base pair long homeobox is decoded into a 60 amino acid long structure called the *homeodomain* (proteins are made up of amino acids). The homeodomain is what makes a given homeoprotein a *transcription factor,* that is, a protein that can attach itself to DNA and activate a particular gene. Homeoproteins activate homeotic genes. Over the course of the 1990s, just when the critical importance of homeoproteins for the embryogenetic formation of the brain was being established, it was discovered that homeoproteins are also expressed in neurons of the adult brain, where they seemed to keep nerve cells in a plastic—embryonic—state. Could it be, therefore, that homeoproteins induce a silent embryogenesis in adult human brains?

The fourth entry in my list of technical terms concerns less a term, strictly speaking, than a grammatical oddity: my frequent refusal to use the word *about* where proper English would demand it. For example, I frequently write that the emergence of plastic reason changes how one can *think the brain* (rather than how one can think *about* the brain). The reason for this is an analytical one: the major focus of this study is on thought (understood as practice) and on how the work that went into elaborating a new way of thinking—plasticity—has made the brain into a new, a different kind of, object (one that did not as such exist before).

Were I to use the word *about* in relation to thinking, however, I would sever the practice of thinking from the object of thought. I would suggest that the brain is a given, that it is an obvious object out there, independent from the way it is, well, thought. More than that, I would ultimately suggest that the world is organized in discrete objects waiting to be discovered and described by science. And that would be grossly misleading. I am far from suggesting that the brain is just a human invention (a construct) or that what the brain is and how it functions were actually contingent on how humans talk or think about the brain. That would be a naïve overinterpretation of the significance of human words or knowledge. However, it would be equally naïve to unwittingly decouple the brain from the work that has been necessary to single it out from an undifferentiated real and to constitute it as an object; it would be naïve to decouple it from the history of the nonlinear, conceptually fragmented, and experimentally often incommensurable ways in which it has been known. By dropping *about* I endeavor to make visible that the brain (just as well as homeoproteins or neurons) is not so much found as constituted. And I want to make visible that a major change in the ways in which *the brain can be thought* is much more than a change in the way in which one can think *about* the brain: it is a reordering of the real, is a reconstitution of an object.

Thought doesn't create matter—but it constitutes it.

The last technical formulation to mention is owed to my interpretation of anthropology as (among other things) the study of *the human*. What I mean by this phrase *the human* is not that there is some unchanging essence to being human of which anthropology would be the guardian. On the contrary, I understand the human as an open question and as such as an analytical tool that can be applied to different domains to find out how, at a given time in a given domain, the human is conceptually configured. The implication here is that the human is not a given but a concept, one that often remains hidden in everyday life; that is nowhere clearly articulated but that nonetheless configures the possible—how humans can live and can think about themselves and the world; one that has often undergone dramatic changes.

In the late eighteenth century, in the work of the Viennese physician Franz Josef Gall, the claim first emerged that what is constitutive of humans, what sets the human apart from all other beings, is their brain. In this book I am concerned with this grounding of the human in the brain. More specifically, I am concerned with a far-reaching conceptual reconfiguration of what the brain is—the discovery of its homeoprotein-induced embryogenetic plasticity—and with how this reconfiguration unwittingly upsets and mutates the conception of the human that had been inscribed in the cerebral organ since the term *neuron* was first coined. I am concerned with the human in motion.

ACKNOWLEDGMENTS

It is through relations—through exposure to the world—that ideas emerge and mature (and not just ideas). I am thrilled to have the chance to make visible to the world how very grateful I am for the relationships that have given potential to my thinking and writing.

First, there were those who welcomed me and patiently engaged me in conversations that opened up spaces of marvel and surprise, conversations that opened questions I had not even known one could ask. I still blush when I think about the gifts I received during my years at Berkeley.

Paul Rabinow introduced me to the art of "fieldwork in philosophy" and helped me to see—and enjoy—the beauty of a philosophically inclined anthropology focused on *Vernunft*. It is thanks to our countless conversations in his office, on walks through Berkeley, in the Jardin and the Rostand, in Texas, on airplanes, and on trains that I first came to think of my research as an empirical study of a moment in which the philosophical presuppositions that silently, in nonabstract ways, organize everyday life mutate.

Let's think about thinking.

As much I owe to my admired teacher and friend Lawrence Cohen. Lawrence's adaptation of *philia,* his quest for exuberance, his wild realism, his adamant insistence on not reducing scenes of life to academically convenient arguments and on instead following the intricate, often broken lines that escape just these arguments, were form-giving to my anthropological ventures. It was in conversations with Lawrence (about the total book) that I first came to wonder whether perhaps one (of the many) challenge(s) of fieldwork as realism could be the accumulation of a surplus of questions, ideas, curiosities, associative flights—surfeits of the unexpected. Not as a means toward an end, but as an end: a surplus of questions one could never exhaust.

Your friendship means the world to me.

Irina Paperno's response to my work, the response of a literary scholar to an anthropologist of science inspired by the dreams of early-twentieth-century German *Kulturwissenschaft,* has opened up new horizons to me. Our conversations about Tolstoy and Dostoevsky, about Zola and Flaubert, about Auerbach and Warburg—about life and science—were most inspiring. And her strict insistence on *Sachlichkeit,* her reactions against the anthropologist's self-centered descriptions of his field experience, have been invaluable correctives for me.

Sharon Kaufman has provided keen intellectual guidance throughout my research adventures, for which our conversations about conceptions of life itself have proven extraordinarily helpful. Her wisdom has helped me to understand that, and to what degree, science is a lived space, even (or especially) where life itself has become the object of science. And once I was writing, Sharon's insistence that I not let concepts get in my way spared me from many mistakes.

I miss you both dearly.

Then I left Berkeley for Paris. Here the first to mention is—again and again—Alain Prochiantz, and not only because he opened up his lab to me (and made me learn how to produce neuron cultures and watch them grow). Alain taught me more than I can list here. Two lessons, however, ought to be mentioned: the beauty of a biology that wants to do full justice to the irreducible richness of life, and the joy of a science of movement in terms of movement. As anyone who has read anything I published on the idea of anthropology as a field science must recognize after reading *Plastic Reason,* I owe him more than he can be aware of. And then there are the members of his lab: Bernadette Alinquant, Isabelle Cailé, Edmont Dupont, Alain Joliot, Stéphane Nedelec, Michael Tassetto, Alain Trembleau, Michel Volovitch, and especially Brigitte Lesaffre, who took care of me, who walked me around, took me out, shared her life's stories with me. Her, in particular, I wish well.

I would also like to thank Philippe Ascher, Jean Pierre Bourgeois, Jean François Brunet, Jean Pierre Changeux, and Christo Goridis for the time they spent with me.

While in Paris, I had the great privilege of sharing some of my unruly thoughts with senior colleagues in the human sciences. I gained much insight from the Wednesday lunches with Ian Hacking; from a walk with Bruno Latour through the Jardin du Luxembourg; from tea hours with Michel

Callon; and from Claude Imbert's introductions to the history of French thought. Gratitude is also due to Claude Debru and Michel Morange.

And then there are the walks through Paris with Aude Milet; the croissants beure every morning with Isabelle Brunet; the many, many evenings with G. F.; the countless Sunday afternoons with Corentin La Magueresse, who became my *prochain* and reminded me of just how difficult it is to be an object; and the flights with Jean François Peyret, who has opened up venues of thought that would have otherwise remained hidden from me. He—his plays—provided me with a first sense of what I hoped to achieve.

Like every fieldworker, the anthropologist of science is confronted with the difficulties and pleasures of becoming part of a foreign society. Intimacy is the shameless but hilarious method.

I also would like to thank Frédérik Keck and Joëlle Soler for their friendship.

Once I began writing, a whole new set of challenges and concerns emerged on the horizon. Michael Hagner has generously commented on chapters and provided important insight. George Marcus's insistence on design found in the field has proven invaluable to me—as a guiding principle and equally as a suggestion of what the art of fieldwork could consist in. Thank you, George, for being there, for listening, for talking back, for giving advice, for your friendship. Conversations with Sarah Franklin, on plasticity and on the future, have not only sustained but furthered my interest in plastic matters. The same is true for the wonderful exchanges with Hannah Landecker about plasticity, *The Island of Doctor Moreau,* and the biological human. My work has gained immensely from Hannah's exceptionally fine mind. Nicolas Rose listened and gave advice when I was most insecure. Finally, I had the privilege of working with and listening to Fritz W. Kramer. Our conversations about ethnography past and present have been wonderfully inspiring and have opened up new possibilities, new ways to travel. And, almost as important, he offered moral and intellectual support when it was most needed in my struggles with the (written) wor(l)d.

Three friends, Carlo Caduff, Nick Langlitz, and Janet Roitman, have read and commented on several versions of chapters presented here. Nick's associations were more than once helpful in finding a better form for the things I tried to say. Carlo's enthusiasm, coupled with his thorough listings of my various mistakes, provided solace and support. In fact, without Carlo's often immediate response to my worries, my despair in writing would have been unbearable. And Janet's extraordinary sense for the poetic quality of dry ethnographic language—and her hot chocolate—kept my imagination going.

Comments along the way were provided by Nima Bassiri, David Bates, Stephen Casper, Gabriella Coleman, Debbie Cohen, Stefan Ecks, Fred Gage, Stefanos Geroulanos, Delia Gravus, Anne Harrington, Stefan Helmreich, Adrian Johns, Eric Kandel, Gerd Kempermann, Kenton Kroker, Andy Lakoff, Katherine Lemons, Catherine Malabou, Emily Martin, Martin Pickersgell, Joelle Abi-Rachid, Rayna Rapp, Eugene Raikhel, Robert Richards, Beatrix Rubin, and Miriam Ticktin.

I am especially grateful to Peter Redfield for helping me understand the practice of provocation; to Vincanne Adams for her wisdom; to Alberto Sanchez for being my best friend in the world; to Warwick Anderson for his encouragement (and a Sunday roast); to Miriam Ticktin for her complicity; and to Stephen Collier for our continuous conversations about concept work.

You are my family.

Once I joined McGill's Department of Social Studies of Medicine (SSoM), in 2009, a new adventure began in my intellectual life—and again new venues of thinking and orienting oneself opened up. There are the conversations with Allan Young about foreign moons of reason and about anthropology as a rigorous intellectual endeavor; the explorations with Margaret Lock of the complicated relations of the social and the vital; Alberto Cambrosio's consistent challenge to consider concepts as practical configurations and his invitations to explore the possibilities of a postdisciplinarily science; the discussions with Thomas Schlich about practices and plastic surgery; the wondering together with Andrea Tone whether neuroscience has moved "after" neurochemistry and what that could mean; and the debates with George Weisz about France, the French, and French epistemology.

And then there is—always, every day—Abraham Fuks. Thank you, Abe, for being there and for always having your door open.

SSoM also opened up for me the joy of working with students—with Dörte Bemme, Raad Fadaak, Kristin Flemons, Fiona Gedeon Achi (Quentin Stoeffler!), Julianne Yip, Adam Fleischmann, Nicole Rigillo. Your questions—and answers—have been a gift, and our Friday afternoon "thought collective," one of the most enriching aspects of my intellectual journey thus far.

It was at SSoM that I first learned how much it matters to actually tend the intellectual environment one is part of—to foster it, to intervene in it, to build it.

At the University of California Press I want to thank Reed Malcolm and Stacy Eisenstark, for taking me on and for enduring my questions as well as my countless worries, and to Kate Hoffman, who shepherded me through the production process. I am also grateful to the two reviewers who provided comments on an earlier version of this manuscript. One of them was anonymous, and the other was Stefan Helmreich, whose generosity has prevented me from quite a few mistakes. The other reader's name remains unknown to me. Special thanks goes to Kerry Tremain, my exceptionally gifted writing coach. I hope that at least some of the projects we envisioned for the future come true.

Finally, though by far most important, my gratitude goes to my family. The one that was home, M. and P., and the one that has become home. To be surrounded by K., J., and C., to have the chance to be part of their lives, to share mine with them, has meant a joy indescribable in words.

On Growth and Form

Not long after I arrived in the lab—it was concerned with the embryonic formation of the brain—I noticed that its director, Alain Prochiantz, frequently walked
into the cell culture room, where he placed a seemingly randomly chosen petri
dish of growing neurons under a microscope. Then he just watched for a little
while.

I found that curious. "What is he doing there?" I eventually asked Brigitte
Lesaffre, a senior researcher who had taken care of me during my first months
at the lab.

"Alain?" she said. "He watches how neurons grow."

I wasn't sure whether this was an answer. But Brigitte's voice—or perhaps it
was the way she looked at me—suggested that she had given a most meaningful response. And so I decided to leave it at that.

Only much later did I realize that Brigitte's reply was just the beginning of an
answer—that my whole fieldwork was in fact one long, multifaceted, emergent
response to my question, a question the stakes of which I hadn't been aware of
when I first asked it.

In any case, during my time in the lab, hardly a day passed without a
conversation about cellular growth. I learned about the deeply moving—
aesthetically, ethically, intellectually—observation of the coming into existence of form where before there was none. I was engaged in conversations
about the exquisite, always changing forms that cellular growth gives rise to.
I was introduced to forms in motion and initiated in the art of following this
motion. I was told that "form" is perhaps the wrong word, for it suggests continuity, something stable, whereas in reality there is only becoming and hence
movement. In short, I was introduced, in so many different ways, to the beauty
of cellular growth.

And during one of these conversations, I, for the first time, understood that
while the lab was officially dedicated to embryology, its actual aim was to
show that embryogenetic growth continues in the adult, where, counter to the

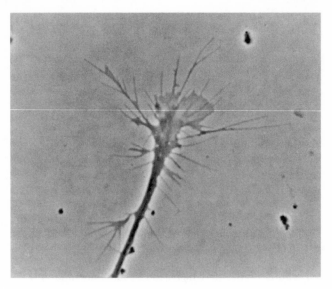

A growing neuron. Courtesy of the American Association for the Advancement of Science.

established conception of the brain as a fixed and immutable structure it gives rise to new, not yet specified and hence plastic (formable) tissue. What is more, I understood that the lab's work was grounded in the possibility that this embryogenetic generation of plastic tissue in the mature brain might be the decisive cerebral process—the one that is constitutive of the human.

ONE

Entry

Il s'agit de prouver que les phénomènes du développement n'existent pas seulement dans l'état embryonnaire, mais qu'ils se poursuivent dans l'état adulte.

CLAUDE BERNARD

The beauty of fieldwork is its unpredictability. What one will discover, if anything at all, cannot be known in advance. The challenge is to submit to the outside, to become part of a foreign milieu, to drown in it—and to stay alert to the unforeseen story that is gradually emerging.

The unforeseen story that has been emerging in the course of my fieldwork among Parisian neurobiologists, that intrigued me and involved me and carried me away in unexpected directions, was the story of what I came to call *plastic reason*—the story of the sometimes intensely contested effort by people such as Brigitte Lesaffre and Alain Prochiantz to prove that was a "silent embryogenesis" keeps the adult human brain plastic.[1] In this introduction I trace how I became a part of this story, this effort, and to provide a first sketch of what is at stake in it.

UNFORESEEN

I had never planned to do work on the brain, let alone its retained embryogenetic plasticity. When I arrived in Paris in early 2002, I wanted to study French biology. To be more precise, I had prepared to inquire into the belated emergence of French—as compared to American or British—biotechnology. Why was there this delay in France? I had wondered whether it had something to do with the late and controversial French institutionalization of molecular cell biology. Could it be that the belated emergence of biotechnology was a reflection of the predominance, in France, of a different, a nonmolecular biology? Different not just in its conception of the living but also in its practice?[2]

In addition, I hoped to explore the relationship between two things often said to have no relationship at all: life and science. "Science," Max Weber famously quoted Tolstoy in the early twentieth century, "is meaningless because it gives no answer to our question, the only question important for us: What shall we do? How shall we live?"[3] What, I wondered, is the relationship between life and science a century later? How is life lived where life itself, in the form of biotechnology, has become the object of scientific knowledge and intervention? How do organisms living their life relate to new knowledge about living organisms?

Once I arrived in France, however, things developed in unforeseen ways. Gaining access to biotechnology centers turned out to be arduous and slow. Weeks passed, and I made little progress in securing a site for my research. But while my frustration with biotechnology labs grew, an unexpected opportunity opened up. I was offered the chance to work in the laboratory of Alain Prochiantz, located at the École Normale Supérieure (ENS) and concerned with the evolution and development of the nervous system.[4]

In conversations with Alain, I learned that he had a plan.[4] "Until September," he explained, "you will work in the lab and learn how to practice at the bench. From October onward, you will then participate in a DEA, a yearlong program in neuropharmacology, and conduct your own research under my supervision."[5] I could thus gain a practical and conceptual understanding of neurobiology, he went on, and that would allow me, perhaps, to do better anthropological research. Was I interested?

I was overwhelmed by this unexpected opportunity—and felt ambivalent about it. Not only was I unsure if I actually wanted to learn how to dissect and experiment on brains, but more important, my visits to the lab made clear that the work of Prochiantz's group did not speak to the curiosity I had so carefully fostered. I wanted to learn about biology, about biotechnology, and about life and science in France. What would I do in a developmental neurobiology lab? I had never read any article, let alone any book, about the brain. I knew nothing about neuroscience.

If, despite my severe concerns, I soon began working in Alain's lab, it was because I quickly became enamored of the intensity that radiated from it—by the movement that seemed to grip everyone who came near it. I could not make sense of this movement, of this intensity, but it intrigued and engaged me, and it carried me further and further away from the questions I had set out to study.

I began, if still hesitantly, to do fieldwork in neurobiology.

The lab was located on the seventh floor of the nine-story Science Building of the ENS, in the Rue d'Ulm, in the Fifth Arrondissement of Paris. I began working in the lab in March 2002, and my first few months were dominated by practice. I learned how to dissect brains; how to distinguish shapes of neurons taken from diverse brain parts; how to grow neurons in cultures and how to feed them, infect them, and crash them with a centrifuge. In parallel, I began to make sense of the movement that had attracted me to the lab in the first place. Gradually, I could reconstruct the following, somewhat unlikely story.

In the late 1980s, Alain began experimenting with homeotic genes. At that time homeotic genes—and the proteins they code for, homeoproteins—were known to coordinate the formation of the basic body structure in animal development. Alain's idée fixe was that homeoproteins, transcription factors that regulate which part of DNA is activated and when, might also be involved in the cellular formation of the central nervous system.[6] Perhaps homeoproteins determine whether a cell becomes part of the gut or of the brain? Perhaps they even coordinate whether a cell becomes a hippocampal, rather than, say, a striatal, neuron?

In experiments Alain Prochiantz conducted with Alain Joliot, a graduate student who had become a senior researcher in his unit by the time of my fieldwork, he made three observations: that homeoproteins, at least in vitro, appear to slide between cells; that this sliding seems to cause a powerful morphogenetic outgrowth even in already differentiated neurons; and that homeoproteins are found not only in the embryonic but also in the adult human brain.[7]

To Prochiantz and Joliot these observations were exhilarating. Quickly they went public and informed their peers that they might have identified a not yet known developmental mechanism—the cell-to-cell migration of homeoproteins—that is active not just in the developing but also in the adult brain, where it appeared to engender embryogenetic-like processes.

Perhaps, they speculated, drunk by the possibilities opened up by their experiment, the adult human brain is the locus of a "silent embryogenesis."[8]

To their colleagues, both suggestions were absurd. First, at the time, it was held that cells are strictly autonomous, that each cell acts according to the genetic information it carries in its nucleus. That there could be a protein-based, rather than a cell-based, organization of embryogenesis, that is, a non-cell-autonomous mechanism was at best fantastic. Second, it was a well-established experimental fact that transcription factors exist somewhat exclusively in the nucleus and that, should they ever travel across the cytoplasm and cell membrane, they would degenerate. That homeoproteins would slide from cell to cell, whether in the embryo or in the adult, was utterly absurd. Third, generations of histologists had shown that the birth, migration, and differentiation of neurons occur exclusively in the course of embryogenesis and that, once adulthood is reached, the myriad connections that build up between neurons during development hardly change. The adult human brain was known to be a fixed and immutable structure, with synaptic communication as the only true dynamic element.[9] To claim, as Prochiantz and Joliot did, that homeoproteins would keep up basic embryogenetic processes in the adult was a ridiculous idea to be laughed at, *the* statement beyond the scope of (neuronal) reason.

Alain's reaction to the laughter of his colleagues was seriousness. With cool restraint he insisted that he and Joliot had indeed discovered a little-understood developmental mechanism—the cell-to-cell sliding of homeoproteins—that is critical for the embryogenesis of the nervous system as well as for a silent embryogenesis occurring in the adult. Plasticity, he maintained in talks, radio shows, articles, and popular science books, is the very perspective from which one has to think the brain.[10]

With his staggering suggestions, Alain outraged his peers. In the eyes of many of his Parisian colleagues, he had gone too far, beyond what a good neuronal researcher could reasonably say about the brain. When, despite his colleague's severe protests, he decided to devote his lab exclusively to the role of homeoproteins in the developing and the adult brain, French neuroscience had its scandal, and its enfant terrible.

The consequences were severe. Alain—his lab—was increasingly isolated, with no collaborators to speak of. If he and his researchers had not been in France, where the budget for civically funded research is (almost) independent from the actual research being done, their lab would have disappeared.

And then the unexpected happened.

In the late 1990s, after Alain's lab had worked in isolation for almost a decade, two American groups published reports documenting the birth of new neurons in diverse parts of the adult primate (1997) and the adult human brain (1998).[11] These reports established decisively that at least some embryogenetic processes continue in the adult human brain. And they reinforced the spectacular possibility that Prochiantz and his co-workers had sought to elaborate for almost a decade: that the adult human brain is a plastic organ.

For Alain's lab, the discovery that new neurons are born in adult brains marked a turning point in the reception of its work. It now seemed conceivable that he and Joliot had indeed made an important discovery—that homeoproteins are plastic forces active in the mature nervous system. For isn't it precisely the role of homeoproteins during embryogenesis to trigger and then organize the birth, differentiation, and migration of neurons? Could it not be, then, that this is also their task in the adult? Perhaps the cell-to-cell migration of homeoproteins is a kind of signal that regulates adult neurogenesis? Perhaps they provoke the birth of new cells, which they then shape and guide?[12] Perhaps the adult human brain is plastic.

It was as if Alain and colleagues had elaborated an answer to a question that was only now becoming conceivable. What had seemed ridiculous had become avant-garde.

In France Alain's sudden international recognition as an avant-garde thinker and most prominent voice of the newly emerging field of plasticity research caused an intense revival of the polemic that had surrounded his work since the late 1980s. Many of his colleagues angrily insisted that a transfer of homeoproteins is impossible, that plastic changes occur only in minor centers of the brain, that the brain, after all, is an immutable chemical machine, and that Alain was a postmodern out there to destroy science. At home, Alain was not a genius, but a provocateur, and his work on plasticity not a breakthrough, but a scandalous attack on science.

When I traveled to Paris in 2002, I arrived amid these debates about Alain and his work. Hence, the intense motion that surrounded him, his lab, and almost everyone who came close to it.

OF MOTION

Once I understood that the motion that surrounded the lab in which I had accidentally arrived was provoked by a possibly far-reaching metamorphosis of the neuronal conception of the brain, and once I understood that Alain's lab was an exemplary site for thinking about the brain from the perspective of its retained embryogenetic plasticity, I became incredibly excited by the possibility of an anthropology of knowledge—of thought—in motion.

The distinct beauty of the situation I found myself in, or so it seemed to me, was its openness, its no-longer-not-yet quality—after fixity, yet on the way to plasticity.[13] I was thrilled by the idea that a new, not yet fully elaborated way of thinking and knowing the brain was emerging, one that would likely change what the brain "is." In addition, there was the clear sense, conveyed by countless conversations I had in the course of my fieldwork, that what was at stake in the turmoil surrounding me was less the brain per se than the brain as the locus of the human.

What was at stake was a shift from a conceptualization of the brain—the human—as a neurochemical machine largely determined in its basic design, fixed in its being, toward a conceptualization of the brain—the human—as a ceaselessly emerging cellular organ, an organ that never stands still, that is defined by an irreducible openness. At stake was a shift from neurochemistry to plasticity.

Gradually, I began to recognize the opportunity: as anthropologist of Alain's lab, a lab that many of my interlocutors held responsible for the scandalous advent of plasticity, I could study the conceptual and experimental work that goes into the formulation of a new way of thinking and knowing the brain (and the human). And as an anthropologist of the Parisian neuroscientific community, with its intense reactions to Alain's work, I could study the relational, conceptual, and institutional motion that paralleled the emergence of plasticity—the battles, the debates, the gossip, the affirmations, and eventually, if plasticity would stabilize, the gradual transformation of the institutional landscape, including the emergence of new grants for plasticity research and the subsequent establishment of new research groups, new journals, and new prizes. In short, it seemed to me as if there were the exhilarating possibility to document and analyze a profound metamorphosis in the neuronal order of knowledge while it was taking place, a metamorphosis in which the brain, and with it the human, was changing its form and becoming plastic.

And so I let go, if still hesitantly, of my preconceived questions about life and science (and about biology and biotechnology in France) and began to follow the story unfolding around me, which in many ways, if only in retrospect, turned out to be a story of life and science.

I wanted to be the anthropologist of the sweeping and multifaceted motion initiated by plasticity.[14]

This book is the result of my endeavors. It is a fieldwork-based analysis composed of anecdotes, observations, and anthropological trouvailles, interspersed with historical excursions and philosophical reflections of the gradual, tentative, continuously contested effort by Alain and his colleagues to think and know the brain from the perspective of its retained embryogenetic, homeoprotein-induced plasticity. It is an anthropologist's account of the emergence of *plastic reason*.

ON FORM

Finally, a word on form. As I had never prepared to study neuroscience and hence had no concrete research question to guide me when I entered Alain's lab, my research assumed a somewhat curious form. Ultimately, my time in Paris was one long and at times frustratingly nonlinear discovery process. Literally everything about "my" lab's work, and about past and present brain research, came to me in the form of fieldwork-based discoveries.[15] It is only a slight exaggeration to say that every day of fieldwork put things in a new light, changed my understanding, and added an insight or prompted a question that had never before occurred to me.

I initially found this contingent, emergent quality of my fieldwork rather disconcerting. All too frequently, my will to find a topic was undermined by yet another observation that changed my comprehension of what my fieldwork was or could be about. At one point, however, my perception of fieldwork began to change—when I first realized, about seven months after I had begun working in the lab, that plasticity was potentially a major event in the history of brain research and that Alain's lab was a key site of this event.

Was this my topic, plasticity?

Reading through my field notes, I realized that the overwhelming majority of the fairly dispersed and contextually unrelated observations and associations I had collected in my notebooks related in one way or another to Alain's effort to document that the brain is an organ undergoing a continuous, ceaseless morphogenesis. Gradually, I was gaining confidence. And the more confidence I gained, the more I fell in love with the idea that anthropology could be a radical field science. And by "field science" I not only mean that a kind of data production happens in the field. Rather, I mean a practice directed by the outside, a practice at the core of which are accidental encounters, chance observations, and contingent events that eventually give rise, as if by themselves, to an unforeseen, always tentative, emergent story.

In my case, the emergent story my research brought into being coincided temporally and locally with the emergent effort to know the brain from the perspective of its plasticity. It was as if my fieldwork and plasticity literally coevolved.[16] I still marvel at the fact that what had at first seemed a chaotic assembly of anecdotes gradually gave rise to a coherent if multifaceted story utterly impossible to foresee, a story that, without providing closure, gained stability and a certain equilibrium even as I was still, every day, making new discoveries. At the end of my research, fieldwork had become much more than a data-producing method for me. It had become an intellectual as well as aesthetic practice that allowed contingency to give rise to a form where before there was none.

While writing this book, I wanted to capture at least some of the beauty of the emergent quality of my fieldwork—and of the emergent story of plasticity. My ambition (if that is not too ambitious a term) was to involve the reader in the spectacle of the emergence of a form (or story). For that reason I have composed *Plastic Reason* in five chapters, each of which is organized around one or several fieldwork scenes that have been shaping my understanding of the neuronal sciences in general and the emergence of adult cerebral plasticity in the work of Alain's lab in particular.[17]

Plastic Reason, then, is organized around the surprises my research produced. The (kind) reader should, thus, not expect coherence, but surprise.[18]

I title the chapters "Relational" (a relational account of plastic reason); "Conceptual" (an effort to sketch the conceptual challenge at stake in plasticity research); "Nocturnal" (Alain's work on the possible); "Experimental" (the challenge of inventing plastic experiments); and "Ethical" (the difference an ethos of plasticity makes). Every chapter is followed by a digression (at times short and at other times not so short).

Observation

Let's begin in 1948. That year Sien-chiue Yu, a graduate student in genetics at Caltech, found a fruit fly mutant whose antennas had been replaced by legs. Aptly, he called the mutation Antennapedia.[1]

Yu's supervisor, Edward "Ed" Lewis, was an expert in fruit fly mutations, specifically those in which one body part appears in place of another, structurally similar one.[2] Over the years, Lewis had learned to use these so-called homeotic mutations to give experimental contours to the initially somewhat abstract concept of a gene—to define what a gene is, how it functions, how it evolves.

In the late 1950s, prompted in part by Yu's discovery of Antennapedia, Lewis had an idea. Wouldn't it be possible, simply by studying homeotic mutations, to identify at least some of the genes that control the developmental formation of a fruit fly?[3] Over the following twenty years, Lewis identified eight genes that control the development of the chest and the wings. He called these homeotic genes *regulator genes* and, in a 1978 paper, wondered aloud if not all homeotic genes, including the most famous of them, Antennapedia, have such a regulatory function.

Were homeotic genes "master control genes" of fruit fly development?[4]

Inspired by Lewis's question, Christine Nüsslein-Volhard and Eric Wieschaus, then at the European Molecular Biology Laboratory in Heidelberg, Germany, launched a large-scale experimental effort. They began to collect all known fruit fly mutants in the hope that such a collection of curiosities would allow them to systematically identify those genes that, when mutated, alter the usual segmental arrangement of the fruit fly larva. (Each body part emerges from a single segment.) Were their efforts successful, they could identify the proper function of each gene and would eventually be able to list all the genes necessary to build the body of the insects. Already by 1980 they published a first draft of a list that affirmed Lewis's speculation: all genes involved in building a fruit fly body are controlled—regulated—by homeotic genes.[5]

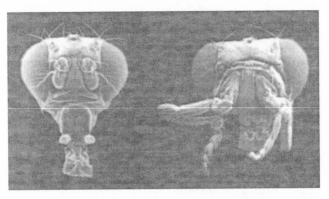

When mutated, the Antennapedia gene causes the growth of a leg in
place of an antenna. Courtesy of Rudi Turner, FlyBase.org.

The discovery that Antennapedia & Co. are indeed master control genes of
fruit fly development gave rise to a new question: how exactly do homeotic
genes control development?

At the time Nüsslein-Volhard and Wieschaus published their first draft list,
their previous supervisor, Walter Gehring, was busy transforming his lab in
Basel, Switzerland, into a fruit fly gene bank.[6] The plan was to sequence all
known fruit fly genes and to thereby facilitate understanding of how the insects
get built. In 1983, while sequencing Antennapedia, Gehring, together with his
postdoc William McGinnis, noted that it shared a DNA sequence with a homeotic gene they had sequenced before. Further experiments followed and
showed that in fact all homeotic genes of the fruit fly share one almost identical, 180 base pairs long DNA sequence. They called this highly conserved
region the homeobox and later discovered that the homeobox codes for precisely that part of homeoproteins that makes them transcription factors; that
is, that allows them to attach themselves to DNA and thereby control when
which part of the genome is activated. They called this part of the proteins
their homeodomain.

Gehring and McGinnis's work suggested that it is the homeobox that makes
homeotic genes master control genes of drosophila development. And it
opened up a spectacular possibility: as homeotic variations were reported for
a large number of animals, could it perhaps be that each one of these mutations was due to a mutation of—homeotic genes? Could it be that all of these
animals actually have genes containing a homeobox?[7]

The possibility seemed spectacular because up to this point it had been
assumed that the development of a mouse, a fruit fly, or a human had very little to do with one another—each animal had its separate, individual line of
development. Now there was the possibility that the development of all these
animals is related, that all known animals are descendants of one single ancestor, and that the evolutionary emergence of different animal forms results

from mutations of homeotic genes and their activation patterns. Only a year later, in 1984, Gehring and his co-workers established that indeed all animals have genes that contain almost exactly the same DNA sequence— the homeobox.

Homeotic genes, it turned out, control the body building not only of fruit flies but of every known animal, including humans.

At this point, in the mid-1980s, Alain enters the story. He was interested in whether homeotic genes play a role in the embryonic formation of the cellular brain. If homeobox-containing genes are body-building genes, if they control the formation of body parts, then could one not assume that they are also brain-forming genes? Perhaps homeotic genes tell cells what kind of nerve cell they should become, which kind of brain center they should build up?

Prochiantz asked Gehring if he could have a copy of the plasmid he had used to clone the Antennapedia gene, and then he recruited Alain Joliot and asked him to study, on the one hand, up until what time in the cellular emergence of the organism Antennapedia is expressed and, on the other hand, the impact of Antennapedia proteins on not yet differentiated neurons in vitro. Imagine their surprise when Prochiantz and Joliot found that Antennapedia is expressed throughout life, in the developing as well as in the already mature brain—and that the Antennapedia protein slides between neurons and causes a powerful morphogenetic outgrowth.

The questions opened up by their experiments gripped them. What are these proteins doing in the adult brain? What is it that these powerful form producers—these plastic forces that form or deform entire organisms—are doing in the mature nervous system? Is there some kind of developmental process going on? In the form of a cell-to-cell sliding of homeoproteins? Is the mature nervous system undergoing some continuous, never ending formation process? Is the brain a form in motion? The locus of a silent embryogenesis? Could it be that the brain is plastic—and embryology the science adequate to the adult human brain?

Add that brain researchers had known for over a century that the adult brain is devoid of developmental processes, that it is an essentially fixed and immutable structure; and add that Prochiantz and Joliot next found that homeotic genes are also expressed in the adult human brain—and their sense that they had made a sweeping observation becomes tangible.

TWO

Relational

The final goal, of which an ethnographer never should lose sight.
This goal is, briefly, to grasp the native point of view, his relation
to life, to realize his vision of his world. We have to study man,
and we have to study what concerns him most intimately, that is,
the hold which life has on him.

BRONISLAW MALINOWSKI

"Have you noticed that Joliot is almost always among the loudest in our meetings?" Brigitte asked when we returned to our bench.

Every Wednesday at noon the whole lab met to discuss the work of one of the four research groups in the laboratory. Brigitte led one of these groups, Joliot another. In addition, there were the teams of Michel Volovitch (like Brigitte and Alain, in his late fifties) and Alain Trembleau (like Joliot, in his early forties). Each group had two or three graduate students and a postdoc.

In the lab meeting that had just ended, Stéphane Nédélec, a student of Trembleau, had presented. (Joliot and Trembleau were usually called by their family names.) And Stéphane's presentation had left everybody excited: he provided some of the first in vivo evidence that a homeoprotein called Emx2 is responsible for continuous axonal sprouting in adult mice.[1]

Most of the scientists directed the questions about Stéphane's report to his supervisor, Trembleau, who had designed the experiments. At one point, however, when Alain was asking Trembleau yet another question, Joliot, who sat in another corner of the room, did an imitation of Trembleau and gave a silly answer that made fun of Emx2 as well as of Stéphane and Trembleau. Everybody laughed. When Michel Volovitch posed a follow up question, Joliot repeated his playful imitation and gave another silly response. The scene was repeated several more times until the lab meeting dissolved into wholehearted laughter.

Such joking held a special place in lab life. Quite frequently our weekly lab meetings became a joking contest, with each participant trying to trump a previous joke or come up with an even more ludicrous association. By far the most common way of joking was to endow homeoproteins with the character traits or gender of the researcher presenting. Often this playful back-and-forth between person and protein got so wild and frivolous that I lost track of who we were talking about (person or protein), a confusion from which a new round of more serious conversation would almost always emerge.

"Yes," I replied to Brigitte, "Joliot is always among the loudest. And among the funniest. He really has a great sense of humor."

Indeed, Joliot was a master of associations. It was almost always he who began blurring the surprisingly thin line between the serious and the silly.

"Do you know about the Curie-Joliot family?" Brigitte went on.

I shook my head.

"You should really know about these things," she smiled.

"What things?" I wanted to know. "And why?"

"Social things, because they matter."

She was adamant that I learn systematically where people come from, what their families are like, with whom they worked, under whom they studied, who their friends are, whom they married and had affairs with, and so forth.

"If you don't," she insisted in the sincere tone of the already initiated, "you won't understand anything at all."

And then, as if to underline what she had told me, she opened the family album.

FAMILY ALBUM

The story begins with Maria Sklodowska. Born in 1867 in Warsaw, Poland, she arrived in Paris in 1891, where she studied physics and math at the Sorbonne.[2] In 1894, the year of the Dreyfus Affair, she met Pierre Curie. The two married only a year later. The year Marie Curie gained her doctor of science degree, 1903, she was also awarded the Nobel Prize for Physics, along with her husband and Henri Becquerel, for the discovery of radioactivity. Following the death of Pierre Curie in 1906, she succeeded him as professor of physics in the faculty of sciences at the University of Paris, the first woman to hold this position.

In 1911, Marie received a second Nobel Prize, this time in chemistry, for the isolation of radium. The same year, she was appointed director of the

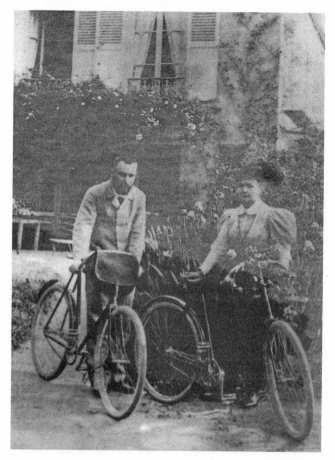

Pierre and Marie Curie on their honeymoon, 1895. Courtesy of the Musée Curie.

Curie Laboratory in the Radium Institute of the University of Paris, founded in 1910. Marie Curie died in 1934—and was the first woman to be buried in the Panthéon.[3]

Marie and Pierre Curie had two children, Irène (1897–1958) and Ève (1904–2007). Ève, inclined toward the fine arts, married Henry Richard Labouisse Jr. (1904–1987), an American diplomat who was the long-standing director of UNICEF and who received, on behalf of UNICEF, the Nobel Peace Prize in 1965. Ève and Richard lived most of their lives in the United States, where she became a well-respected writer and journalist. Ève also made herself a name as a pianist and was, people say, the most glamorous member of the family.

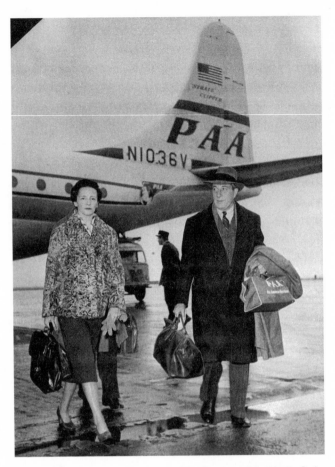

Henry and Ève Labouisse (née Curie), 1954. Courtesy of the Musée Curie.

Irène followed her parents' path—she became a physicist and married a physicist, Frédéric Joliot (1900–1958), whom she met in her mother's laboratory. In 1935, a year after Marie's death, Irène and Frédéric received the Nobel Prize for Chemistry, for the synthesis of new radioactive elements. Two years later, Frédéric was appointed professor at the Collège de France, the most prestigious academic institution in France.

Irène and Frédéric were perhaps the most influential scientists in twentieth-century France.[4] Even before the Second World War they became involved in the political organization of science. In 1934 Frédéric became a member of the Socialists around Leon Blum, who succeeded in uniting the various socialist and communist parties and led "the Left" to an

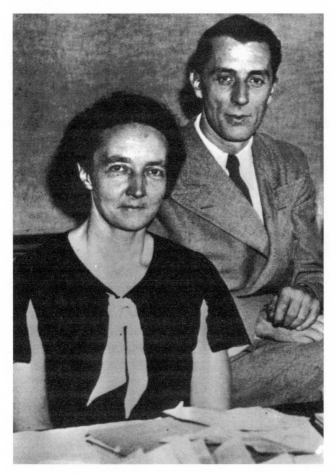

Irène and Frédéric Joliot, 1935. Courtesy of the Musée Curie.

electoral victory in 1936.[5] As prime minister of France, Blum then helped Frédéric to build the first cyclotron in Western Europe, and appointed Irène undersecretary of state for scientific research, with the mandate that she facilitate women's entry into science. And when the Nazis occupied France, Blum managed to move Frédéric's scientific apparatus and data to England.

During the occupation, Frédéric Joliot took an active part in the *résistance*. He became president of the National Front and was centrally involved in the formation of the French Communist Party.

After Hiroshima and Nagasaki, at the beginning of what was to become the Cold War, physics became a central concern in state politics, not least in

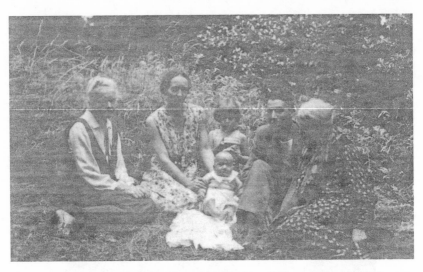

Irène and Frédéric Joliot with their mothers and their children Hélène and Pierre, 1932. Courtesy of the Musée Curie.

the France of General De Gaulle, who sought to establish his country as an important military power. The Joliots played an active role in the construction of a scientifically informed Cold War France. In 1944 Frédéric was appointed director of the Centre National de la Recherche (CNRS), an institution created by the Vichy regime in 1939. His main task was to work out a national plan for the organization of research.

Frédéric Joliot envisioned a *nouvelle politique de la science:* the state should organize and finance scientific research, and researchers should be state civil servants.[6] In 1946, the same year Irène became director of the Radium Institute, he was appointed the first high commissioner for atomic energy. Together they directed the construction of the first French atomic pile, which was launched in 1948. Irène then worked out the plans for a large center for nuclear physics at Orsay; Frédéric continued its construction after her death in 1956.[7]

Irène and Frédéric had two children, Hélène and Pierre. Both became scientists and married scientists from other scientific dynasties. Hélène Langevin-Joliot followed the family tradition, studied physics, and became a professor at the center for nuclear physics at Orsay that her parents had helped found.[8] Pierre, today professor emeritus at the Collège de France, opted for what might be described as the new science of the day, biology.

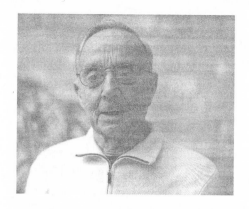

Pierre Joliot, 2015. Courtesy of Mattias Pettersson.

With his wife, Anne Joliot, he has specialized in the bioenergetics of cells and is today one of the great old men of plant biology.

Early on in his career Pierre Joliot, continuing the institutional labor of his father, took part in or presided over several CNRS committees. In the 1970s and 1980s, he had been an important advocate of the molecularization of the biological sciences in France. He was also the first director of the newly created Department of Biology at the École Normale Supérieure in the late 1980s, when Prochiantz got his lab there.

Pierre and Anne have two children, both scientists and both married to scientists. Their son, Alain Joliot, was the graduate student who observed in 1989, along with Alain Prochiantz, that homeoproteins travel in vitro from cell to cell and are expressed in the mature nervous system. In short, Joliot, who was always the loudest (and funniest) in our lab meetings, was the great-grandson of Marie and Pierre Curie, grandson of Irène and Frédéric Joliot, and son of Pierre and Anne Joliot.

RELATIONAL SELVES

Brigitte's introduction to the family album gripped me. During the previous months I had struggled to make sense of the apparent obsession my interlocutors had for relational matters. They had a seemingly inexhaustible curiosity for what they called *des chose sociales* (social things). Busy scientists who rarely had time to answer my questions between experiments were almost always ready to discuss any aspect of life and science in terms of who relates to whom how, how a particular relation came into being, how it was prefigured by other relations, how it led to new ones. The contrast with the few American and German labs in which I had worked—where the exchange of social information was almost entirely absent—could not have been sharper.

At first I ignored these elaborations of things social. I regarded them as a form of gossip. However, the seriousness and persistency with which my interlocutors continuously elaborated on social relations made it difficult to maintain this attitude. Evidently, the theme was dear to them. But why? It was of a relevance, a necessity, that I did not understand—not until Brigitte opened the family album for me. Wasn't her story of the Curie-Joliot history providing me with a suggestive answer? I had the impression that Brigitte was introducing me to something that I came to call, without much conceptual grace, a relational conception of the human, according to which what one is cannot be separated from the relations one has—and doesn't have.

Is this perhaps why they constantly talked about relations? I wondered.

Once Brigitte had shown me the family album, I noticed that it was rather frequently alluded to, if to quite diverse ends. Brigitte had told me the history of the Curie-Joliot lineage to explain "Jojo's" way of being. On other occasions, I heard the same history, or a version of it, to explain why Joliot was given, immediately after earning his PhD, a position as CNRS researcher (because of his family relations); why Alain got a lab at the ENS in 1989 (Pierre Joliot was director of the Department of Biology); and why he might or might not get a job at the Collège de France (again because of Joliot's father), and so forth.[9] Each time the story was told, it was used to elaborate on a person's way of being or to probe why he or she occupied a particular academic position.

The longer I stayed in Paris and the longer I was exposed to conversations about relations, the clearer it became to me that the genealogy that ran from Marie Curie to Alain Joliot was not only not exceptional but in fact exemplary: virtually every one of my conversations about relations, inside as well as outside the lab, traced lines of descent (familial or, more often, through affiliation), explored alliances, discussed them, took them apart, turned them upside down, and then looked at them a second and a third time, thereby illuminating the relational web in which my friends and colleagues lived and worked.

It was by listening to such relational stories, by observing how they choreograph everyday life in Paris—in the *métro,* the café, the classroom, the street, the lab—that I eventually arrived at the assumption that *des choses sociales* were the constitutive ground of the world inhabited by those I spent my life with. They perceived themselves and others as existing in relations.

I am inclined to say existing *exclusively* in relations, for when the self is relational, one exists and gains contours by way of association with others. There is no outside, no independent or individual autonomy, no sovereignty of the subject. All there is are relations. Talking about relations, and locating oneself or others, or both, in a relational field, was, literally, an existential practice, in which the people I lived with gave contour to themselves and others and elaborated the world that surrounded them.

I came to think that everyday life in Paris is choreographed by an ongoing relational game in which one continuously locates oneself in a relational field by talking about relations or establishing them. And I learned that science, like all other aspects of life, is subject to this relationality.[10]

A cultural historian of France would likely describe this relational organization of life as the distant echo of a court society: as the flip side of La Rochefoucauld's *homme honnête,* and his *politesse* and *galanterie*—a relational field characterized by deception, intrigue, by the artful masking of one's intention in a ceaseless strategic game characterized by the forming of alliances, the search for influence and power, a *faible* for wit and clever hints and, above all, for seduction and flirtation.

Perhaps I exaggerate the degree to which French life is grounded in relationalism. Perhaps, there is no stable "native point of view," no common disposition of thought. And perhaps it is an exaggeration to say that science takes place entirely in a relational field, in which success is inseparable from the art of telling stories about relations, inseparable from the art of establishing (or refusing) relations. But exaggeration can be a device to help make visible aspects of life that would otherwise go unseen. To understand relationalism, not as one aspect among others of French academia, but as the distinct form of life in which academia happens, may be the presupposition for understanding anything about French academia at all. And this, in turn, may be the presupposition for understanding anything about the turbulent history of plastic reason.[11]

A RELATIONAL ANTHROPOLOGY OF (PLASTIC) REASON

In the course of my fieldwork the relational gaze emerged as one of my key analytic tools for understanding the work of Alain's lab. It was by listening to relational stories, by slowly beginning to reflect on myself in relational terms, and by enjoying or being shocked by relational games that I came to think that the only appropriate way to present the at times simply ignored, at times aggressively contested story of Alain and his colleagues' effort to think of the brain as characterized by a silent embryogenesis was to write the turbulent history of his lab in terms of the relationalism constitutive of Parisian life. And the more I thought about such a relational chronicle, the more it thrilled me. It was as if the field had suggested to its anthropologist its own means of understanding it—a relational anthropology of plastic reason.[12]

Such a relational anthropology does not reject the focus on reason—on the work of thought—but it asks of the anthropologist to look at reason, to comprehend it, from the perspective of relations and relational events. The challenge is to relate every movement in the production of truth to the movements in relational events that parallel it—flirtation, hatred, seduction, reproduction, strategic alliances, and love, requited or not.

This, then, is what this chapter is all about, a chronicle of plastic reason, written in a local idiom of relational realism that I learned from my interlocutors—Brigitte, Alain, Joliot, and many others.

BORN TWICE (1985–1989)

Plastic reason was born twice: first as an idea, an attitude, a way of thinking about organisms, in 1985, at New York University's School of Medicine; and then again, experimentally, in the form of an obscure but evocative observation in Paris, in 1989 at the Collège de France.[13] If the first was an outcome of Alain's effort to escape the relations that nourished him, the second was a straightforward departure from them.

A Chemist of the Brain

In 1985, Alain had worked for almost a decade in the lab of Jacques Glowinski, professor of neuropharmacology at the Collège de France and a major figure in French brain science.[14] In the 1960s Glowinski had been a postdoc in the lab of Julius Axelrod at the U.S. National Institutes of Health, who would later receive the Nobel Prize for his contribution to the chemical decoding of synaptic communication. When Glowinski returned to Paris in 1965, he quickly emerged as one of the key authors of the then still novel chemical, or pharmacological, description of the brain, which he managed to institutionalize on a large scale in France.[15]

Glowinski was the central figure through which the web of the neurochemists was woven.

At the Collège, Alain quickly became a celebrity. His esprit, wit, and vigor made a great impression on his colleagues. Independent of their personal judgments—which varied from deep admiration to deep contempt—they got to know him as an exceptionally smart scientist of almost frightening energy, skilled in bench work and driven by boundless curiosity. What is more, they remembered him as a virtuoso of flirtation, able to transform any conversation—high or low, serious or not—into a play of seducing and being seduced.

Alain was relationally skilled—and seems to have made ample use of this skill. I was told countless stories of how he—master of relations—literally seduced Glowinski, that the senior fell in love with the junior, with his intellect, with his skills, with him. While some of these stories were told with the bitterness of disappointed love—unrequited either by Glowinski or by Prochiantz—others suggested that the relation between the junior and the senior was more than a mere relation: it was about affect, care, love.

Be that as it may, Glowinski was much taken by the newcomer. He adopted him, and soon invited him to form his own small subgroup focused on how the interaction of neuronal subpopulations in the course of embryogenesis give rise to the pharmacological topography of the human brain.

"I was a chemist of the brain," Alain told me, summarizing his early years at the Collège.

Protected and positioned by Glowinski, he flourished. Within a few years, he had made himself a name as the inventor of pure neuron cultures—at the time, a spectacular methodological innovation that allowed the study of neuronal growth in vitro. In addition, he had become something of a world expert on the embryogenetic emergence of the dopaminergic system.[16]

Relationally speaking, Alain, who held a PhD in molecular biology, had become a member of the community of neurochemists.

Despite his success, however, Alain was ready to move on. After a decade at the Collège, he no longer wanted to be part of a relational web evolving around someone else's ideas. He did not want to be defined by his relations with Glowinski. Rather, he wanted to be a center himself and to begin weaving a new web, one that would evolve from ideas and curiosities he was excited about and that seemed urgent to him. Relationally speaking, though, the only way to become someone himself was to break with Glowinski and the ideas that held the network of the neurochemists together and to come up with other, with different, ideas that would be attractive enough to allow for the emergence of a new web of affiliation. In 1985, therefore, Alain took a year off and left Paris for New York, where he hoped to formulate his own independent research project.

For his year in New York, Alain set himself two goals. The first was to understand the concept of development. Alain wanted to better grasp something that had most fascinated him during his research into the cellular emergence of the brain—developmental growth, or the coming into existence of form where before there was none.

"Have you ever watched how an embryo grows?" he replied when I first asked him why he wanted to shift away from chemistry. "To see how cells grow, how they give rise to forms where before there simply was nothing: this is one of the most spectacular experiences one can have. I needed to understand this better."

As a former student of the French historian and epistemologist Georges Canguilhem, Alain approached his fascination historically and conceptually.[17] When was it first suggested that organisms "develop"? When was it first "thought" that organisms are the result of growth? By whom and why? When were such growth patterns first analyzed? How did the emergence of the concept of "development" reconfigure biology?

Alain's second goal was to learn more about the recently discovered homeotic genes. Perhaps these genes, also called developmental genes, would allow him to formulate a project concerned with development.

What Is Development?

When Alain read through the classics of embryology—from Caspar Friedrich Wolff to Wilhelm Roux, from Wilhelm His to Hans Spemann, Ross Harrison, and Hans Driesch—he encountered a concept of development that had emerged and gained contour through two battles. The first of these battles occurred in the late eighteenth century and was fought by the young Caspar Friedrich Wolff (1733–1794) and the older Albrecht von Haller (1708–1777).

In 1744, Abraham Tremblay (1710–1784), a naturalist from Geneva, published a book in which he reported his discovery of the regenerative quality of sweet water polyps (Hydra), and specifically of the polyp's reproduction through regeneration (they regenerate after dissociation). Tremblay's book prompted von Haller, a Swiss anatomists who had studied under Hermann Boerhaave (1668–1738) at Leiden (The Netherlands), to take up the older question of whether humans are preformed in the uterus and to study the reproductive processes in a variety of animals (mainly chickens and humans). In 1757, then a widely recognized authority in physiology and a professor at the University of Göttingen (Germany), von Haller published the first volume of his *Elementa Physiologiae,* a book full of drawings, with which he sought to prove that the human organism is indeed preformed as a miniature organism in the female egg and that, once a woman becomes pregnant, this miniature organism merely gets bigger. Von Haller's work was circulated widely and quickly emerged as the definitive answer to the question of reproduction. Two years later, however, in 1759, the young Caspar Wolff published his dissertation, "Theoria Generationis," which challenged von Haller's view. According to Wolff, Haller's drawings were inaccurate and preformationism untenable. What he found under the microscope were not preformed little humans but a process he termed *epigesis,* a phrase he later translated as "*Entstehung*" (becoming) and "*freies Wachsthum*" (free growth). With enthusiasm Wolff reported that he had found a *Keimblatt*—literally, "germ leaf"—from which an embryo would gradually grow, just as a plant grows.

What was at stake for Wolff was becoming understood as free growth—and he borrowed the language to explain the free growth of the human organism from descriptions of the natural world and its seasonal changes. At least retrospectively, his concept of epigenesis marks the formal origins of the idea of development.

The second battle occurred in the 1920s and 1930s and was in many ways a modernization of the first. Over the second half of the nineteenth century, embryology had become an independent, autonomous discipline. In the aftermath of Wolff, Karl Ernst von Baer (1792–1876) and Christian Heinrich Pander (1794–1865) offered exquisite descriptions of embryogenetic growth. And in the final decades of the nineteenth century Wilhelm His (1831–1904), Wilhelm Roux (1850–1924), Hans Driesch (1867–1941), and Ross Harrison (1870–1959) began to articulate the first mechanical and experimental understanding of the different stages of embryogenetic development. By the 1920s, the sheer aesthetic and intellectual spectacle of cellular becoming had convinced most experimental embryologists, as they called themselves in the aftermath of Roux, that the growth processes that shape the embryo were radically incommensurable with any kind of preformationist understanding of the living. In the mid-1920s, however, Thomas Hunt Morgan (1866–1945) and his students, notably Alfred Sturtevant (1891–1970) and Herman Muller (1890–1967), challenged the embryologists. Their work on fruit flies had established, they argued, the chromosomal theory of inheritance, which showed that each trait of an adult organism is determined by a particular corpuscular gene located on a chromosome. Development, they concluded, must be thought of as determined in a physicochemical way by genes. Hence the study of development should focus on genes rather than, as the embryologists had it, on dispositions (so-called *Anlagen*) in the tissue layers of the developing embryo.[18]

The embryologists, enthusiasts of free growth in the tradition of Wolff, felt intensely provoked. Collectively—and ferociously—they opposed the geneticists' venture. Not that they were against the study of genes, then still largely a hypothetical construct (they were not). Not that they rejected the significance of genetics for understanding heredity (they did not). The affront to which they reacted was what they perceived as the wholly inadequate conception of development put forth by Morgan and his followers, which suggested that the becoming of the organism was simply a mechanical, physicochemical realization of preformed traits embedded in genes. Indeed, most embryologists seem to have understood their debate with the geneticists through the lens of the debate between Haller and Wolff; that is, as a debate between *preformationists,* who believe that the developing organism is preformed and thus determined down to its tiniest detail, and *epigeneticists,* who see development as a living, open process that cannot be reduced to any determinants.[19]

Although the debate between the embryologists and the geneticists gave rise to many exquisite journal articles and reflections, one of them stood out at the time: Gavin de Beer and Julian Huxley's textbook, *The Elements of Experimental Embryology,* first published in 1934. What makes Huxley and de Beer's volume so remarkable is that it distills more than 150 years of embryology into a single, coherent endeavor, as if all embryologists at all times and in all places had been struggling with just one question: What is development?

Scrupulously, Huxley and de Beer review the then-available embryological literature. They compare countless, often temporally and geographically dispersed experiments, set various observations and speculations in relation to one another as if they were concerned with similar issues, and go back and forth in time, consistently ignoring context, in order to arrive at suggestive conclusions. The outcome of their reading adventures was what had never existed before: a single, unified embryological conception of development.

According to Huxley and de Beer, development is a process and a reality sui generis that requires its own, autonomous discipline—experimental embryology.

> The kernel of the problem [of embryology] is the appearance during individual development of complexity of form and of function where previously no such form existed. [...] This coming into existence of new complexity of form and function during development is styled epigenesis. [...] The modern view is rigorously preformationist as regards the hereditary constitution of an organism, but rigorously epigenetic as regards its embryological development. [...] There is no way of saving the view that the adult is preformed in the egg [...]. It is impossible to imagine any theory of preformation, however elastic, which will explain the fact that an egg normally develops into a single embryo, and yet can be made to give rise to two or four whole embryos. The inevitable conclusion is that development involves a true increase of diversity, a creation of differentiation where previously none existed, and that the interpretation of embryonic development must be sought along the lines of some epigenetic theory.[20]

The challenge, in Huxley and de Beer's view, was to avoid the mistake of the geneticists, who conceived of the organism almost exclusively in terms of its adult form and assumed that this form was somehow already contained in genes. Rather, one would have to understand the adult organism in terms of its developmental history. And this developmental history was ultimately an undetermined, irreducibly open process, a process of the coming into existence of genuinely new and, in their particular realization, always singular forms (while the young of a chicken is always a chick, no chick equals any other one)—forms that cannot be explained by any previous stage of development.[21] What Huxley and de Beer somewhat pejoratively called "neo-Mendelism" was to them merely the most recent episode in the long but ultimately futile history of preformationist theories, and thus an inadequate and illegitimate endeavor.[22]

A concept that figures most prominently in Huxley and de Beer's textbook is "the plastic." Time and again they speak of the generation of new, still-"plastic" matter. They write about "formation processes" in the course of which the still-"plastic" organs and organisms are "molded" or "shaped." According to them, all life is plastic, and they and thereby argue that the living is plastic and development the process that "shapes" or "molds" or "sculpts" the open, undetermined—plastic—organism and thereby "gives form."

For Alain, who carefully studied *The Elements of Experimental Embryology,* the encounter with the history of ideas and arguments that had given rise to this plastic, developmental conception of life was a powerful opening. More than that, it was his hoped-for opportunity for a departure from the chemists.

"When I left for New York," he told me in one of our conversations about the history of his lab, "I found myself increasingly frustrated with my chemical work and the conception of the brain the chemists allowed for." The image of an immutable structure, of a chemical machine organized in fixed synaptic networks, governed by chemical compounds, ran counter to the developmental growth he saw in his Petri dishes at the Collège. "Though I could not articulate this frustration well back then; it was only with my discovery of development that I learned to put this frustration positively in words."

What Alain learned in New York reading through the history of embryology, was to self-consciously claim that the only plausible way to understand the brain was to study how this plastic organ gets developed—how it assumes its form.

"I now could see that I wanted to understand growth," Alain went on. "And I could see that neurochemistry did not provide an answer to this question. It was not, is not, itself concerned with the emergence of cellular form, with cellular motion. Growth and form are not its actual object."

Alain's way of severing himself from the relational web of the neurochemists, from Glowinski, had been to enroll himself in another relational web, one largely composed of dead embryologists.

A Kind of Plastic Force

In 1985, homeotic genes were still a spectacular novelty. Only a few years earlier, in 1978, Ed Lewis had published the paper in which he introduced the idea that homeotic genes are master control genes of development. The publication of Nüsslein-Volhard and Wieschaus's draft of all the genes necessary to build a drosophila body dates from 1980. And Gehring and McGinnis had identified the homeobox only in 1984. When Alain left for New York, biologists were only beginning to explore the spectacular implications of these discoveries, notably the possibility of thinking about evolution in terms of development.[23] The enthusiasm surrounding homeotic genes was extraordinary: editorials were written, comments published, prizes announced.

Alain was hardly immune to this enthusiasm. Though influenced by his readings in experimental embryology, his excitement took a somewhat unexpected form. While most biologists celebrated the discovery of the homeobox as an achievement of genetics and a confirmation of the genetic view of life— DNA makes RNA makes proteins, and proteins make us—Alain was excited about homeotic genes because they potentially made development central to the understanding of organisms. And by "development" he meant precisely the irreducibly open, plastic conception of becoming that the embryologists of the early twentieth century had described.

The contrast was striking. In their publications, Gehring and his colleagues suggested that homeotic genes contain a plan of the body, thereby implying that development is largely the execution of a genetic plan. For Alain, however, development was a process sui generis, one that was plastic, always individual, and impossible to reduce to genetically coded information. It was an open-ended process with a singular dynamic, which had to be understood in its own terms.

Alain was less interested in plans to be executed, which from his perspective amounted to a negation of development, than in the possibility of rendering visible the beauty of cellular becoming that he had seen in his Petri dishes and that he had learned to conceptualize while reading Roux, Spemann, von Dürken or Huxley and de Beer.

Could he use homeotic genes to conceptualize the brain in terms of development? Could he explore the role of homeotic genes in such a way that they would not so much confirm a mechanical as a plastic conception of adult organisms? Weren't homeotic genes an opportunity to experimentally explore a radically embryological philosophy of life?

Alain's bold move was a shift in scale. Perhaps, he wondered, homeoproteins, coded for by homeotic genes, are critical not only for the formation of the basic body axis but also for the cellular emergence of the brain. Perhaps homeoproteins tell a cell where to travel (the brain), how to differentiate (become a neuron), and what position to assume (which part of the brain). Perhaps this cellular emergence of the brain is a plastic, always individual process of becoming.

Are homeoproteins plastic forces, rather than master genes? Do these plastic forces sculpt—like a sculptor sculpts—the plastic material they in part trigger themselves?

For Alain, homeotic genes were an opportunity to devise his proper research project: a study of the development of the brain, focused on the role of homeoproteins at the single-cell level. Would this project—a genetic approach to development that rejected the mechanical philosophy of life developed by geneticists—allow him to move away from the chemists and justify starting his own lab and web?

Jeopardy

With his new project Alain was putting himself, relationally speaking, in jeopardy.

> c.1300, *ioparde* (13c. in Anglo-French), from O.Fr. *jeu parti,* lit. "a divided game, game with even chances," from *jeu* "a game" (from L. *jocus* "jest") + *parti,* pp. of *partir* "to divide".

His turn toward homeotic genes put him inevitably in the camp of those studying the brain in genetic terms. That was unfortunate. First, there was a numbers problem. In the mid-1980s the effort to apply the tools of molecular cell biology to the study of the nervous system was still avant-garde, especially in France, where angry electrophysiologists sought to prevent the molecularization of their discipline.[24] Aside from Jean Pierre Changeux's pioneering work on allosteric proteins and the genetics of synaptic communication, which was vehemently rejected by the electrophysiologists, there was little use of molecular biology in the neuronal sciences. Alain was still among the first to turn toward genetics—and there was not much of a support network yet to defend him or his project against the numerically dominant electrophysiologists.

Second, Alain's embryogenetic interpretation of homeotic genes made him an oddity among the geneticists. After all, his developmental approach, even if centered on homeotic genes, amounted to a thorough critique of molecular biology.[25] Against the genetic approach to life he articulated a developmental comprehension of the living organism.[26] In several publications of the late 1980s, at a time when the Human Genome Initiative was launched and the enthusiasm about genetics somewhat unbroken, Alain emphatically declared that molecular cell biology was a mere tool—not a discipline, or a theory of life, or an explanation of cerebral processes. He lamented the "epistemological poverty" of molecular biology, which, he claimed, did not allow thinking about "the inevitable plasticity of living processes," that is, of an "adapting, developing, and evolving organism in a complex milieu." In several of our conversations Alain told me that he thought molecular biology suffered from the absence of what his dead embryological interlocutors taught him to call "genuine biological questions"—questions about the emergence of cellular form as the key to understanding cellular function.[27]

So Alain not only successfully alienated himself from the numerically dominant coterie of electrophysiologists, who refused to work with the molecularists, but also from the small number of geneticists of the brain.

Third and most significant, however, was that his work on homeotic genes amounted to an open departure from the chemists of the brain and, in particular, from their key figure Jacques Glowinski. With his turn to development Alain broke with the relational web of which, up until that point, he had been a member.

His alignment with the experimental embryologists of the 1920s and 1930s thus left Alain potentially isolated from all three of the relational webs that then structured the French neuronal sciences. For the geneticists at the Institut Pasteur, the developmental approach was counterintuitive. The electrophysiologists, all descendants of the Institut Marey, were unhappy with the prominence of genes; and the neurochemists at the Collège de France were not ready to lose one of their most promising juniors (Glowinski had openly talked about making Alain his successor).

Getting a lab to work on the brain in terms of development thus proved difficult. Neither his wit nor his talent for transforming almost any situation into a flirtation, neither the art of seduction nor the power of thought amounted to much without a relational other open to being impressed, willing to flirt, ready to be seduced. Alain had to stay with Glowinski, with the neuropharmacologists, as a chemist of the brain, whether he wanted to or not. In his free time, though, he silently began to conduct experiments with homeotic genes.

Perhaps he would get results that would enroll others in his curiosity?

Experimental Reality (1989)

By early 1988, Alain's clandestine experiments had indicated that homeotic genes indeed could play a role in the cellular emergence of the brain. He thought these promising results justified assigning a PhD student to work on the role of homeoproteins for neuronal morphogenesis. His choice fell on a graduate student who had recently joined his group—Alain Joliot, great-grandson of Marie Curie, member of the legendary Curie-Joliot clan, and son of Pierre Joliot, professor at the Collège de France and director of the Biology Department at the ENS.[28]

Alain and Joliot worked along two lines. The first concerned time. Could they come up with a time line of gene expression? Of when which homeotic genes were expressed by what kind of neurons in the course of development? And could they correlate the timing of particular homeotic genes with the emergence of particular brain regions? Could they draw up a time-sensitive topography of homeotic gene expression in the brain? The second line of inquiry concerned function. Alain asked Joliot to synthesize a peptide (a chain of amino acids) that resembles that part of homeoproteins that binds to the consensus-binding motif of homeotic genes (the homeodomain) and thereby causes their expression (the chosen peptide was pAntp, which corresponds to the homeodomain of the Antennapedia protein). Could they determine the effect of pAntp on live cells in culture?

In early 1989, the second line of research led to a curious observation. When Joliot added pAntp to a Petri dish full of cultured rat neurons, it was internalized, without degradation, into the nucleus of the cells, where it seemed to cause a dramatic morphogenetic outgrowth. At first Joliot was ready to discard the finding. As cells were known to be autonomous, and as transcription factors were hardly ever found outside the nucleus and certainly never outside of cells, he thought the internalization of pAntp was an artifact, the result of a technical error in the experimental setup.

"Experiments go wrong rather often," he told me. "At times the medium is congested; at other times the cells are old, the protein doesn't have the right size, et cetera."

But when Joliot reported to Alain that pAntp had caused a powerful outgrowth on the level of axons, dendrites, and spines, Alain asked him to repeat the experiment.

"I had an intuition," Alain said when I later asked him why he thought it worth redoing the experiment. "Do you know Bergson's work?"

Over the course of my fieldwork I had heard Alain more than once give brief lectures about Bergson's philosophy of intuition.

"Anyhow," he went on before I could give an answer, "I had this vague idea that perhaps the morphogenetic outgrowth Joliot observed could be more than an artifact. And besides, it was just a matter of repeating an experiment."

"And what about the intuition?" I asked.

"You know," he smiled, "many intuitions turn out to be wrong."

Joliot repeated the experiment—and retrieved the exact same result. Next he repeated it with different cells, a different medium, under different temperatures. Each time he observed that pAntp was internalized and caused drastic morphogenetic effects, even in already differentiated (that is, mature) neurons. The repetitiveness of Joliot's results left Alain enthusiastic. Wasn't Joliot's observation suggesting the possibility that homeoproteins were a kind of plastic force, that because of a yet unknown mechanism—the sliding between cells of homeoproteins—they coordinated the emergence of the brain at the single-cell level? When, shortly thereafter, Alain and Joliot found that homeotic genes were also expressed in the adult human brain, Alain's effort to think the brain in terms of development assumed a spectacular, if utterly unexpected, form. There suddenly was the concrete experimental possibility that development—embryogenetic growth—continued in adult brains.

Could it be that a silent embryogenesis occurs in the adult human brain? Could it be that homeoproteins, their sliding between cells, not only sculpted the embryonic but also the adult brain? Could embryology perhaps be the science adequate to the adult mammalian brain in general and the adult human brain in particular?

Falling in Love

When, in May 2003, I asked Alain what he had felt when he was first struck by the possibility that the internalization of homeoproteins could be more than just an artifact and when subsequent experiments seemed to confirm his intuition, he told me the following story.

> Listen. Suppose you are in the *métro*, okay? You have a very nice wife and children. You go home every night, you have dinner, you have sex with your wife, she is very charming, and everything is good. On Sundays you go to your mother-in-law and [...] I mean, you know, happiness. And one day you take the *métro* and there is this blond coming by. And instead of going home, you follow the blond, okay? You take the chance of your life. And everybody says you're crazy. But you do it because you could not do otherwise. It could or couldn't work with the blond, but you quit everything for the blond. It is something like that, you know? At some point you see something really exciting and you feel—I mean this is intuition!—you feel that there is something important. And you cannot just let it go, just like that, saying it is an artifact, it doesn't matter, it cannot happen. So that's it. You take your big chance.

Sexual encounters in the *métro* have surfaced in many conversations I had in Paris. They are a central, ubiquitous element of the cultural repertoire of Parisian life, and as such almost a cliché.[29]

"A blond?" a friend later remarked. "He could at least have said a bird! A bird flew by and I just couldn't help but follow it."

Indeed, given that Alain had freely alternated between male and female partners and had a profound disgust for the bourgeois, there is some irony to his story about the blond. However, taking it simply as a (sexist) cliché overlooks that Alain also told me a story of how he thinks about science and how he thinks science should be lived and practiced. He told me something about what he thought of as the overwhelming beauty of ideas (and things) and about the fact that he fell in love. Science requires one to find one's demon and to live with it—and for it.[30] The passion and the curiosity involved are endless, for what's at stake is not just an experimental result but oneself.

At the same time, Alain's story was tailored for a specific audience, namely, the anthropologist. He engaged me (talk about relations!) in an erotic conversation in which everything was at stake, a conversation about falling in love and leaving everything behind. Such was the adventure of science. Would I be ready?[31]

RELATIONAL DEATH

In early 1989, amidst the excitement about the prospects introduced by Joliot's work with pAntp, an opportunity arose to open a lab in the newly created Department of Biology at the École Normale (directed by Alain Joliot's father). Prochiantz applied, and after the summer he and his little group left the Collège for the ENS.

Ironically, Alain was recruited as what he no longer wanted to be—a chemist of the brain. He was offered the lab as the former protégé of Glowinski, as a promising next-generation neuropharmacologist, as the inventor of pure neuron cultures, and as an expert of the embryological formation of the dopaminergic system—not as the experimental embryologist of the adult human brain that he now aspired to be.

Alain, though, was hardly troubled by this mismatch between expectation and aspiration. As soon as he was at the ENS, he successively made homeoprotein research the only focus of his laboratory. From now on, as anyone should see, he ceased being a chemist of the brain. His lab and research would evolve solely around the idea that the brain is a plastic organ, that even the adult brain is the locus of silent embryogenesis, that the key to the brain's plasticity is homeoproteins and their nonautonomous transfer between neurons, and that embryology is the science adequate to understanding the (adult) brain.

The reactions Alain earned for his turn to homeoproteins were overwhelmingly negative. And that was only consequential. The relational jeopardy he encountered upon returning from New York had hardly been resolved. Now, as then, Alain was in between the three major relational webs that constituted French brain research: genetics, electrophysiology, and chemistry.

He had thought that once he had his own lab, the reception of his effort to describe the brain in terms of development would improve. But the electrophysiologists, the geneticists, and the chemists were less than interested in his research. Why would they support a project that ultimately implied that their work was grounded in a misconception of the brain? For the Parisian geneticists, electrophysiologists, and chemists the idea that the mature nervous system is plastic was ridiculous. What is more, geneticists simply shook their heads when they heard Alain suggest that homeoproteins could travel between cells and undermine cell autonomy. Within months, Alain had alienated himself from the complex webs of affiliation that were constitutive of French neuronal research. And his former colleagues in neurochemistry regretted that he had been granted his own lab.

If reason is relational, then Alain had become utterly unreasonable.

Going Public

As if unfazed by the relational trouble that surrounded them, Alain and Joliot went ahead and wrote up their findings in a paper. They were eager to share what appeared to them as a most exciting possibility, a silent embryogenesis in the adult brain. And they were curious to learn what colleagues elsewhere, outside France, would make of their discovery.

Their journal of choice was *Development,* perhaps the most prestigious journal for developmental biology. Alain's hope had been that the editor, Walter Gehring, discoverer of the homeobox, would, given his special interest in homeotic genes, be sympathetic to their research.

They began their article,

The homeobox sequences have been highly conserved during evolution and genes containing homeobox sequences are present in all vertebrates, including mammals. In vertebrates [...] homeobox gene expression is not limited to the period during which the general features of body organization are established. In particular, a number of these genes are expressed in the nervous system rather late during development and, in some cases, through adulthood. [...] We demonstrate that the presence of pAntp produces dramatic and rapid morphological modifications of the cultures. In addition, we show that pAntp added to already differentiated neurons enters into nerve cells, accumulates in their nuclei, and further enhances morphological differentiation. Our results demonstrate that neurons possess an efficient uptake system for the Antennapedia homeobox peptide and suggest that binding of pAntp to consensus motifs present in nerve cell nuclei influences neuronal morphogenetic programs.[32]

In prose carefully worded so as to avoid provoking anyone, Alain and Joliot stated the implications of their observation: the brain is a plastic organ; it is characterized by a lifelong morphogenesis; homeoproteins (as plastic forces) and their nonautonomous transfer (a plastic event) are the key to this lifelong plasticity. None of the peer reviewers, however, even bothered to engage their carefully stated sketch of a plastic brain. The very idea of a continuation of embryogenetic processes in the adult was so absurd to them that every one of the referees classified the nonautonomous transfer as an experimental artifact.

The first reviewer wrote to Gehring:

The largest problem of this paper is that the conducted experiments have little to do with biological phenomena. [...] Furthermore, their claim that pAntp applied to cells in culture enters the nucleus is unconvincing. [...] It is well possible that pAntp is simply sticking to the cell surface and that addition of the oligonucleotide prevents sticking by binding to the peptide.

The second reader report was much shorter and more explicit: "This referee does not think this paper should be even seriously considered by any journal."

Gehring agreed with the assessment of his referees. He informed Alain that "your claim that pAntp enters the nucleus is unconvincing and your photographs are poor." He went on to list a series of control experiments that he suggested Alain run, adding, "You have no chances if you resubmit the paper before all the major criticisms listed by both reviewers are taken care of."

Alain was angry. "We had done most of the experiments he listed before we submitted the paper," he said. "Is there a point in publishing a paper about control experiments?"

After an exchange of faxes, Alain and Joliot gave up and sent their paper to another journal, and then to another one, and then to yet another one. In every case, the journal turned them down with the argument that their work amounted to the careful description of an experimental artifact. Finally, after more than two years of shopping around, their article was published by the *Proceedings of the National Academy of Science (PNAS)*.[33]

Still, the 1991 publication of "Antennapedia homeobox peptide regulates neural morphogenesis" hardly meant that their research had been accepted. It hadn't been. Throughout the 1990s and early 2000s (when I arrived in the lab) they got reviews such as the following:[34]

The authors state [...] that "to our surprise, we have observed [...]." This is also the general feeling in the scientific community at large where I have heard these experiments being discussed recently. I would recommend that the present paper [should] not be published.

It doesn't seem like a useful method anyhow; and the author's glib assertions that little is known about homeobox genes is simply nonsense. [...] There is nowhere any evidence [...]. As it is, there is simply no rational basis for any further discussion. [...] In the present paper they attempt to propagandize this unfounded claim for significance [...]. This paper should not be published under any circumstances.

In Drosophila, [...] all of the homeotic genes appear to function in a strictly autonomous fashion. Thus, at least in Drosophila, there is no reason to believe that homeoproteins, or even homeodomain peptides move from one cell to another. Indeed, there is every reason to believe the opposite is, and normally must, be the case.

These experiments appear to be done with reasonable care, but almost certainly consist of the careful description of a cell artifact. There is no previous evidence that homeopeptides are secreted from cells *in vivo*. In addition, the contention that pAntp homeopeptide is having a "strong" effect on neurite outgrowth is ridiculous.[35]

Provocation

Alain reacted with provocative perseverance. Not only did he stick to the focus on the nonautonomous transfer of homeoproteins, he also gave a series of public talks in which he insisted his lab had made an important and far-reaching observation. The mere fact that one could not use the established terms and concepts of neuroscience to describe a nonautonomous transfer or adult cerebral plasticity, he informed his listeners, did not in any way negate the importance of what he and Joliot had observed.

"To many it was simply outrageous," one senior biologist remembered the debates of the early 1990s. "Alain drove them nuts. He seriously—and publicly, in front of colleagues—claimed to have pity for his peers. He explained that he understood how hard it must be for them to give up their established ways of thinking. He told them that they were objectively wrong. It was inevitable for Alain that neuroscientists had to give up their assumptions about what proteins do and what brains are and to begin making sense of an observation difficult to make sense of, a silent embryogenesis in the brain. People were outraged. And Alain calmly explained to them that what was required now was thinking along new lines, and this was, of course, not everybody's business, for thinking along new lines was risky and required intellect."

Alain took intense pleasure in challenging the established—concepts, morals, people, truths. I could observe this many times in my fieldwork. Indeed, his joy was so intense and visible that at first I wondered whether what he liked most about his work was the opportunity to provoke. But whenever I tried to engage him in a conversation about his provocations, he smiled and changed the subject. If I insisted, he would either cite Claude Bernard—"When we meet a fact which contradicts a prevailing theory, we must accept the fact and abandon the theory, even when the theory is supported by great names and generally accepted"[36]—or tell me with a wink: "There was little I could do for them. It is a pity that they were so stupid."

Eventually, though, I came to view Alain's provocations as a form of flirtation. Alain was provoking in order to be provoked. Provocations were for him an invitation to a contest of wit and words. He was thrilled when an interlocutor talked back to him—and he was disappointed, almost sad, when the other turned away without response.

Je Me Tire une Balle dans la Tête

The speed with which Alain was isolated was spectacular. In 1989, he had been celebrated as a most promising chemist of the embryonic brain. He was successful, internationally recognized, a rising star of French neurochemistry, a potential candidate for the Collège de France. From the perspective of relations and strategic alliances, doors were wide open. Only two years later, in 1991, all these doors were shut, the relations cut.

A glance at how severe the effect of the exclusion was—of the despair and the doubts that ensued—is offered by an interview Alain gave to Jean François Peyret, a well-known French playwright and theater director, in the early 1990s.[37] At one point, Peyret, who had the conversation videotaped, asked Alain what he regards as "pathetic." Without hesitation Alain responds that there are forms of suicide, which are for him not pathetic at all. They may even be beautiful, a form of dignity. The example he gives refers to his own life and work:

> Si on dit "J'aurais voulu être très bon mais finalement je suis mauvais donc cela ne vaut plus le coup de continuer et je me tire une balle dans la tête," c'est n'est pas pathétique. C'est même bien. On souhaiterait que cela arrive plus souvent. [...] Il est possible qu'un certain nombre de mes collèges pense que je suis mauvais et que je n'en suis pas conscient et donc éprouve pour moi un sentiment de pitié et de compassion. Parce que ce sont des gens qui sont chrétiens et donc ils éprouvent la compassion. Tandis que moi non. Mais je suis certain que certain auront beaucoup de compassion pour moi, en pensant à quel point je suis mauvais. Il y en a qui m'ont conseillé d'arrêter. Au mois de Septembre dernier, à la fin d'une conférence, un collègue m'a dit: "Si j'étais toi, j'arrêterais de faire ces choses-là. Tu te ridiculises. Tout le monde pense comme moi et personne n'ose te le dire. Arrête. Tu es en train de ruiner ta carrière." Comme je suis un être fragile, j'ai failli vomir. Cela m'a rendu malade pendant au mois quelques heures. Il m'a dit d'ailleurs: "Je ne te dis pas ça parce que je ne t'aime pas mais parce que je t'aime bien et je pense que tu pourrais être un bon scientifique. Ce que tu veux démontrer est absurde et comme aucun de tes amis ne t'aime suffisamment pour te le dire, moi qui ait de la compassion pour toi, je préfère t'en informer."[38]

At this point Alain turns away from Peyret and toward the camera. "I have been working now for so many years on a fact nobody believes," he said, with a most disconcerting gaze. "If I am wrong, I kill myself."[39]

THE DECADE OF THE BRAIN (1991–2000)

Instead of growing, Alain's lab shrank. Once he had decided to narrow the research to homeoproteins in general and their nonautonomous aspects in particular, several of his researchers left. Alain reacted to the loss along two lines. On the one hand, he recruited friends. In 1989 Alain hired Michel Volovitch to his lab, a specialist in molecular cell biology who was, like

Alain himself, a former *thésards* (graduate student) of François Chapeville. And in 1991 Joliot, who was by now a close friend and anyhow inseparably related to the work on homeoproteins, joined them. On the other hand, Alain recruited people from elsewhere who had little stake in Parisian relational turbulences. In 1992, Daniele Derossi arrived from Italy, and three years later, Alain could hire Alain Trembleau, an expert in electron microscopy and neuroanatomy, who after several years in San Diego had just returned to France and was looking for an opportunity to work in Paris.

Each of the early lab members—Alain, Michel, Joliot, and Danielle (who later left science to become a writer)—remembered the early years as a period of intense isolation and unusually strong friendship. Independently from one another, they talked to me about how the doubts that surrounded them glued their lives together. They were alone with one another—and with their nonautonomous homeoproteins.

Determining Internalization (1991–1996)

The challenge the lab faced in these early years was to provide evidence—evidence that a nonautonomous transfer occurs, that it is biologically important for the cellular emergence of the brain, and that it renders the brain plastic. This challenge was enormous, not only relationally but also materially and experimentally.

Materially, because the four friends recognized early on that, as a lab working on an observation that lay outside mainstream research, they could not rely on commercially available cell mediums, antibodies, or electrophoresis gels. "The materials of laboratory science," as Joliot put it, "are tailored toward dominant experimental questions. If you work on other questions, things get complicated." Alain and his friends had to spend a lot of time developing materials suited to their work.

Experimentally, insofar as the question "What is the biological function of the nonautonomous transfer of homeoproteins?" did not make any sense in 1991. Without any knowledge of the actual mechanisms of how homeoproteins slide between cells and cause a morphogenetic outgrowth, no one could design experiments that would interfere with these mechanisms in such a way that the actual physiological role of the transfer could be determined.

How, because of which capacities, by way of which mechanisms do homeoproteins travel between cells? What properties allow them to cause morphogenetic reactions?

Alain, Michel, Joliot, and Daniele, sought to address these questions by transforming the journey of homeoproteins into two sets of technical events: secretion (from the nucleus into the cytoplasm and from the cytoplasm across the membrane) and internalization of homeoproteins (from the exterior milieu across the cell membrane and from there to the cytoplasm and into the nucleus). And then they began to chemically build the homeodomain, amino acid by amino acid, at each step trying experimentally to determine which part of the homeodomain is sufficient for internalization (they focused first on internalization).

At the time they began their work, they had all four been made aware that no scientific fact is ever relationally neutral. And the hope that guided their daily work at the bench was that if they were to discover the molecular mechanisms of the transfer—that is, if they could show that homeoproteins actually slide between neurons—this would help make their research perhaps attractive to other neuronal scientists—whether from genetics, electrophysiology, or chemistry.

After five years, Alain and co. had published a series of papers (all accompanied by doubtful comments from their peers) showing that the neurotrophic factor of pAntp depends on its specific DNA-binding properties; that this factor effectively has gene-regulating properties; that the third helix, sixteen amino acids long, is responsible for internalization; and that internalization is receptor independent (that is, that internalization is a process independent of cell autonomy).[40] Internalization thus began to come into view as a well-preserved mechanism, at least in cells in vitro.

And *des choses social?*

Becoming a Chemist (Again)

The work on internalization was a big relational success, if for somewhat unexpected reasons. For although no one seemed to care in the least about what Alain and his small circle of friends had to say about homeoproteins and brain plasticity, a good number of their readers cared a lot about the sixteen–amino acid strain that allowed pAntp to slide between cells independent of cell autonomy.

Under normal circumstances, a cell's membrane is almost impermeable. It consists of a lipid bilayer that is hydrophobic, making it (largely) impossible for hydrophilic compounds (like proteins) to cross the membrane. The potential of the sixteen-amino-acid–long peptide, insofar as it bypasses cell autonomy, was that it could be used as a vector to deliver almost any protein (or other biologically active substance) directly to the cytoplasm and the nucleus without destroying either the compounds or the cell. After much discussion the lab members chose to call the peptide—which corresponds roughly to the third helix of Antennapedia, a three-helix protein—Penetratin.[41]

Shortly after they had identified the third helix as responsible for internalization, they synthesized several variants of Penetratin, smaller and shorter ones, each with different functions and differently suited for specific cargoes and destinations. Some cross the membrane but do not accumulate in the nucleus; others are specifically made for delivering large proteins straight to the nucleus; and so forth. By 1996 they had designed an entire cascade of what they called cell-permeable peptides (CPPs).[42]

Penetratin made the lab relationable; it made a small, underfunded, and utterly isolated research group internationally recognized and the lab sought-after for the design of CPPs. And precisely insofar as CPPs were widely used to administer drugs, or chemical compounds, to specific brain cells, Alain now emerged as what he no longer wanted to be—a successful pharmacologist. Something quite appropriate for a former protégé of Glowinski.[43]

After five years of near-complete isolation, Alain, Michel, and Joliot cared little that they were recognized for the wrong reasons, that is, as pharmacologists rather than as embryologists of the adult brain.[44] What mattered at that moment was that they were relationally better off—and that the work on Penetratin, due to collaboration with industry, brought in money that the lab urgently needed.[45]

"Penetratin," Alain put it, "saved us."

But there was never any doubt as to the lab's goal. Some of the revenue Alain used to recruit lab technicians to whom he would then assign almost all CPP work. The by far bigger part of the new revenues, however, he spent on recruiting new postdocs, who researched what really mattered to the lab, plasticity as induced by homeoprotein signaling.

Understanding Secretion (1995–2001)

When it became clear in 1995 that they were able to control internalization, Joliot began working on secretion. After some initial hesitation about which protein they should focus on, they settled on Engrailed (hereafter Eng), a homeoprotein involved in the patterning of the midbrain-hindbrain region, as their experimental model.[46] Already in 1997, amidst the hype around CPPs, Joliot and Trembleau published evidence that Eng is not only present in the nucleus of neurons, as the classical assumption had it, but also in (caveolae-like) vesicles that are primarily transported into the axon, where they are integrated into the cell membrane. Only a year later, in 1998, they had identified a signal sequence necessary for the nonautonomous secretion of Eng in vitro. Another year later, they published a description of the nuclear export mechanism, which diffuses Eng from the nucleus into other compartments of the cell.[47] And by 2001, combining the lab's work on pAntp and Eng, Alain and co. could provide the first detailed molecular account of the secretion and internalization of homeoproteins in vitro.[48]

Shortly after the turn of the millennium, the task Alain and Michel had worked out ten years earlier—the experimentalization of the nonautonomous transfer of homeoproteins in vitro—was achieved.[49] The challenge now was to go in vivo and to prove that homeoproteins are indeed plastic forces and that their nonautonomous transfer is a plasticity-inducing event that occurs throughout life.

ALTERNATIVE RELATIONS

Before discussing the shift from technology to physiology that occurred around 2002, just when I arrived in the lab, I briefly turn to another relational aspect of Alain's project, one that was for many of his colleagues a source of outrage—his reaching out to the worlds of arts and letters.

To be sure, many scientists are interested in the arts (Jean Pierre Changeux, for example, is a well-known, if controversial, expert in eighteenth-century paintings). However, scientists usually maintain a clear boundary between fact and fiction, especially in France, a country characterized by a rather rigid divide between science and art (a divide partly due to an educational system that forces high school students to choose either arts or science). Alain—and this was the provocation—blurred the boundary. He did not speak across the divide. He inhabited and bridged it.

Alain's foray into the worlds of arts and letters proceeded along three lines. The first and least controversial one was a solitary endeavor. Between the late 1980s and the early 2000s, Alain published a whole series of popular science books, each of which is a partly historical, partly scientific effort to think the adult brain in embryogenetic terms. In 1987, two years after his stay in New York and while still in Glowinski's lab, he published *Les stratégies de l'embryon* (an effort to understand homeotic genes as the key to an embryogenetic understanding of the central nervous system). In 1989 and 1990, books number two and three followed, *La construction du cerveau* (which argued that the way to study the brain is to figure out how it gets constructed, that is, as a living, changing, emergent organ) and *Claude Bernard: La révolution physiologique* (an introduction that analyzes Claude Bernard's oeuvre as an effort to think through his discovery that the liver produces sugar, which was rejected as impossible by many of his peers). In 1997, Prochiantz published his fourth popular science book, *Les Anatomies de la Pensée: A quoi pensent les calamars?* (a biological study of thinking, defined as the adaptation of an organism to its environment—an adaptability made possible by homeotic gene–induced plasticity). And after the turn of the millennium, in 2001, he presented his fifth book, *Machine-Esprit* (an effort to articulate, with the help of D'Arcy Thompson and Alan Turing, an embryology of the adult human brain).[50]

The second and more provocative venture into the worlds of arts and letters was a radio show Alain produced with fellow biologist Jean Didier Vincent. The aim of their unruly show, which ran throughout the 1990s, was to be provocative—and was to question the boundaries that usually separate science from the arts. Wasn't it time to let go of the everyday conception of science as a neutral and sober undertaking? Alain and Vincent invited scientists as well as artists on their show to discuss controversial experimental findings, the challenge of exploring the yet unknown, how researchers and artists nourish their imagination, what they thought about art or, inversely, science, and other "frivolous" things.[51]

The third and, for many, most provocative line was by far the most important and productive for Alain—a multiyear, multi-relational venture into the theater world. In 1992 and 1993, he took part in a play by Jean François Peyret, who had invited several (in)famous Parisian intellectuals to participate in his *Traité de Passion*—among them Baudrillard, Derrida, and Alain (whose thoughts on a nonpathetic suicide, quoted above, are taken from this play). Two years later, in 1995, Alain published his own play, *La biologie dans le boudoir* (a Sade-inspired piece that described the indebtedness of the plastic brain to a living, feeling body and mocked several of his Parisian colleagues). And in the late 1990s, he entered into an intense, still-ongoing working relationship with Peyret, which to date (2015) has resulted in five plays (all revolving, directly or indirectly, around the work of Alain's lab) and two books.

Once I understood the extent of Alain's entanglement with the arts, I began to wonder how to explain that a busy scientist, struggling to show that the things he works on are not just fiction or artful imaginings, could spend so much time and energy in collaborations with artists. During my fieldwork I learned that there are several complementary answers to this question, all of them suggested by Alain himself, though at different times and in different contexts.

Occasionally, for example, Alain would describe himself as a "boundary subject." "I know," he once remarked about himself, "Prochiantz travels across different domains just as his proteins travel from cell to cell, in a nonautonomous fashion."[52]

The metaphor, if meant ironically, is intriguing. Alain takes pleasure in *se jeté à travers champ* (his words). He enjoyed transgressing boundaries and the possibilities and provocations these transgressions create.

I also heard him explain with some regularity that reaching into the art world was for him simply a longing for conversation. In the neuroscientific community, his opportunities to converse were fairly limited. Running a radio show and working with Peyret was a kind of substitute.

Most often, however, Alain explained that the arts, and here especially his work with a playwright, are simply where his research (*sic!*) led him. Put differently, in his books, during talks, or in interviews, Alain was adamant that his exchanges with, for example, Peyret, just like his excursions into the theater world more generally, were not external to his research. On the contrary, he insisted, "My collaborations with Jean François, are for me ways to explore my work. Our conversations are instructive to me. I learn something from listening to him. I learn new ways of thinking through the nonautonomous transfer of homeoproteins and to conduct experiments that document that the brain is a plastic organ."

The relationable quality of his work was such that it largely excluded conversations (relations) within the world of neuroscience, where his project was rejected, but opened up the possibility of conversing (having relations) with artists.[53] The curiosity and passion Alain and many of his artist friends shared was their interest in forms, in the appearance of form, in forms in motion. In their conversations, they learned from each other by exploring further how to think about (in the words of de Beer and Huxley) the "appearance of form [...] where before no such form existed."[54]

In the decade of the brain, then, Alain had found, for himself and his lab, two relational niches. One was the industry–applied research nexus and evolved around CPPs. The other was the world of theater, which revolved around the effort to understand the brain as an emergent, continuously changing form. Whereas plasticity—as form/event[55]—did not matter to the first, it was central to the latter. In the art world, Alain had the liberty and the duty to think through the irreducible plasticity of the brain.

RETURN (2001–2006)

In late 2001, the laboratory began to shift from experimenting with cells in culture to experimenting with living organisms (mostly mice and rats). It was a critical moment. What, if anything, would they find? Would there be an in vivo function of the nonautonomous transfer? Would the transfer turn out, as Alain had provocatively claimed for more than ten years, to render the brain plastic?

Given the relational turbulences, and the provocations, the stakes were extraordinarily high. And yet the researchers in the lab were optimistic. Not least because there was now a growing number of neuronal researchers who were genuinely interested in the lab's work—at least outside France. This had little to do with their in vitro work. Rather, a new and unanticipated relational web had begun to emerge.

A Revolution Elsewhere

Reports about the birth of new neurons in old brains had been circulating in the margins of the neuronal sciences since the 1960s. It was only in the early 1980s, however, that adult neurogenesis was sufficiently stabilized—experimentally, conceptually, relationally—to seriously challenge established conceptions of the brain as fixed and immutable. The work that led to this stabilization was largely carried out by Fernando Nottebohm, then at Rockefeller University. In the late 1970s, Nottebohm, who was by training an ornithologist, had made a stunning discovery: when he was trying to correlate song behavior of adult male canaries to their brain physiology, he found that their brain undergoes marked seasonal changes. Over the late summer and early fall, when the mating season is over and the birds no longer sing, their brains shrink by more than 80 percent. Over the winter months, then, just when they are about to begin learning new songs, their brains regrow.[56] Canaries, Nottebohm concluded, have a brain for all seasons. But how was he to explain this massive disappearance and reappearance of brain mass? At first he speculated, in accordance with the then-dominant conception of the brain as a synaptic machine, that the seasonal variation was caused by a massive loss and eventual regrowth of synapses (after all, synapses were held to be critical for learning and what seemed at stake for the canaries was the learning of new songs). In the early 1980s, however, together with his postdoc Steven Goldman, Nottebohm then made a second spectacular discovery: what actually accounts for the seasonal changes was not the death and regrowth of synapses but of nerve cells. Nottebohm and Goldman's 1983 paper on the production, migration, and differentiation of new neurons in the adult brain marked the emergence of an unanticipated possibility, one that had the potential to trouble the neuronal sciences for the coming years: are human brains also undergoing seasonal changes?

For a brief moment, in the mid-1980s, the neuronal sciences seemed to enter into a period of massive conceptual turbulences. Was the conception of the adult human brain as a fixed and immutable machine wrong? The explosive potential of Nottebohm's canaries, however, was defused in 1985 when Pasko Rakic, at the time president of the American Society of Neuroscience and the world's foremost expert on the neuronal growth and composition of the primate brain, published a paper on the "limits of neurogenesis." Rakic reported that he had cut his way through the brains of ten rhesus monkeys and that the slices he prepared from them established beyond doubt that in primates "all neurons [. . .] are generated during prenatal and early postnatal life." He concluded that the brain of primates as well as some other species may be uniquely specialized in lacking the capacity for neuronal production once in the adult stage. One can speculate that a prolonged period of interaction with the environment, as pronounced as it is in all primates, especially in humans, requires a stable set of neurons to retain acquired experiences in the pattern of their synaptic connectivity."[57]

After all, the mature nervous system was the fixed and immutable cellular structure it had been known as. Or was it?

In the late 1990s, after a small group of researchers had silently expanded Nottebohm's work from canaries to mice and rats, two reports were published that powerfully undermined Rakic's "no." First, in 1997, Elizabeth Gould of Princeton University reported that she found new neurons in the hippocampi of adult primates. And then, in 1998, Fred Gage (Salk Institute), with whom Alain had worked since the 1980s, released a paper that document the birth of new neurons in adult humans.[58]

The impact of these two discoveries on the neuronal sciences was extraordinary. A whole field exploded into an intense, at times ferocious controversy.[59] Is the adult human brain really plastic? Or is plasticity, in the form of adult neurogenesis, a negligible phenomenon? Are new neurons born in all brain areas, or in only some of the more ancient parts of the brain, such as the hippocampus? Does adult neurogenesis occur in the cortex? Do other forms of cellular plasticity exist? Is adult neurogenesis, as Alain wondered, perhaps simply the most visible form of plasticity? Would other forms soon be discovered? How does a plastic brain allow for memory, for learning, for behavioral changes? What is the role of synaptic communication in a plastic brain?

The consequences of the emergence of adult neurogenesis research were twofold. On the one hand, it powerfully undermined the old comprehension of what the brain "is" (an immutable structure) and how one has to study it (as a neurochemical machine with the synapse as the only dynamic element), without actually giving rise to a coherent new way of thinking about the brain. On the other hand, it meant the emergence of a new relational web that evolved around the effort to think the adult human brain in terms of development.

For Alain, the simultaneous breaking open of the established conceptual horizon and the emergence of a new web amounted to a breakthrough—for it brought about a situation in which it could seem as if he had been struggling with questions most neuronal researchers only now began to appreciate, questions about the continuity of basic embryogenetic processes in mature human brains. Could it be, for example, that homeoproteins guide the production, migration, and differentiation of new neurons not only in the embryo but in the adult as well? And could it be that their capacity for a nonautonomous transfer is critical for especially the adult form of neurogenesis? The emergence, around the early 2000s, of adult neurogenesis research liberated the lab and its research from the margins and opened venues for international collaborations that were not focused on CPPs but on plasticity.

Alain's vision of a silent embryogenesis made him an avant-garde thinker who had been ahead of his time. His hardship and perseverance made him a star of the newly emerging relational web.

Enfant Terrible, Still

In Paris, however, things were different. At home, many of his colleagues still regarded Alain as an *enfant terrible.*[60]

In informal settings, for example, many people I talked to were eager to tell me "the truth" about Alain. They described him as a "trickster," a "sexist," a "homophobe," a "homosexual," or a "communist." Some explicitly held him and him alone responsible for the advent of plasticity and described him "and his postmodern friends" as traitors of reason, out there to destroy science.[61]

"How come so many colleagues are being taken for a ride by him?" on senior electrophysiologist asked me. "I know that he is charming, a great seducer. And yet, don't they see that he is not a serious scientist? That he makes claims that are unfounded and simply wrong? All this talk about plasticity—from a neuroscientific point of view it is ridiculous."

A more elaborate and indirect form of criticism I encountered was the enthusiastic praise of his work on Penetratin. Alain, I was told, must be seen as a formidable pharmacologist who had invented an excellent tool. This emphasis on *invention* and *tool,* I quickly learned, was a courteous way of saying that Alain is primarily a technician, not a biologist, and that the non-autonomous transfer of Antennapedia is a technique he has invented, not an in vivo phenomenon he has discovered. This critique most often accompanied a comment about Alain's company, Elistem Biopharmaceuticals (which he founded with friends and colleagues in 2002), as if mentioning his company would reveal what he really is, namely an *applied* scientist. A business-man could not possibly be a *real* scientist.

The most widespread critique, however, focused on Alain's ventures into the domain of the arts. In both informal and formal settings, for example, when someone introduced him before a lecture, Prochiantz was described as a brilliant thinker and theoretician. What appeared to be appreciation was in fact a polite way of refusing to call him a brilliant scientist. A distinct form of this dismissal was to call him in passing a *homme de science* and then to explain at length that he is as well a *homme de lettre* and a *homme de théâtre.* In almost every conversation, such an "appreciation" was a way of saying that there was something dubious about him, that he had a penchant for specula-tion, for ideas, and that I should not take his talk all that seriously.

"How do you deal with such criticism?" I once asked Alain when we were walking home together after he had given a talk.

"Their critique doesn't bother me much," he smiled. "I am not responsible for their stupidity. I mean, I don't know if the nonautonomous transfer has an in vivo function. But at least I can think. I mean, seriously, what hurts me is not that they criticize me. Criticism is important. What hurts me is how stupid their critique is. I feel sorry for them."

After a few minutes' silence he added in a fragile, silent voice: "Of course critique hurts. One learns to ignore it, you know. Perhaps one learns to live with it, to the degree this is possible."

Return to the Collège de France?

When I left Paris, in the summer of 2003, the lab was—despite the still intense turbulence that surrounded it—doing well experimentally as well as relationally. Experimentally, it was busy moving from technology to physiology, from the technical in vitro work to the critical question of whether or not the non-autonomous transfer had a physiological function. The mood was cautiously optimistic. There were several indicators that the projects under way would succeed. Particularly promising was the work of Stéphan on the importance of the nonautonomous transfer of Emx2 for axonal sprouting in the adult (briefly mentioned at the beginning of this chapter); a close collaboration with Christine Holt at Cambridge, largely focused on the role of Eng for growth and guidance of axons during embryogenesis and in the adult (specifically, the development and transformation of the retino-tectal topographic map); a study of the significance of the nonautonomous transfer of Eng for the repro- duction and maintenance of dopaminergic cells in the substantia nigra; and a project concerned with the role of homeoprotein Pax6 for the formation and reformation of function-specific areas of the central nervous system.

Relationally, too, the lab was successful, with collaborations in France, the United Kingdom, Germany, Japan, and the United States. This relational success was remarkable. In 2003, strictly speaking, there was no more evi- dence for an exchange of homeoproteins in the living brain than there had been in 1989, when Alain and Joliot's first paper was so vehemently rejected. Nevertheless, what had been a scandalous claim back then, a silent embryo- genesis in the adult brain controlled by the nonautonomous transfer of homeoproteins, seemed now possible and even plausible.[62] What a neuronal researcher could reasonably say about the brain had changed. Even at home, among his Parisian colleagues, Alain seemed to gradually be appreci- ated (especially by a more junior cohort). The most powerful hint for this appreciation was a rumor that began to spread just at the time of my depar- ture—that Alain might get elected to the Collège de France and replace Glowinski.[63]

That Alain was positioning himself in a strategic game I could observe throughout my stay. A whole series of events suggested that he was refashioning himself as neuro-bio-pharmacologist and hence as a successor to Glowinski. In 2002, he took over the directorship for the DEA in neuropharmacology and launched Elistem Biopharmaceuticals; in 2003 he changed the name of his lab from "Evolution and Development of the CNS" to "Neuropharmacology and Development"; and in 2004 he became a member of the Académie de Science, an institution he had previously smiled at ("Still smiles at," he commented on an earlier draft of this chapter). Throughout my time in his lab he had what could be called relation-building dinners with professors of the Collège (Peyret, his most important collaborator, accompanied him on some of these occasions).

In fall 2004 the decision about the position at the Collège was made. Perhaps because I had been thinking of Alain's work as a success story, I assumed he would get the job. But there is no logic to history—at least no apparent one, not to this one. In fall 2004 Stanislas Dehaene, a protégé of Changeux, got the job. I thought that this would be it for Alain and that he would leave France altogether, accepting an offer he had received from Columbia University. But I was wrong. When I met Prochiantz in May 2005, he explained, with a big smile, that nothing was decided yet.

"First Glowinski retired," Alain told me. "And now it is Changeux's turn."

In 2006, he indeed was elected professor at France's most elite academic institution, the Collège de France. And as the relational information goes—which is, I now know, very different from gossip—Alain was elected with the support less of the scientists than of the arts and humanities (though Alain vehemently disagrees with this story).

What had begun with an obscure observation in Paris (1989)—or with a reading adventure in New York (1985)—had grown into one of the key sites of the new, still-emerging conception of the brain as plastic.

Reason and relation had mutated together.

Regional Rationalities

Shortly after I left Paris, I began to read the work of the French historian of science Gaston Bachelard. Alain had told me that he had been taking seminars with Georges Canguilhem, and this made me curious. If Alain had been a student of Canguilhem, and Canguilhem had been a student of Bachelard, could I perhaps recognize elements of Bachelard's conceptualization of scientific knowledge production in Alain's way of producing scientific knowledge?

While reading Bachelard, still under the impression of the relationalism that silently choreographs Parisian life, I soon found myself wondering about a whole other question, one that was to me as exciting as surprising: Could it be that Bachelard was actually a nativist? Couldn't one say—wouldn't one have to say—that his analytical tools were relational ways of sense-making, insofar as he decoded scientific facts into relational ones? Didn't Bachelard—and with him a whole series of French thinkers, from Bourdieu to Latour—assess the world from the natives' point of view?[1]

Gaston Bachelard, who was born in 1884 in Bar-sur-Aube and died in 1962 in Paris, was a French historian of science. In France, the history of science is not just any subject. At least since the early nineteenth century it has been a topic of broad and general importance to disciplines ranging from philosophy to ethnology to science itself.[2] If one asks for the reason for the prominence of a field that in many other countries is at best confined to the margins of academic life, one is usually referred to Auguste Comte, the French Hegel, who fought energetically for the creation of a chair for the history of science at the Collège de France. Given his theory of a three-stage evolution of the human mind—theological, metaphysical, positive—he regarded the history of science as a sort of philosophy of the contemporary state of the *esprit humaine*.[3] Bachelard claimed membership in this tradition. Indeed, his work is as much a philosophy of the contemporary as it was a history of science.[4]

The main theme of Bachelard's work concerns what he called the epistemological rupture between everyday conceptions of the real and the scientifically real. More specifically, he was concerned with how the *nouvelle esprit scientifique,* the emergence of which he dated to Einstein's 1905 sketch of the theory of relativity, amounted to a whole new kind of the scientifically real. The theory of relativity, and the subsequent emergence of quantum physics, Bachelard argued, escaped the two epistemological schools that had thus far explained how scientists get to know things in the world—constructivism (the idealists) and realism (the materialists). The challenge Bachelard set for himself was to articulate a new epistemology, one that would do justice to the *nouvelle esprit.* In twenty-three books published between 1929 and 1962, he sought to elaborate this new epistemology. One of them, *Le Rationalisme Appliqué,* is of special interest here.

Bachelard opens *Le Rationalisme Appliqué* with an analysis of the way cyclotrons (one of the first was constructed by Frédéric Joliot) produce isotopes and how these isotopes are identified by mass spectrometry. On many condensed pages he is at pains to make comprehensible the idea that the atoms a cyclotron allows a physicist to know cannot actually be found as such in nature, not as actually out there as discrete objects, just too tiny to be seen. Instead, he suggests, they are technically materialized theoretical phenomena. Not that they were, he explained, a mere arbitrary invention of a speculative mind. And yet, they ultimately exist only because "abstract rationalities" have made them thinkable and, translated into technological apparatuses, visible and thus available to experimentation.

For Bachelard, scientific concepts are scientific when they are technical: "Les trajectoires qui permettent de séparer les isotopes dans le spectroscope de masse n'existent pas dans la nature; il faut les produire techniquement. Elles sont de théorèmes réifiés."[5] And precisely insofar as they are "reified theorems"—produced through a coming together of the conceptual and the technological that he called an *"acte épistémologique"*—Bachelard could conclude that neither constructivism (scientific objects are constructed) nor realism (scientific objects a real entities) is an approach that suffices for comprehending the *nouvelle esprit de la science.*[6]

Bachelard's alternative was what he called "applied rationalism," or "technical materialism," by which he meant that scientific objects or truths are a form of technically materialized—occasionally he said, "realized"—rationalities, which are always in an "emergent state."[7]

Scientific objects—he was adamant about this—never stood still.

An important consequence of the *nouvelle esprit de science* was for Bachelard that it would inevitably cause a fundamental "regionalization" of knowledge production.[8] Inevitably, scientists working in their own labs would develop their theories, with ever more detailed and refined technologies to materialize these theories. Each laboratory would thus, necessarily, have its own rationality and hence its very own kind of knowledge.

And Bachelard pushed his concept of a provincialization of science even further. He vehemently insisted that each one of these regional rationalities—Bachelard occasionally spoke of "cultures"—would have hardly any relevance for other regions insofar as those regions' objects of knowledge are the result of different theories and different methods to reify them. Sooner or later, he speculated, different regions might even become "incommensurable" to one another.[9]

With his insistence on "regional rationalities," Bachelard sought to replace the more traditional philosophy of science, according to which all science is characterized by a single, universal rationality. Bachelard's programmatic message was that epistemologists had to give up the futile task of finding and naming such a universal rationality. Rather they should study the increasingly multiple and incommensurable regions of scientific knowledge productions. They should understand the different, always emerging "rationalities" that organize them, and analyze the *acte épistémologique* specific to each one of them. What mattered were epistemological ruptures, jumps, breaks, and displacements—not a unified rationality that would never be found.[10]

> La question ne se pose donc plus de définir un rationalisme général qui recueillerait la partie commune des rationalismes régionaux. On ne retrouverait dans cette voie que le rationalisme minimum utilisé dans la vie commune. On effacerait les structures. Il s'agit tout au contraire de multiplier et d'affiner les structures, ce qui du point de vue rationaliste doit s'exprimer comme une activité de structuration, comme une détermination de la possibilité de multiples axiomatiques pour faire face à la multiplication des expériences.[11]

It was precisely Bachelard's idea of "regional rationalities" that made me first wonder whether one could call him a nativist. Couldn't one say that Bachelard's description of science mirrored the relational organization that constituted the world of which he was part? Couldn't one say that Bachelard, product and astute observer of French science, took one of the basic features that structured the world that surrounded him, relations, and used it to think through the implications of the emergence of the new spirit of science? Wouldn't one have to argue that when Bachelard writes of a "city of knowledge" and its different "regions," "cantons," "districts," "areas," and "domains," he relies precisely on the relationalism characteristic of Parisian life in general and of academic life in particular?[12]

If Bachelard is approached not only as the brilliant epistemologist he is usually remembered as but also as the native he was, then his concept of epistemic ruptures opens up a whole new, unexpected way of understanding his oeuvre.

Couldn't one say that for Bachelard epistemic ruptures were at least as much a conceptual as a relational event? If every region has its own rationality with its own questions and problems, and thus its own technically reified and materialized objects, wouldn't the logical conclusion be that the expansion of one's relational web, the sweet search for allies and the brutal elimination of competitors, is the way to make one's own work matter?

This is precisely what Bachelard means when he writes that the "emergent quality" of scientific objects is socially constituted: "Ces émergences sont effectivement constitue socialement."[13]

More relations, more truth. That is why the history of science has to be written as a history of relations.

Note, though, that Bachelard, at least as far as the natives' point of view is concerned, does not speak here about ruthless individuals who seek to maximize power. Rather, Bachelard's speaks about *the last métro*—about seduction, love, wit, sex and death.

Differently put, guarding one's relations is a matter of such exquisite passion—and art—not only, perhaps not even primarily, because of one's work, one's own rationality, one's own vision of science. All of this would presuppose that humans are individuals, monads, who merely use relations. Instead, it is a matter of such intensity precisely because humans—in Paris, at least—are relational. Bachelard thus adds an existential edge to science—or makes science one of the venues of the art of living.[14]

And the other French authors mentioned above? I began to draw up a list of (some of) the French thinkers who have so brilliantly taught us to think about the world in relational terms, from Saint Simon and Durkheim to Tarde, Dumont, Bourdieu, and Latour.

Couldn't one—wouldn't one have to—argue that they were all, just like Bachelard, nativists? Wouldn't one—couldn't one—actually understand the analytical categories they use—such as—"the field," "the social," "relations," "reproduction," "distinction," "actor network theory," "mediation"—as different interpretations of the natives' point of view, as abstractions from and generalizations of the relational organization of the world to which they belong?

That is, as nativism?[15]

THREE

Conceptual

The neurosciences have experienced an expansion matched only
by the growth of physics at the beginning of the century and of
molecular biology in the 1950s. The impact of the discovery of
the synapse and its functions is comparable to that of the atom
or DNA.

JEAN PIERRE CHANGEUX, *L'homme neuronal*

"For the anatomist I am," Jean Pierre Bourgeois explained, "the cortex is a
thoroughly fixed and immutable structure."

It was January 2003. We were sitting in a corner of the cafeteria at the
Institut Pasteur (IP), where Jean Pierre, then in his early fifties, was a senior
researcher.

"Changes," he went on, describing the basic anatomical structure of the
human brain, "can be observed only on the level of the synapse."

We had gotten to know each other only a couple months earlier when Jean
Pierre had been teaching the anatomy section of my one-year DEA in neuropharmacology. Once he learned that I was an anthropologist interested in
the brain, he was determined to make me familiar with the anatomical basis
of things human. "We should have a conversation," he said, approaching me
in the middle of a lecture. "I am interested in anthropology."

For a few months, beginning in early 2003, we met in the IP cafeteria,
where he, always equipped with pen and paper, drew shapes of different neurons to explain the structural composition of the central nervous system—
and to elaborate how these shapes allowed for the possibility of the human.
On that day in January, we had met to talk about the cortex.

"These changes on the level of the synapse," Jean Pierre continued, "are the
expression of adaptation and individuation, learning and memory, and thus
the locus of an openness constitutive of the human, as opposed to other animals. Everything distinctly human can be found, in fact it can *only* be found,
on the level of the synapse."

"Distinctly human?" I asked.

"By 'distinctly human' I mean all that which is not determined by nature. A space of liberty and freedom that is constitutive of culture and hence the human."

This was the lesson Jean Pierre had prepared for me and that he repeated, in so many different ways, in almost all of our conversations: "The existence of culture is the direct result of synaptic plasticity. Synapse," he emphatically but not without irony declared, "synapse is liberty!"

Jean Pierre knew what he was talking about. For almost a decade, from the mid-1980s to the mid-1990s he had studied—as a postdoc of Pasco Rakic at Yale—the development of the nervous system in macaque monkeys and other primates.[1] The two fixated (killed) animals at different developmental stages, from before birth to old age. They then froze their brains, cut them in thin slices, and analyzed, with electron microscopes, the gradual cellular formation of the central nervous system, with a particular focus on the cortex.[2]

In eight classic papers Jean Pierre and Rakic established that primates (human and nonhuman) are born with a definite number of neurons, that after birth no new neurons are added to the nervous system, and that post-natal brain development consists largely of a massive increase in synaptic connectivity. In humans this increase begins in the uterus and continues until puberty is reached, at roughly the age of fifteen or sixteen. Next, an astonishing decrease of synaptic connectivity sets in. Until the age of twenty to twenty-five a huge part of the established connections irreversibly die and disappear.[3] From the mid-twenties onward, the pattern of synaptic connections remains almost stable—almost, because there is a silent but accumulative loss of synapses that can eventually result in old age senility.[4]

"And liberty?" I wondered when we discussed the papers he had written with Rakic.

"Given the essential fixity of the brain we have observed," Jean Pierre replied, "the synapse is the only plausible locus of liberty. This is my take-home message for you: culture, that is, liberty, is ultimately an anatomical and, as far as synaptic communication is concerned, a chemical condition."[5]

Alain's work, about which we spoke rarely, neither challenged nor changed Jean Pierre's synaptology of the human. The idea of a silent embryogenesis in the adult was to him little more than a counterintuitive speculation, and the nonautonomous transfer of homeoproteins was less a phenomenon in vivo than a potentially valuable technology. For Jean Pierre, the birth of new neurons in the adult—the event most decisive for the eventual emergence of a morphogenetically plastic brain—was a dramatically overvalued.

"Adult neurogenesis," he commented regarding a paper we both had read, "is restricted to fairly ancient parts of the brain, namely to the dentate gyrus (part of the hippocampus) and the olfactory system, and hence cannot account for the distinctly human."

For Jean Pierre, the brain was composed of distinct layers, each with a different evolutionary point of origin. As the oldest of these layers were widely shared in the animal kingdom, they could not account for the distinctively human, which he associated largely with the most recent layer, the neocortex. (This hierarchical and historical interpretation of the brain goes back to the British physician and neurologist John Hughlings Jackson [1835–1911]).[6]

"I fully understand that people are excited about adult neurogenesis," he went on. "This is an expression of their desire for liberty and human freedom. I share this desire. But from a strictly anatomical point of view, these are minor phenomena that do not impact the fact that our brain and, hence, we are to a large degree determined. Only the synapse is plastic."

And then Jean Pierre smiled, raised his finger, and repeated his favorite sentence: "Synapse is liberty!"

A BRAIN BEYOND THE SYNAPSE?

Jean Pierre's synaptology of the human set in motion my understanding of Alain's work. Until I met Jean Pierre, I had assumed that plasticity was such a scandal because it undermined the widely shared assumption that the adult brain is an immutable cellular structure (and because of Alain's provocations). This impression was confirmed, I thought, by conversations with electrophysiologists and chemists who either explained (in the case of the former) that "the brain is already wired" or (in case of the latter) that "the brain is a chemical machine."[7] However, Jean Pierre's anatomy lessons made me wonder if fixity was perhaps only half the story?

I often came away from our conversations with the impression that Jean Pierre had much less investment in fixity as such than in the synapse—as if plasticity was somehow threatened to undermine his synaptic conception of the human. Didn't he frequently juxtapose the plastic with the synaptic brain, as if the two were mutually exclusive—two different, conceptually incommensurable brains? Gradually, I began to wonder whether Alain's work was scandalous not because it undermined fixity, but because by undermining fixity it threatened the synaptic conception of the nervous system. Could that be?

Were the other critics of plasticity also synaptologists?

I went over my notes again, broadened my conversations, and worked through the articles that rejected plasticity of the brain. What I found was that indeed almost all of the critiques—whether by electrophysiologists, chemists, molecular biologists, or cognitive psychologists—rejected plasticity in favor of a synaptic, neurochemical conception of the brain. Consistently, they argued that synaptic communication, and not the growth of new or the disappearance of old neuronal tissue, had to be seen as the key to mental disorders, to memory and learning, to the self, to social behavior, and, as Jean Pierre had it, to the distinctively human.

"The fixity of our brain," one electrophysiologist told me, "guarantees the continuity of memory and hence a sense of self. The death and birth of new neurons would be deleterious for humans. Understanding the wiring and firing of synapses is the only way to plausibly understand cerebral function."[8]

I was overwhelmed—shocked—by the implications of my findings. Indeed, Alain's work was much more provocative than I thought! If he and his colleagues—Brigitte, Michel, Joliot, and Trembleau—were to be able to show that the nonautonomous transfer of homeoproteins effectively keeps the nervous system in a continuous embryonic (plastic) state, they would have effectively called into question the significance of the synapse for understanding the brain. They would have subverted the very conception of the brain that seemed to tacitly organize neuronal research.

Slowly my discovery of the egregious magnitude of Alain's insistence on plasticity mutated into a nervous excitement—and a whole new appreciation of Alain's work began to take form. At stake in the battles that surrounded Alain's lab, or so it seemed to me now, was not at all whether or not the brain is plastic. At stake was instead how one would have to think the brain and how it functions. At stake was the effort to overthrow how the majority of neuronal researchers understood the brain. At stake was the suggestion that their understanding was wrong, that one would have to invent a whole new, different way of thinking the central nervous system. At stake was what Jean Pierre called the "distinctively human."

Could that be?

Amidst my rising enthusiasm about the sweeping metamorphosis of the brain—of the human—my lab seemed to hope to achieve, I began to wonder when the brain was first described as a synaptic organ. "If it were true," I scribbled in my notebook, "that the synapse was already identified in the 1890s as the key to understanding the brain, as most books on the history of neuroscience had it, then wouldn't that imply that the experiments meant to prove an ongoing silent embryogenesis in the adult brain were putting in question a century of neuronal research?"

I went to the library of the ENS determined to figure out when it was established that the adult brain, except on the level of synapses, was essentially a fixed and immutable cellular structure. How was the synaptic conception of the brain brought into existence? By whom? Where? Was this conceptualization controversial at the time? What were the alternatives it proved wrong? Was it ever challenged after it became dominant? Has fixity throughout served as the condition of the possibility of the synapse?

Were Alain and his researchers really up against a century of neuronal research?

REPORT FROM THE LIBRARY: A CENTURY OF NEURONAL KNOWLEDGE PRODUCTION

As it turned out, fixity and the synapse have closely intertwined histories yet they belong to different epochs. Fixity, first authoritatively asserted in 1897 by the Spanish histologist Santiago Ramón y Cajal (1852–1934), was the culmination of the nineteenth-century effort to understand the brain in terms of its cellular coming into existence. The synapse, however, a term coined by Sir Charles Scott Sherrington (1857–1952), also in 1897, marks the beginning of the twentieth-century functional (physiological) interpretation of the fixed cellular anatomy drawn up during the previous century. Fixity marks somewhat of an end, the synapse a beginning.

Fixity: The Brain Enters Cell Theory

In the 1830s, thirty years after Franz Josef Gall's localization theory had established the brain as the organ constitutive of the human, a new line of brain research emerged in Germany. The nervous system was being enrolled in the theory of the cell. Already two decades later authors such as Jan Evangelista Purkynjě (1787–1869), Theodor Schwann (1810–1882), Robert Remak (1815–1865), Rudolph Virchow (1821–1902), and Albrecht von Kölliker

(1817–1905) had well established that the nervous system is, like any other organ (like any other plant, as Schleiden had it), composed of cells—and had thereby prepared the grounds for the emergence of a novel branch of research: the inquiry into the cellular composition of the nervous system.[9] One could now study cells—and draw conclusions about the human.[10]

The problem that dominated early histology was largely a methodological one: finding a way to order the seemingly chaotic cellular composition of the brain. Of what kind of cells is the brain composed? Can one, morphologically speaking, set apart different kinds of cells? Are different kinds of cells found in different regions of the brain? And how does this cellular organ give rise to the distinct human faculties?

Among the researchers who addressed these questions was a physician and embryologist little remembered today named Richard Altmann (1852–1900). Around 1880, working under the guidance of Wilhelm His at the University of Leipzig, Altmann applied Walther Fleming's then-novel method for staining mitoses to the human brain. What he found was rather curious: there was no single mitotic figure after birth. Humans, he concluded, are born with a definite number of nerve cells. Curious Altmann's finding was insofar as it presented histologists with an unexpected antinomy: If there are no new nerve cells after birth, how, then, could one explain the postnatal growth of the brain? And how was one to explain distinctive human capacities that seem to emerge only much after birth, like reasoning, memory formation, and language? Altmann summarized his observation in a privately printed 1881 article that he sent to a few select researchers across Europe, many of whom repeated his experiments and confirmed his argument, and thus the predicament.[11]

At the time Ramón y Cajal began his anatomical work in the mid-1880s, two mutually exclusive responses were given to Altmann's antinomy. On the one hand, there was the Italian histologist Camillo Golgi, inventor of the *reatione nera,* one of the most powerful staining methods of the late nineteenth century. By drawing on his stains and on the earlier work of Joseph Gerlach (1873), Golgi argued that nerve cells form a reticulum, that is, that the whole brain is a single, giant multinucleic cell that is fully in place at the time of birth and then merely gets bigger.[12]

On the other hand, there was the work of Wilhelm His (1831–1904) and Auguste Forel (1894–1932), both Swiss, the former working in Leipzig and the latter in Zurich. His, a world-famous embryologist and Altmann's academic supervisor, concluded that if Altmann was right, if indeed no new cells are formed after birth, then the only plausible key to understanding the cellular composition of the brain was embryogenesis. In his research, he then set out to follow the emergence of nerve cells in the course of embryogenesis and to map how they gradually found their place. What he found was that nerve cells are actually independent units, that nerve fibers are the outgrowth of single nerve cells (at the time, some speculated that the fibers grew independently of cells), and that while this outgrowth becomes more complex over the course of embryogenesis, it remains, at least up until birth, discontinuous.[13] The nerve fibers of one cell don't touch those of another cell.[14]

Auguste Forel's work was more inspired by His than by Altmann (it is unclear whether Forel even knew of Altmann). To be more precise, Forel was intrigued by a finding that was somewhat of a by-product of His's analysis— the contiguity of nerve cells. Was His right? Are nerve cells really contiguous? And was this also true for the adult? Forel, working in Zurich, repeated and expanded His's work. In a random, nonsystematic manner he cut through embryonic and mature brains and found that his Leipzig colleague had gotten it right: nerve cells are contiguous throughout life. Consequently, Forel concluded, Gerlach and Golgi were wrong.[15]

Ramón y Cajal's early morphological studies convinced him that His and Forel had gotten it right. Like them, he followed the growth of the nerve cell and concluded that projections grow from the cell body and are continuous. And like them, he became a ferocious opponent of Gerlach and Golgi.[16] Unlike His and Forel, however, Ramón y Cajal was systematically inclined. Where the two Swiss had eclectically followed one nerve cell at a time, the Spaniard wondered about the whole brain. If there are no new nerve cells after birth, and if nerve cells are independent and contiguous, then wouldn't a comparative study of when and how nerve cells emerge, of how and where they migrate, and of how their fibers and their distinct forms grow make possible a systematic cellular comprehension of the brain?

Over the course of the 1880s, Ramón y Cajal cut his way through bird, chicken, and cat embryos and systematically followed the cellular development of the brain over the course of embryogenesis (and, in a few cases, also after birth). In each species he found that development follows a similar plan: individual nerve cells emerge during embryogenesis; by the time an animal is born, they have given rise to the basic anatomical structures of the nervous system; and postnatal development essentially consists of the growth of the fine structure, that is, the smaller branches of the neuronal tree.

From these studies he concluded that the growth of axons and dendrites had to be the key to understanding the storage of experience and hence the brain and human.[17] It had to be, because the growth of the fine structure seemed the only true dynamic element of the emergent brain; hence, it was the only plausible way to understand the nervous system.[18]

By the late 1880s, his work on the cellular emergence of the brain had made Ramón y Cajal one of the most prominent histologists of his times. The major breakthrough to fame, or so he reflected in his autobiography, came in 1889 at the Anatomical Congress in Berlin, where he succeeded in convincing some of the major figures in the cellular study of the nervous system that he was right—and Golgi and Gerlach wrong.[19]

Among those who had fallen to Ramón y Cajal was also the German histologist Wilhelm Waldeyer (1836–1924). Indeed, Waldeyer was so much taken with the young Spaniard that he published a review about state-of-the-art brain science that made Ramón y Cajal a major reference to histologists across Europe. He suggested calling Ramón y Cajal's individual nerve cells "neurons" and then went on to provide a sketch of what he referred to as Ramón y Cajal's "neuron doctrine," which he contrasted with Gerlach and Golgi's "reticularism." Soon thereafter, the work of the Spanish histologist was translated into German, French, Italian, and English. It was discussed in anatomy journals and Ramón y Cajal toured Europe to give talks and receive honorary degrees (and, in 1906, the Nobel Prize).

Amidst the furor that increasingly surrounded him, Ramón y Cajal then embarked on a new, even more ambitious project: a multivolume atlas of the human nervous system in its entirety, composed of detailed maps of the cellular becoming and composition of the various brain regions. He carefully documented the kind of neurons constitutive of each center and provided drawings of their typical form and distinctive pattern of connection. To this day, or so Jean Pierre assured me in one of our conversations, Ramón y Cajal's *Textura del sistema nervioso del hombre y vertebrados,* published between 1897 and 1904, forms the basis of our anatomical comprehension of the brain.[20]

Jean Pierre was the proud owner of a stained slice of cerebral tissue produced by Ramón y Cajal, from whom he as an anatomist traced descent.

It was in the opening pages of the *Textura* that I found the earliest explicit and conceptually coherent suggestion that the adult brain is an immutable cellular structure. "In fully grown animals, the nervous system is essentially fixed."[21]

What, though, did Ramón y Cajal mean by "fixity"? How did he arrive at the conclusion that the mature brain is "essentially fixed?"[22] Frantically, I kept on reading, but to no avail. Nowhere in his text does he provide a straightforward answer. However, at the end of the *Textura,* after well over a thousand pages, in the context of a final speculative outlook in which he correlates the brain and the human, there are a few lines that make clear what Ramón y Cajal did *not* mean by "fixity." He writes: "The ability of neurons to [...] create new associations in the adult" is likely to be the physiological basis of "human adaptability and facility to change ideational systems."[23]

When I first read these lines, I was taken aback. New associations? Meaning the growth of new branches on the neuronal tree? How did that fit with fixity? I began to systematically read Ramón y Cajal's work from the 1880s onward and found that already in 1894, in a lecture at Oxford, he had suggested that "mental exercise facilitates [...] a multiplication of the terminal branches of preexisting connections between groups of cells," potentially even "the formation of new collaterals and protoplasmic extensions."[24]

His decade-long work on development, from the early 1880s to the early 1890s, had convinced him that the space available for the growth of new tissue in the adult brain is greatly limited. Once sexual maturity is reached—once the cellular trees have fully branched out—the growth of the fine structure, constitutive of storage, could occur only within already existing, preformed connections among neurons. The scale was tiny.

In lectures and conversations with students, Ramón y Cajal frequently argued that in the brain of an adult human there is simply no place left for growth (storage)—except perhaps, as he speculated shortly before his death in a letter to his student Rafael Lorente de Nó, on the level of dendritic spines (discovered by Ramón y Cajal).[25] And in old age even this minimal space would eventually be used up, causing the incapacity to form new memories.

Ramón y Cajal's brain was "essentially"—not strictly—fixed.[26]

In sharp contrast to Jean Pierre and other synaptologists of the human, Ramón y Cajal in fact did not formulate the concept of fixity against the assumption of lifelong growth, which for him was obvious. Fixity and plasticity, understood as the growth of new, still-plastic tissue, were to him not necessarily mutually exclusive. But then, Ramón y Cajal, like the contemporary synaptologists I encountered, effectively precluded the possibility of profound structural changes—of the birth of new neurons, axons, or dendrites. To him, such structural changes would have undermined memory and identity, both the result of the neuronal storage of earlier experiences. Ramón y Cajal's work thus simultaneously undermined the concept of fixity regnant in 2003 and confirmed or at least prefigured it.

And the synapse?

The concept of the synapse came from elsewhere, was the product of a different regional rationality.

The story begins with a disagreement, carried out on stage, at the 1881 International Medical Congress in London. On one side was Friedrich Goltz (1834–1902), a German physiologist who argued that the lesion experiments he had conducted since the early 1870s had proven that the brain is devoid of specialized areas. To underscore his argument, he operated on stage, randomly cutting lesions in a dog's brain, so that everyone could observe that none of his incisions caused any obvious functional impairment. Hence, Goltz concluded, the idea of a function-specific anatomy had to be wrong.[27] On the other side was David Ferrier (1843–1928), a gentle Scot who operated on a monkey, right after Goltz, to show that the German was wrong: of course the brain was compartmentalized in task-specific regions.

Reading through the debate that ensued between the two, it seems as if Ferrier thought of Goltz as a relic of an earlier time. He judged the German's tools as too crude and his conclusions as too sweeping. Politely seeking to escape a confrontation, Ferrier suggested that, as lower animals, dogs may not actually need a highly refined function-specific cortex. But for monkeys, as his surgery had shown, this was obviously different: the cortex of higher animals is organized into functionally specific areas.

In the aftermath of the conference, Charles Sherrington, then a physiology student at Cambridge, was charged, along with John Newport Langley (1852–1927), a young Cambridge professor, with studying the brain of Goltz's dog.[28] What they found was that Goltz's lesion had actually resulted in the death of a great many neurons—but only of those that Goltz had actually managed to damage.

It was while working on Goltz's dog and wondering why the cuts of the German physiologist had not visibly affected the dog's behavior, that Sherrington first found himself gripped by a set of questions that would not let go of him for his entire scientific career: What path actually leads from the brain to the rest of the body? How does the brain control the body's movements? And how does information travel from the body to the brain?

Sherrington's answer to these questions was the spine—and his ambitious hope was that he could use the electrophysiological instruments recently invented by Emil du Bois-Reymond (1818–1896) and Hermann von Helmholtz (1821–1894) to map how electric impulses flow from the brain through the spine to the periphery and thereby organize the movements of an organism.[29]

In 1890, after half a decade of rather disappointing research, Sherrington began to wonder if he had addressed the problem of the cord from the wrong end. Instead of approaching the functional role of the spine top-down (from cortex to cord), wouldn't it be more promising to try a bottom-up approach (from the skeletal muscles and nerves to the cord and from there to the cortex)?[30] He began to work on the knee-jerk reflex and quickly made several discoveries. First, he identified the cellular substrate of what he called the reflex arc, from muscle to cord and brain and back. Then he used the tools of electrophysiology to measure how electricity flows through the arc. And eventually he learned to refine his instruments to such a degree that he could, by playing with the intensity of the stimulus, vary the muscle's reaction.

In the mid-1890s, when Sherrington began to emerge as one of the best-known physiologists of the nervous system, Sir Michael Foster (1836–1907), Cambridge's inaugural professor of physiology, invited Sherrington, his former student, to rewrite the brain section for a new edition of his *Textbook of Physiology* to be published in 1897. To Sherrington, Foster's invitation was an honor—and an opportunity to pause and abstract from his experimental findings a coherent conceptualization of the nervous system. It was in his contribution, that Sherrington first introduced the concept of the synapse.[31]

"So far as our present knowledge goes," the passage goes, "we are led to think that the tip of a twig of the arborescence is not continuous with but merely in contact with the substance of the dendrite or cell-body on which it impinges. Such a special connection of one nerve-cell with another might be called a synapsis."[32]

When I first read these lines, I was taken aback: Sherrington's distinction between the anatomical fact of contiguity—"not continuous"—and the "special connection [...] called a synapsis" radically defies the history of the synaptic brain as it is told by most histories of brain research (and certainly by all of the neuroscience textbooks I had read). According to these histories (and textbooks), it was precisely "the tip of the twig of the arborescence" that Sherrington defined as synapse. But this is, well, wrong. For Sherrington, the synapsis was neither the twig of an arborescence nor the space separating axon from dendrite or soma. Instead it was a physiological, electrical event that occurred in that space—in his words, "a special connection." The primary role of such a special connection, his text continues, is to transmit an electronic impulse from one cell to another:

In the ordinary action of the cell, nervous impulses pass along the axon centrifugally from the cell, and along the dendrites centripetally to the body of the cell surrounding the nucleus. Hence we may suppose that nervous impulses or influences sweeping along the axon of one cell are brought to bear through the terminal arborization of the axon or that of a collateral, on the dendrites of another cell, setting up in those dendrites nervous changes, which passing to the body of that cell issue in turn along its axon.[33]

However, Sherrington adds, it would be wrong to think of a synapsis as a mere transmission event. Rather, one has to understand it as a modulatory event: "The lack of continuity between the material of the arborization of the one cell and that of the dendrite (or body) of the other cell offers an opportunity for some change in the nature of the nervous influence as it passes from the one cell to the other."[34]

What led Sherrington to his conception of synapses (plural) as modulatory events was part observation, part speculation. He had noted that whenever he ran an electric current through nervous tissue, there was an inexplicable delay of about two milliseconds in the time an electrical impulse needed to travel from the site of stimulation to the site of measurement. Why this latency? Sherrington imagined that a marvelous event must take place in the gap that separates neurons from one another, an event in the course of which an incoming stimulus is not just transmitted but also interpreted and adjusted. And it was precisely these transmitting and interpreting synapses—later he would describe a synapsis as a "mode of nexus"—that Sherrington assumed must be key to understanding the work and action, if not of the nervous system, then at least of the spine. In Sherrington's own words:

> The delay in speed occurs whenever the impulses pass through the grey matter. [...] The delay in the grey matter may conceivably be due to slower conduction in the minute, branched, and more diffuse conducting elements— perikarya, dendrites, arborizations, etc.—found there [...]. The delay in the grey matter may be referable, therefore, to the transmission at the synapse. And if the delay occur at the synapse, the possibility suggests itself that the time consumed in the latent period may be spent mainly in establishing active connexion along the nervous-arc [...]. The latent time would then be comparable with time spent in closing a key to complete an electric circuit [...]. The key once closed [...], the transmission is as expeditious there as elsewhere.[35]

A few years later, in his 1904 Silliman Lecture, published in 1906 as *The Integrative Action of the Nervous System,* Sherrington spelled out the kind of nervous system his graphs of electric flows and reactions would give rise to. Abstracting from his work on the spinal cord, the skeletal muscles, and the cerebellum (a center for locomotion), he depicted the brain—the human—as a gigantic "reflex machine" made up of a definite number of discrete, if related, reflex arcs. The main task of this reflex machine, he explained, is the integration and coordination of the diverse electronically coded stimuli from the peripheral to the central nervous system and back. These stimuli travel, first, by way of synapses between cells (thereby enabling the organism to function as a unified whole) and, second, by way of the spinal cord—between "me" (the organism) and "not me" (the environment).[36]

Sherrington referred to humans as the "spinal animals."

Perhaps one has to pause for a moment to recognize the beautiful if accidental complementarity between the work of Ramón y Cajal and that of Sherrington.[37] The former's anatomical descriptions appear as a precondition for the electrophysiological inquiries of the latter. Only once Ramón y Cajal had described the adult human brain as essentially fixed—no new neurons, (almost) no new connections, no regeneration—could Sherrington succeed in thinking of Ramón y Cajal's anatomical drawings as electronic circuits, with the synapse as switch. Yet the difference between the two could hardly have been more radical. Sherrington's functionalization of the brain was a sweeping departure from Ramón y Cajal's histological drawings. For Ramón y Cajal, the brain was a freely growing (anatomical) assembly of cellular trees, and the gap between neurons was primarily an argument against Gerlach and Golgi—an anatomical detail of no further functional relevance. For Sherrington, however, the brain was an electrical machine, and the gap between neurons not just some empty space but a key site for understanding how this electrical machine functioned. Sherrington literally electrified the nervous system. And this electrification had far-reaching consequences for the concept of fixity. For Ramón y Cajal, minor growth in the adult was still possible. But once the brain had become an electrical machine, once axons and dendrites had become wires, there was no space for growth anymore, not even on a modest scale. How could a switchboard grow?

Strikingly, the radicalization of fixity brought about by Sherrington is best documented by the only passage in his writing in which he explicitly speaks about plasticity:

The more complex an organism, the more points of contact it has with the environment, and the more frequently will it need readjustment amid an environment of shifting relationships. These nervous organs of control being organs of adjustment will be more prominent the further the animal scale is followed upward to its crowning species, man. And these organs which give adjustability to the running of the reflex machinery, as such, seem themselves [. . .] to be among the most plastic in the body.[38]

A few sentences later Sherrington then explains what he means when he writes of the plasticity of nervous centers of control: "Mere experience can [. . .] mould nervous reactions insofar as they are plastic."[39]

For Sherrington, it is no longer the cellular tissue that is plastic. In his reflex machine, neither is there space for the growth of new cells nor can existing cells alter their form. Rather the "nervous reaction," that is, the ease with which electrical impulses are transmitted from axon to dendrite—from periphery to center—is plastic.

If Ramón y Cajal's brain was "essentially fixed," allowing for at least a minimal degree of free growth (and hence plasticity), Sherrington's was "strictly fixed." Fixity had become a conceptual presupposition of the synapses. No fixed brain, no synapsis.

Multitude—No Synaptic Brain Yet

According to the histories of neuronal research I read during my first months in Alain's lab, Ramón y Cajal and Sherrington established that the brain is a synaptic organ. What followed was merely refinement. In the wake of the two big men of the neuronal sciences, all serious brain research revolved around understanding how synaptic transmission organized nervous action and hence the human brain. However, reading the articles and books published in the aftermath of Ramón y Cajal's *Textura* and Sherrington's *Theory*, I found that this origins story is rather misleading. In the early twentieth century, there actually was no synaptic brain, not for Sherrington, not for his contemporaries.

Not for Sherrington, because he never actually suggested that the brain is synaptic. It was in his lab that the idea and concept of a synapsis was introduced and refined, but not, as popular history has it, as a universal fact of the brain. Rather, Sherrington assumed that synaptic organization is probably limited to certain nervous regions (neuromuscular junction, spinal cord, cerebellum) and functions (integration). As he explained in his Silliman Lecture:

> As to the existence or the non-existence of a surface of separation or membrane between neurone and neurone, that is a structural question on which only histology might be competent to give valuable information. In certain cases, especially in invertebrata, observation indicates that many nerve cells are actually continuous with one another.[40]

Not for his contemporaries, because outside of Sherrington's lab few people cared about the synapse. Instead of a coherent synaptic brain, one rather finds a wild and colorful diversity of differently conceptualized brains. For example, there were those who doubted contiguity altogether. The most prominent among the second-generation reticularists who succeeded Gerlach and Golgi included István Apáthy (1863–1922), a Hungarian microscopist and the German anatomists and neurologists Albrecht Bethe (1872–1954), Hans Held (1866–1942), and Franz Nissl (1860–1919). In a series of papers published between the 1890s and the 1910s, this Hungarian-German collective claimed—and documented with novel staining techniques (Nissl staining)—that the neuron doctrine was in fact wrong: neurons are not individual building blocks. Instead, tiny neurofibrils (Apáthy and Bethe) or intercellular gray (Nissl) or tiny leglike fibers called *Füsschen* (Held) maintain the continuity between nerve cells.

Neither Ramón y Cajal nor Sherrington had defeated reticularism. On the contrary, reticularism was alive and well and even expanding.[41]

Then there were the many groups, each a somewhat autonomous regional rationality, that supported contiguity but had no investment in Sherrington's concept of the synapse. Take the Cambridge school, which revolved around Keith Lucas (1879–1916) and Edgar Adrian (1889–1977). Sherrington's famous Cambridge colleagues both studied the nervous system in terms of electrophysiology. For them, as for Sherrington, the brain was an electrical organ. Unlike Sherrington, however, Lucas and Adrian never claimed a special reaction would occur in the space between axon and dendrite.[42] What mattered in Cambridge was less the synapsis—Lucas and Adrian had little interest in the speculative concept of contiguity and its functional role—but rather the more general proof that nerve cells send systematic signals to one another and thereby communicate.[43]

On the Continent, not only the synapse was absent, but the electrical brain as well. In Spain, for example, neuronal research was almost entirely untouched by the British debates. Ramón y Cajal and his students, most notably Pío del Río-Hortega (1882–1945) and Fernando de Castro, continued to analyze the brain in terms of its stages of cellular growth and to map the cellular composition of function-specific structures.[44] In Germany, as in Spain, the focus on cellular anatomy prevented a sustained interest in neuronal electrophysiology in general and in the concept of the synapse in particular.[45] But whereas the Spaniards focused on cellular growth, German histologists such as Oskar Vogt (1870–1959) and Cecile Vogt (1875–1962), and Korbinian Brodmann (1868–1918) were interested in classifying neurons according to their form and in understanding how that form was linked to their function.[46] In France, neither the synapse nor the study of the cellular composition of the brain were much present (histology was marginal in France until the early twentieth century).[47] After Jean-Martin Charcot, the field was dominated by a potpourri of the physiology of motor movement, localization theory (in the form of ablation experiments in the tradition of Broca), and psychiatry.[48]

As this brief tableau shows, before World War II, brain research was hardly organized by a single methodological challenge posed by a conceptually coherent synaptic brain that somehow emanated from the works of Ramón y Cajal and Sherrington. The exact opposite was the case—different local fragments of research gave rise to very different, somewhat incommensurable kinds of brains (anatomical brains, electronic brains, morphological brains, brains to operate on, etc.). Sherrington's synaptic reflex arcs were of little more than provincial relevance.

Neurochemistry, or the Emergence of the Synaptic Brain

The reason I stress the conceptual and methodological heterogeneity of neuronal research is that it is only against the background of this heterogeneity that one can appreciate the sweeping event the emergence of a synaptic brain after World War II actually was: it effectively ended the colorful diversity of brain conceptions that had characterized the neuronal sciences since the mid-nineteenth century. What brought about this end were three intertwined yet separate events that occurred in close temporal succession.

First, the problem of the synapsis was globalized (institutionally as well as relationally). Until World War II, the most prominent sites of brain research were England, Spain, and Germany. With the war's end and the defeat of Germany and Spain, the students and postdocs of Sherrington and Adrian, who were primarily concerned with the electrical transmission of nervous impulses, succeeded in securing important professorships in the United States, Europe, and Australia. Several launched major research centers concerned with what was increasingly referred to (especially among Sherringtonians) as synaptic communication. Among them were Bernhard Katz in London, Alexander Forbes at Harvard, John Eccles in Canberra, Hodgkin and Huxley at Cambridge, Alfred Fessard in Paris, Wilder Penfield in Montreal, Giuseppe Moruzzi in Pisa, and Frédéric Bremer in Brussels.[49]

Second, in the late 1940s and early 1950s, the synapsis was chemicalized. The story of the discovery of the chemical nature of synaptic communication is usually told as the battle between "the soups" and "the sparks"—that is, between chemists who argued that synaptic communication is a chemical event and electrophysiologists who insisted with Sherrington that synaptic transmission is electrical.[50] The chemists were organized around Henri Dale (1875–1968), Otto Loewi (1873–1961), Wilhelm Feldberg (1900–1993), Alfred Fessard (1900–1982), Bernhard Katz (1911–2003), and Stephen Kuffler (1913–1980). The main protagonists among the electrophysiologists were John Eccles (1903–1997), Alan Hodgkin (1914–1998), and Andrew Huxley (1917–2012). However, if one reads through the primary sources, it appears that the debate between chemists and electrophysiologists wasn't actually a debate about the nature of synaptic communication at all. The reason for this is that the chemists had no stake in the concept of the synapse. After all, a synapsis was an electrical event. To speak of a synapse implied upholding a conception of the brain as an electrical machine. For the chemists, however, the brain was a chemical organ run by chemical reactions that diffused transmitter substances from one cell to another. If anything, the chemists wrote against the very idea of a synapse, emphasizing instead their own concept, namely, diffusion.[51]

Over more than ten years, the chemists and the electrophysiologists—the diffusionists and the synaptologists—vehemently disagreed with one another. By the early 1950s, finally, the electrophysiologists had to give in. The defeat was announced in 1952 when John Eccles, the last student of Sherrington and most ferocious supporter of the synapse, conceded that "synaptic transmission" is indeed a chemical process.[52]

Eccles's 1952 paper was as epoch making as it was brilliant. By chemicalizing the synapse, he allowed Sherrington's concept to live on. And it was by and large only after Eccles's chemicalization of Sherrington's concept that the synapse emerged as a general synonym for the transmission of nervous impulses.[53]

Third, the synapse was universalized. After World War II, the old battle between reticularists and neuronists had faded but had hardly come to an end. There were still researchers who vehemently insisted that the brain is organized in the form of a single syncitium. The discovery of the chemical nature of synaptic communication did little to change this. Almost all of the experiments that had led to this discovery had been conducted either on crustaceans—because mini-electrodes are easily inserted into their large neurons—or on the neuromuscular junction or spinal cord of nonhuman animals. For those invested in continuity, there was no compelling reason to draw general conclusions about the brain as such from the work of a fairly small, institutionally closely related, and thematically somewhat idiosyncratic group of researchers who had conducted experiments on squids and lobsters. In 1952, no one had ever seen the gap Ramón y Cajal insisted was there, and hence no one knew whether all nervous tissue is contiguous, let alone synaptic.

In 1954 this changed. In a series of papers that marked the beginning of electron microscopic studies of the brain, Eduardo De Robertis (1913–1988), George Palade (1912–2008), and Sanford Palay (1918–2002) provided the first visual evidence that all neurons in all areas of the brain are contiguous. They documented presynaptic and postsynaptic terminals, showed synaptic clefts, and even found tiny vesicles that appeared to be the material substrate of neurotransmitter release across the synaptic cleft—exactly as Eccles and his chemist colleagues had assumed.[54]

It is difficult to overestimate the significance of the work of De Robertis, Palade, and Palay for the emergence of a synaptic brain. Their electron microscopic studies prepared the ground for the universalization of the chemical synapse that emerged just a few years earlier from the war between the soups and sparks. Only now, in the mid-1950s, did the whole brain become both contiguous and synaptic—indeed, contiguity and synapse came to mean one and the same thing.

The enthusiasm generated by the convergence of these three events was extraordinary. Out of the multitudinous past, a single conceptualization of the brain emerged—the chemical, synaptic brain machine. In the late 1950s and early 1960s neurochemistry emerged as *the* science of the brain—and already a decade later labs all over the world were busy understanding the brain, its diseases, and its humans in synaptic and chemical terms. Brain chemicals were systematized as neurotransmitters; neurons were classified according to the neurotransmitters they produce; new tools were invented to trace chemical-specific synaptic circuits; and soon the first links between mental and chemical processes were established, most notably with regard to memory and learning. For the first time in history a global, unified science of the nervous system emerged, grounded in a single conceptualization and nomenclature, in shared technologies, apparatuses, machines, and experimental systems.[55]

Despite these massive conceptual, methodological, and institutional changes, however, there was a powerful continuity between the prewar brains (plural) and the postwar brain (singular). The synaptic, neurochemical brain was conceptually still contingent on Ramón y Cajal's nineteenth-century observation of "essential fixity" and Sherrington's early-twentieth-century radicalization thereof. It was precisely the exclusion of embryogenetic, morphological processes from the adult that made the focus on the synapse meaningful. Synaptic communication seemed the only dynamic element of otherwise immutable cellular tissue.

The most beautiful illustration of this constitutive importance of fixity was the first fully worked-out theory of synaptic plasticity.

Concept Work (Linking Synapse and Liberty)

Already in the late 1940s, two psychologists, Jerzy Konorski (1903–1973) and Donald Hebb (1904–1985), embarked on what was at the time a rather provocative endeavor. Independently of each other, the former in Warsaw, the latter in Montréal, they sought to ground psychology in the neuronal knowledge of their day.

In the middle of the twentieth century the status of psychology as an independent discipline was still fragile. Throughout the nineteenth century, as many psychologists knew, psychology had not yet been set apart—on the level either of basic research questions or of methods—from the anatomical and histological study of the brain. On the contrary, they were inseparably intertwined. Psychology had only gradually and clumsily differentiated itself from brain research. To attempt to ground psychology in the neuronal sciences thus seemed to many of the colleagues of Konorski and Hebb hazardous.

While there were arguably many, geographically dispersed and conceptually diverse efforts to set apart psychology from anatomy, the major contribution to the consolidation of psychology as an autonomous discipline came from the behaviorists.

Although behaviorism has largely been an American affair, its origins lie in Russia. Beginning in the 1890s, the physiologist Ivan Pavlov (1849–1936) carried out a series of experiments showing that a formerly neutral stimulus, if frequently given in close temporal proximity to either a physiological or psychological stimulus, can come to stand in for the physiological or psychological stimulus itself. Pavlov then abstracted from his conditioning experiments a sketch of a psychology that would no longer revolve around the old philosophical vocabulary of introspection, consciousness, or feelings, but instead around concepts such as stimulus, inhibition, reward, punishment, and excitability. In the early twentieth century, the Americans John Watson (1878–1950) and Burrhus Frederic Skinner (1904–1990) then deduced from Pavlov's "other psychology" the idea of behaviorism—the scientific study of outward, observable behavior in terms of stimuli, response, and adaptation. As Watson wrote in 1913:

> Psychology as the behaviorist views it is a purely objective experimental branch of natural science. Its theoretical goal is the prediction and control of behavior. Introspection forms no essential part of its methods, nor is the scientific value of its data dependent upon the readiness with which they lend themselves to interpretation in terms of consciousness. The behaviorist, in his efforts to get a unitary scheme of animal response, recognizes no dividing line between man and brute. The behavior of man, with all of its refinement and complexity, forms only a part of the behaviorist's total scheme of investigation.

Neither Watson nor Skinner was opposed to neuronal research. However, both consistently and continuously argued that the cellular study of the brain had never given rise to any knowledge that was even remotely useful to explaining the behavior of animals, and that therefore it seemed best to understand the experimental and psychological study of behavior as an autonomous, somewhat independent branch of science.[56]

Konorski and Hebb found this delimitation of behaviorism from the neuronal sciences regrettable—and were determined to pull down the walls that separated the former from the latter. However, their critique of Pavlov, Watson, and Skinner was subtle. Neither Konorski nor Hebb ever intended to abandon the behaviorist framework: Konorski was and remained as thoroughly indebted to Pavlov as Hebb to Skinner and Watson. Rather, their ambition was to conceptually prepare the possibility of what they called neuropsychology, that is, the study of behavior in neuronal terms.

Even though they worked independently of one another, the works of Konorski and Hebb are strikingly similar. They both thought that the work on the transmission of nervous impulses as it emerged after World War II had made the partition of psychology from the brain obsolete (they almost exclusively focused on the work of Sherrington and his electrophysiological successors). Years before the electron microscopic studies of Palay, De Robertis, and Sanford showed that all brain tissue is synaptic, they argued that one could now correlate, at least in theory, synapse and behavior.

Konorski's *Conditional Reflexes and Neuron Organization* (1948) and Hebb's *The Organization of Behavior* (1949) offer (the first) fully elaborated synaptic theory of the brain and of human behavior.

Konorski arrived at his synaptic theory by attempting to provide a physiological explanation of Pavlov's conditioning experiments—something Pavlov had never strived to do.[57] And he thought that he could deduce such an explanation from Sherrington's argument that "experience" could "mold" the "nervous reaction":

> The application of a stimulus [...] leads to changes of a two-fold kind in the nervous system [...]. The first property, by virtue of which the nerve cells react to the incoming impulses with a certain cycle of changes, we call *excitability,* and the changes arising in the centers because of this property we shall call *changes due to excitability.* The second property, by virtue of which certain permanent functional transformation arise in particular systems of neurons as the result of appropriate stimuli and their combination, we shall call *plasticity* and the corresponding changes *plastic changes.*[58]

Konorski's coup was the correlation of two Pavlovian key terms—*stimulus* and *response*—with Sherrington's theory of the integrative action of the nervous system, according to which synapses coordinate and integrate incoming stimuli and thereby allow the organism to respond to its milieu.

Hebb's synaptic theory was more ambitious than Konorski's. Whereas the latter had merely aimed to explain the neuronal substrate of conditioned reflexes, the former endeavored to provide an outline of the neuronal organization of behavior as such. The main element of Hebb's outline was what he called "dynamic cell-assemblies":

> Any frequently repeated, particular stimulation will lead to the slow development of a *cell-assembly,* a diffuse structure comprising cells [...] capable of acting briefly as a closed system, delivering facilitation to other such systems and usually having a specific motor facilitation. [...] Each assembly action may be aroused by a preceding assembly, by a sensory event, or—normally— by both.[59]

Starting from the hypothesis that brain function is the result of such cell-assemblies, Hebb explained that use—experience, learning, conditioning—could strengthen the synaptic connections between interrelated neurons; that is, it could increase the action potential of a cell and thus facilitate the transmission of nervous impulses. Hebb further speculated that short-term memory lasting minutes or hours could be the result of reverberation of nervous impulses in closed neuronal circuits—as Forbes (who had worked with both Sherrington and Adrian) and Lorente de Nó (the last student of Ramón y Cajal and later a Spanish émigré to the United States) had argued in the 1920s and 1930s. And continuous use (or stimulation) could lead, as Ramón y Cajal had suggested, to miniscule structural changes that underlie long-term memory. "A reverberatory trace," Hebb wrote, "might co-operate with the structural change, and carry the memory until the growth change is made." Or, in a more formulaic language, "when an axon of cell A is near enough to excite B and repeatedly or persistently takes part in firing it, some growth process or metabolic change takes place in one or both cells such that A's efficiency, as one of the cells firing B, is increased."[60]

Despite the variations in detail and the differences in scope, the sketches of the brain as a synaptic machine offered by Konorski's and Hebb significantly overlap. Both differentiated between a purely functional form of synaptic plasticity, which they viewed as a substrate of occasional use, and an anatomical form of synaptic plasticity, that is, the emergence of new synapses within already existing patterns of connection as a result of persistent use.[61] And both suggested that these two kinds of synaptic plasticity are constitutive of behavior; and both presupposed—relying on the authority of Ramón y Cajal—that the mature brain is "essentially fixed."

A powerful consequence of Konorski's and Hebb's work was that it made ideas that were conceptually thoroughly incommensurable with one another—Ramón y Cajal's freely growing forest, Sherrington's telegraph, Lorente de Nó's reverberation machine—seem to revolve around a single conceptual and experimental problem: the synaptic organization of the brain as key to understanding how an immutable cellular structure would allow for behavioral changes. Konorski and Hebb created a new, previously nonexistent problem in a way that made it seem to have always been the preoccupation of neuronal research. They flattened conceptual incommensurabilities and thereby created the possibility of a straight line of progress from the founding figures, Ramón y Cajal and Sherrington, to the present.[62]

Hebb and Konorski's coupling of synapse and behavior would have likely remained a mere regional rationality, with little or no relevance for brain research, had it not been for the chemicalization and universalization of the synapse in the early to mid-1950s, just a few years after Konorski and Hebb published their works. In the aftermath of Eccles's chemicalization of the synapsis, however, and of the electron microscopists' visualization and universalization of this chemical synapse in the mid-50s, it became possible for this regional rationality to quickly emerge as a general truth. By the early 1950s, this new truth had become the general conceptual scaffold of neurochemistry and had given rise to a new line of research now considered obvious and the apparent telos toward which brain research had always evolved: synaptic plasticity research.

For example, John Zachary Young, a then–well known English zoologist and neurophysiologist, declared in 1951 with reference to Hebb and Konorski: "The most obvious failure of current neurophysiological theory is in providing an account of the changing potentialities or plasticity of the nervous system."[63] And John Eccles explained in his 1952 Waynflete Lectures at Oxford that, justly, "neurophysiologists have been frequently criticized because they have failed to interest themselves in the functional changes that must form the basis of such enduring reactions as occur in learning, conditioning, and memory."[64]

Young, Eccles, and many of their contemporaries were determined to change this state of affairs. But progress was slow to occur. As it turned out, phenomena such as post-tetanic depression (PTP), that is, the synaptic exhaustion brought about by recurrent stimuli, and the endplate potential (EPP) that is, the depolariztion of muscle fibers in the neuromuscular junction caused by neurotransmitters, could hardly account for memory storage or changes in behavior. First, the potentiation or depression brought about by stimulation affected only the presynaptic terminal—but neither affected the excitability of the cell itself nor that of its target neurons. As it could not affect neural circuits, it seemed to be without physiological or psychological consequence. Second, the facilitation brought about by PTP lasted only a few seconds or minutes and could thus not account for the long-term facilitation that seemed necessary for long-term memory. The conclusion was that PTP and EPP were likely to be purely mechanical phenomena without any relation to what they were supposed to explain—the human.[65]

By the early 1950s, the link between synapse and liberty was thus firmly established—but only in the abstract. And fixity was, still, the condition of the possibility of this link.

The first concrete experimental relation between synapse and liberty was established in the 1960s by Eric Kandel (1929–).[66]

While training as a physician at New York University (NYU) in the 1950s, Kandel, who had a keen interest in psychotherapy, became fascinated by the idea that neuronal action would underlie behavior in general and memory formation in particular. As he had no background in neuronal research, Kandel approached Harry Grundfest—a Russian-born American Jew, a professor of neurology at Columbia University, and an expert in the physics of the central nervous system—to ask if he could work in his laboratory and learn the basics of neuronal research. It was in Grundstein's lab that Kandel was first introduced to the electrophysiological study of the chemical, synaptic brain: here he learned about the chemical processes of synaptic communication, learned to use mini-electrodes to chart the release of electrical signals by neurotransmitters, and read the works of Konorski and Hebb.

By the time Kandel graduated from medical school, his time in the laboratory had given rise to an idée fixe that consolidated into a major research program while he was in residency: wouldn't it be possible to use the tools of electrophysiology—specifically mini-electrode recordings—to show that changes in the strength of synaptic firing patterns in hippocampal neurons were the material basis of memory formation?

At the beginning of the 1950s, it had been still unclear if memories are stored in a particular part of the brain, as Hebb had it, or whether the storing of memories would involve the entire brain, as Karl Lashley (1890–1958) had assumed. By the late 1950s, however, a combination of brain surgery, postmortem pathology, and experimental psychology—the reference here is to the Montréal-based surgeon Wilder Penfield (1891–1976), former student of Sherrington; to the American surgeon William Scoville (1906–1984), who worked at Hartford, Connecticut, and admired Penfield; and to Brenda Milner (1918–), a junior psychologist and colleague of Penfield and Hebb at Montréal—had indicated that the temporal lobes and, specifically, the walnut-sized, horse-shaped hippocampus seemed to be critical for memory storage.

In the 1940s, Penfield begun to experiment on the exposed brains of his surgical patients. Once he had opened their skulls, he applied electrical currents to different sites of the cortex and documented the reactions of his patients, who were only locally anesthetized and hence conscious. Penfield found that, when stimulated, different surface areas of the brain evoked very different kinds of psychological and physiological reactions in his patients. For example, he noted that whenever he stimulated the temporal lobes, where the hippocampus is located, memories of a distant past were evoked.

In 1951, after ten years of systematically studying the topography of the cortex, Penfield summarized his results in a comprehensive atlas of the function-specific organization of the human brain (published with the help of Theodore Rasmussen).[67]

A few years later, Scoville, who admired Penfield and knew of his maps, made a discovery that was later followed up by Brenda Milner. In 1953, he surgically removed the temporal lobes from a patient—Henry Molaison (1926–2008), or H.M.—who suffered from severe seizures. The surgery improved H.M.'s condition dramatically but had a side effect that Scoville seems to have noted only in 1955 or 1956: the patient was no longer capable of forming memories. Scoville wrote to Penfield, and Penfield asked Milner, who had just published an article on "The Intellectual Function of the Temporal Lobes," if she wanted to see Molaison.[68]

The articles that emanated from Milner's encounters with H.M.—they first met in 1957—were epoch making. In a series of now classical papers she reported that while H. M. had lost the capacity to remember what had happened just a few minutes ago, he could easily remember scenes from his childhood and use motor skills that he had learned many years earlier. She also found that H.M. could still learn and memorize new motor skills, even though he could not remember practicing them. Milner's conclusion was that the brain must have two different kinds of memory storage systems at its disposal, a "declarative" and a "procedural memory." H. M.'s continued ability to learn new motor skills, she argued, suggests that motor skills— procedural memory—aren't contingent on the hippocampus, but rather rely on some other neuronal circuit that is not part of the temporal lobe. Where the hippocampus is needed, however, is the transformation of skills into conscious or declarative memory.[69]

Kandel's ambition was to experimentalize Milner's conclusions. Could he show, with the tools of electrophysiology, that changes in the intensity of synaptic communication are constitutive of hippocampal—conscious— memory formation? And perhaps even of behavior more generally?

Kandel's ambition proved larger than the potential of the then-available technology. Together with his colleague Alden Spencer (1931–1977), he managed to apply electrodes to hippocampal neurons of cats and to record both transient and long-lasting electrical responses. However, there was no way to draw any conclusions from these recordings about the neuronal basis of memory formation (or behavior). The hippocampus of their cats proved too complex a structure for what Kandel had hoped to achieve: there were too many neurons, too many synapses, and too many far-reaching, topsy-turvy axonal connections; it was therefore impossible to isolate a single neuron, let alone find functionally identical neurons or synaptic circuits in different animals.

Kandel's solution to the predicament he faced was radical reductionism. His model was the work of the discoverers of the chemical synapse. Hadn't researchers like Fessard, Feldberg, Katz, Kuffler and Eccles worked on crustaceans precisely because they had giant neurons that allowed them to measure and analyze the chemically triggered flow of electrical impulses? If the nervous system of cats was too convoluted, what about studying evolutionarily lower animals with a less differentiated nervous system?

Kandel's animal of choice was *Aplysia california,* a sea slug living off the coast of the Pacific Ocean. *Aplysia* had a simple nervous system, made up of only a few nerve cells, each of which could be identified in each animal, each of which was big enough so that one could easily insert mini-electrodes.

In 1962, then, Kandel moved to Paris to work with Ladislav Tauc (1926–1999), a Czech electrophsyiologist who had emigrated to Paris in the late 1940s and who had recently published a series of papers on the spike potential of neurons in *Aplysia*.[70] Tauc introduced Kandel to *Aplysia*, and soon the two found first hints of what Kandel was looking for. When they ran an electrical impulse through a nerve cell, synaptic facilitation changed lastingly. While a major impulse was initially needed for the cell to transmit a signal, the repeated stimulation of the cell sensitized it in such a way that a minor impulse was enough to cause transmission of a strong signal. The facilitations the two electrophysiologists observed often lasted for hours and even days.[71]

Were such changes in facilitation the basis of memory?

Back in the United States, NYU had recruited Kandel in 1965, and he expanded on his work with Tauc and, relying on behavior psychology, began studying so-called primitive forms of learning—conditioning, habituation, and sensitization—at the level of single synapses in *Aplysia*. Again he found what he was looking for. What enabled learning, at least when it came to *Aplysia's* gill withdrawal reflex, were changes in the efficacy with which synapses release, and take up, their action potential.[72]

Aplysia made Kandel famous. During the 1960s, thanks to his work on the sea slug, he emerged as the scholar who, more than anyone else, had contributed to correlating the study of behavior and the electrophysiological and neurochemical study of synapses.[73] Yet *Aplysia* also defined the limits of Kandel's fame. In the early 1970s, no one knew yet whether what is true for a snail—that changes in the intensity of synaptic communication reflect changes in behavior—is also true for other animals, let alone humans.

Was it?

The chance observation that would lead to a tentative answer to this question occurred in Norway. In the late 1960s, Terje Lømo, working in the lab of Per Anderson in Oslo, working on PTP and EPP in hippocampal cells of rabbits, "noticed that the response evoked in the dentate area [part of the hippocampus] by single test shocks to the afferent perforant pathway often remained potentiated for a considerable time"—that is, much longer than classical PTP and EPP patterns.[74] In the early 1970s, then, Anderson recruited the Brit Tim Bliss to work with Lømo. The plan for the two young researchers was to repeat and technically condition Lømo's initial observation. If the hippocampus is central for memory formation, and if the potentiation Bliss had observed was a regular feature of the brain, maybe they could identify the synaptic substrate of at least one kind of memory formation in vertebrates.

Bliss and Lømo used new-generation mini-electrodes to stimulate synapses in the Schaffer collateral pathway—a part of the hippocampus—of rats and rabbits and recorded the responses from different parts of the target neurons. What they reported in 1973 was reminiscent of the work of Tauc and Kandel: a brief high-frequency period of electrical stimulus applied artificially to the hippocampal pathway produced increases in synaptic strength, neuron responsiveness, and speed of response that lasted for hours. When the stimulation was repeated, the increase would last several days and even weeks. They called this type of facilitation *long-term potentiation* (LTP).

Bliss and Lømo established that, at least in principle, mechanisms like those Kandel had shown to be constitutive of memory formation in invertebrates also exist in vertebrates. What is more, they showed that these mechanism occur precisely in the one brain structure associated with memory formation, the hippocampus.[75] It thus seemed likely, in 1973, that synaptic plasticity is the basis of memory formation, in sea slugs as much as in humans. And perhaps not just of memory formation but of cognition as well. And even of a sense of self.

Beginning in the mid-1970s, researchers all over the world began to expand on the work of Kandel, Bliss, and Lømo (with Konorski and Hebb a in the background). What are the precise links between LTP or long-term depression (LTD) and higher cognitive functions? Does LTP or LTD occur only in the hippocampus, or can potentiation and depression of synaptic communication occur in all brain areas, including the cortex? Are changes in the ease with which synapses transmit impulses the key to all forms of behavior?

The sense of possibility that emanated from these new, research-guiding questions quickly made the study of synaptic—that is, chemical or functional— plasticity the fastest-growing and by far the most dominant research field in the neuronal sciences. Finally, the synapse had become the condition for the possibility of liberty.

And fixity?

I quote from a 1982 article by Eric Kandel in which he traced the rise of synaptic plasticity research: "The potentialities for many behaviors of which an organism is capable are built into the basic scaffolding of the brain [. . .]. Environmental factors and learning bring out these latent capabilities by altering the effectiveness of the pre-existing pathways, thereby leading to the expression of new patterns of behavior."[76] For Kandel and many of his contemporaries, the brain was a thoroughly fixed and immutable structure. Amidst the hype about the discovery of the neuronal basis of behavior, the possibility that new synapses appear, which both Konorski and Hebb had assumed, following Ramón y Cajal's correlation of memory formation and anatomical growth, had gotten lost. In the 1980s, the only "plastic" element of the nervous tissue was, as Sherrington had put it in 1904, the "nervous reactions."[77]

From Synaptic Communication to Neural Signaling

In the late 1970s, genetics arrived in the neuronal sciences.[78] The application of the tools of molecular biology to the cells of the central nervous system marked a major event in the history of the relation between synapse and liberty—if primarily for methodological reasons.

Until the 1970s the only techniques available to researchers for transforming the brain into an experimental object came from either electrophysiology or chemistry (with anatomy and histology in the background). The former allowed electrical impulses to be traced; the latter made it possible to classify neurons according to the neurotransmitter they metabolize. The significance of molecular biology was that it added a whole new, previously nonexisting venue of analysis: the study of synaptic communication in terms of genes. Which genes code for which neurotransmitters? How can one use recombinant DNA technologies to identify the molecular processes that organize neuronal metabolism? Can one discover the genetic basis of the neuronal processes—synapse is liberty—that make us human? With the advent of a molecular biology of the neuron, the brain was encoded in the language of DNA, RNA, and proteins.

The key site of the geneticization of the synapse was, again, the laboratory of Eric Kandel, who had left NYU for Columbia in 1974. Again, the model organism was *Aplysia*. In the early 1980s, Richard Scheller, a postdoc of Kandel, succeeded in identifying and cloning the genes that control neuronal signaling in the gill withdrawal reflex of the sea slug—and thereby opened the possibility of studying the process of neuronally organized behavior from the perspective of biological molecules.[79]

The excitement surrounding Scheller's work was enormous: it established that it was possible to identify and engineer the genes that control synaptic communication, whether in the hippocampus or elsewhere. What is more, it opened up the possibility of shifting attention away from the mere neuronal to the molecular organization of the brain. In the words of Eric Kandel, "a new biology of the mind" seemed imminent.[80]

By the 1990s, the genetics of neuronal signaling was gradually being combined with experimental designs taken from cognitive psychology, and with novel functional imaging technologies that, due to their noninvasive character, allowed researchers to enroll humans as experimental subjects in brain research. The hope underlying this fusion of disciplines, designs, and technologies—often described as the rise of "cognitive neuroscience"—was that it would enable researchers to correlate behavior with neuronal signaling in concrete synaptic circuits. This correlation was to be achieved by two different approaches, one focused largely on human, the other focused exclusively on nonhuman animals. In human-centered experiments, research subjects were asked to solve cognitive problems while their brains were scanned either with a position electron tomograph (PET) or with a functional magnetic resonance imaging (fMRI) computer. Such experiments aimed to map the parts of synaptic systems, particularly those of the cerebral cortex, that are active when subjects cognate.[81] The experiments that were focused on nonhuman animals assumed different forms, but almost all of them sought to combine in one way or another tests taken from cognitive or behavior psychology with genetic engineering and imaging technologies (or postmortem brain analysis). For example, researchers would restrict gene expression regionally or temporally, or both, and then explore which molecules were critical for the synaptic organization of a given behavior.[82]

What effects did these new techniques—recombinant DNA and functional imaging technologies—have on the chemical, synaptic conception of the brain that had come to dominance since the 1950s?

On the one hand, the impact was sweeping. The coming together of recombinant DNA technologies, cognitive psychology, and brain imaging enrolled the neuronal brain in the language and apparatuses of genes and proteins, and thereby dramatically changed the terminological and material meaning of terms such as *synapse, synaptic communication, regional organization, neuronal network,* and *functional anatomy.* On the other hand, the conceptual changes brought about by these new technologies were negligible. Genetics, PET, and fMRI hardly changed the basic conceptual grid that had emerged after World War II. The assumption persisted that synapses, and above all synaptic plasticity, are the key to understanding the brain. How else could one understand how an "essentially fixed" cellular structure would allow for the human?

Neither molecular neurobiology (1980s) nor cognitive neuroscience (1990s) marked a departure from the synaptic organization of the brain that had emerged—gradually, sporadically, accidentally—since Sherrington's 1897 contribution to Foster's textbook.[83]

Synapse, still, was liberty.[84]

REINVENTING THE NEURONAL GROUNDS OF THE HUMAN

When I left the library in the basement of the ENS, I was struck by what I had come to think of as the surprising conceptual monotony of neuronal knowledge production. For more than a hundred years the central nervous system had been known as a fixed cellular structure, and for almost five decades it had been understood as a chemical, synaptic machine.

Or had I overlooked something? Had I perhaps missed some authors and their work?

Time and again I returned to the library. With each article I read and each book I worked through, I became ever more painfully aware that the historical digression I offer here does not do justice to a century of neuronal research. Within the roughly one hundred years I cover here (from the 1890s to the 1990s), what the brain is changed many times over. It was conceptualized as consisting of a mass of amoeba-like cells that swim in an ocean; as an anatomical structure composed of discrete, contiguous neurons; as a vast, continuous syncitium; as a kind of muscle that swells when trained; as an assembly of synaptic reflex arcs; as an information-integrating machine; as a switchboard composed of a bewildering complexity of wires and switches (synapses); as a computer; as a soup administered by chemical substances transmitting and releasing synapses; and, with PET and fMRIs, as landscapes to be mapped. I could go on.

Conceptually speaking, each one of these changes mutated what the brain is, and each mutation changed, however slightly, the analytical focus of the neuronal sciences. Yet my visits to the library also convinced me that despite the in part significant conceptual ruptures that constitute the history of neuronal knowledge production, one assumption remained literally unchallenged over the course of the twentieth century: the anatomical fixity of the adult human brain. From at least the 1890s to the 1990s it was consistently assumed that humans are born with a definite number of neurons and that once adulthood is reached the brain is an essentially immutable, unchanging cellular structure.

In the course of the twentieth century, the question of how this immutable structure could allow for behavioral changes (whether styled as learning, memory, experience, individuation, or, with Jean Pierre, liberty) was increasingly answered in synaptic terms. And here, too, change was constant: conceptually speaking, the synapse never stood still. But no matter how often the synapse changed its contours, fixity was and remained the condition of the possibility of all the synaptic brains that have existed since then. What is more, fixity was throughout the one presupposition that made the focus on the synapse as key to understanding the brain meaningful.

I thus came away from my many visits to the library thinking that the scandal of Alain's work was indeed not so much that it undermined fixity as that by undermining fixity, it threatened to subvert the synaptic, chemical conception of the brain. If Alain's work turned out to be true, it would inevitably dissolve the one assumption that organized neuronal knowledge production for a century—or at least for half a century if one counts only the years in which the synaptic brain dominated the neuronal sciences.

It was thus only consequential that the synaptologists of the human (and nonhuman) brain met the suggestion that basic embryogenetic processes occur in the adult—processes that far exceed the minimalist growth allowed for by Ramón y Cajal—with hostility. Plasticity could not be integrated into their conception of the brain without undermining the very principle on which this conception was contingent: the assumption that the synapse, and only the synapse, is liberty.

The challenge Alain and his friends had to confront was thus as huge as the provocation that emanated from his lab. They had to come up with a new conceptual and experimental understanding of the nervous system, of what it is; how it functions; what its functional elements and events are; how these elements and events explain behavior, memory, and disease; how they allow for the possibility of the human.

I wish to avoid any misunderstanding: No one in Alain's lab doubted contiguity, the existence of the synapse, or the "plasticity" of synaptic transmission. But everyone doubted fixity, and thus the idea that understanding the immutable synaptic organization of the brain and the mechanisms of synaptic communication was the only key to understanding the brain. Instead, they dreamed of an organ in ceaseless motion, a motion triggered by the nonautonomous transfer of homeoproteins. New neurons are born while old ones die; axons and dendrites continue to sprout and grow, or dry up and disappear; spines ceaselessly get bigger or thinner or alter their size and form; and synapses appear and disappear.

Conceptualizing such a morphogenetically plastic brain has been a massive challenge. Indeed, Alain, Joliot, Michel, Brigitte, and Trembleau were up against a century-old, firmly established conception of the brain—and of the human. It is only a slight exaggeration to say that Alain and his colleagues, together with other *plasticiens,* had to reinvent the distinctively human.

They had to decouple liberty from synapse.

Histories of Truth

What was I to do with *this?*

Looking for recent literature on plasticity, I found that, over the past decade, since the turn of the millennium, a good number of neuroscientists had published elaborate histories of plasticity research. Working my way through a dozen books and articles, I learned that a genuinely plastic conception of the brain emerged in the 1890s and that plasticity research, which apparently has always been a central focus of neuronal knowledge production, has continuously progressed until now.[1]

I was taken aback. Had I missed something? Why, I wondered, did the authors of these works fail to see what they, as brain researchers, ought to see and know: that a genuinely plastic brain was a spectacular novelty, that plasticity until recently was beyond the neuronally possible?[2]

It was Georges Canguilhem (1904–1995), the French epistemologist of the history of science, who helped me to address these questions.[3] In a talk he gave in Montréal in 1966, Canguilhem observed that every major scientific discovery—that is, a discovery that generates a far-reaching new insight—seems to require the scientists who make it to rewrite the history of their discipline.[4] It is, he explained, as if in moments in which a genuinely novel truth emerges— and a formerly well-established one gets discarded—the history of truth has to be rewritten.

I found Canguilhem's observation most insightful. Indeed, it seemed as if the emergence of plasticity—that is, a major discovery that has generated far-reaching new insights—has caused among neuronal researchers a somewhat competitive effort to rewrite the discipline's history of truth. It seemed as if with plasticity research the brain had outgrown the history of truth that until recently had structured the very idea of progress around which the neuronal sciences evolved. The telos of this history was the synapse. First, Ramón y Cajal discovered contiguity, then Sherrington the synapse, and ever since our knowledge of the chemical, synaptic brain has been refined. As there was now a new (if still-emerging, nowhere fully articulated) telos—plasticity—there had to be new origins and, with them, new histories of truth. I call these histories competing because the various authors (critical of one another's work) insist on different historical origins of "the plastic brain."[5]

For some, the honor goes to American pragmatism and here specifically to William James (1842–1910). They suggest that in his 1890 *Principles of Psychology* he "first introduced the word plasticity to the science of the brain."[6] Others favor anatomy over philosophy and turn to Eugenio Tanzi (1856–1934), who in 1893 offered "the very first hypothesis that associative memories and practice-dependent motor skills depend on a localized facilitation of synaptic transmission."[7] A third set of authors insists that the plastic brain is of French-Romanian origin: "The concept of plasticity was extended and supported for the first time by the Romanian neurologist Ioan Minea," who is said to have learned about the concept from his teacher, Georges Marinesco (1863–1938).[8] Minea, according to this story line, documented "the morphological transformations"—he called them "plastic reactions"—"occurring in spinal ganglion cells surviving trauma to, or transplantation of, their ganglia."[9] A fourth line, finally, favors a German origin, which was then taken up by a Belgian-French connection. The suggestion is that Robert Wiedersheim (1848–1923) and Hermann Rabl-Rückhard (1839–1905) observed in 1890 that parts of "the cerebral ganglion of crustaceans constantly change their volume" (throughout life). Wiedersheim then "proposed that this was in part due to the fact that certain nerve cells were not immobile, but that they changed their shape by undergoing amoeboid-like movements," and Rabl-Rückhard wondered if "psychic processes [. . .] could be explained by their continuous amoeboid movement."[10]

Canguilhem had offered his observation not so much as a critique of the scientists' rewritings of the history of truth—the rendering possible of a linear history of truth is perhaps best seen as an integral (constitutive) part of scientific practice— than as a didactic exposure of the kind of conceptual naïveté that epistemologists could not afford. Epistemologists, he explained, "should not make the error" that amateur historians frequently make, namely, "thinking that persistent use of a particular term indicates an invariant underlying concept."[11] For Canguilhem, there was a significant difference between term and concept. And this difference was constitutive of the work of the epistemologist.

How does a given author conceptualize, say, the organism? How does her particular conceptualization make the organism or parts thereof accessible to thought—to experimentalization—in a new, different way? What methods are invented to address this difference? The challenge of the epistemologist, for Canguilhem, was to study "concepts" and to identify "epistemological discontinuity in scientific progress."[12]

Could I identify the epistemological discontinuities that the four competing variants of the history of neuronal truth were oblivious to—thereby making visible the difference that epistemology makes? Indeed, it turned out that all four accounts of the origins of plasticity research in the late nineteenth century miss the subtle but far-reaching difference between term and concept.

For example, was William James really the first to discover the plasticity of the neuronal brain? How could he, when his *Principles of Psychology* was published in 1890—a year before the term *neuron* was actually coined? James offered a psychological, not a histological, argument.[13] The philosopher, this is to say, inquired into the mind. His tool was introspection, not cellular anatomy.[14]

And plasticity? On five dispersed, unrelated pages out of well over a thousand, James mused that, given the description of the mind his introspection has generated, the brain, insofar as it appears to be the seat of consciousness (he was quite firm about this), must be plastic.[15] Again, his argument was psychological, not neuronal.

Epistemologically, an unbridgeable abyss separates James's psychological reasoning from the anatomical and cellular reasoning that emerged in Europe in the second half of the nineteenth century—and that was a turn away from introspection and psychology.[16] James hardly marks the programmatic origin of neuronal plasticity research.[17]

Certainly the works of Tanzi, Minea, and Wiedersheim are part of the nineteenth-century effort to enlist the brain in cell theory. But their conceptualization of the brain, of what it is and how it functions, makes them as unlikely as points of origins as James. Tanzi understood the central organ as a muscle that, when trained, swells. How could he, in 1893, have provided evidence for synaptic facilitation as the basis of memory formation, half a decade before Sherrington invented the term *synapse,* half a century before Hebb and Konorski came up with synaptic plasticity, and almost a century before Kandel and Bliss and Lømo provided evidence for LTP?[18]

Wiedersheim advanced an oceanography of the brain. He forcefully argued that the skull is full of liquid and that neurons are amoeba-like entities that live in this liquid and store information by swelling. Is there any way from oceanography and amoebas to forestry and arborizations? Or to cables and wires? Or to a constantly renewing tissue?

And Minea, as far as I can reconstruct, worked to identify what exactly prevented the nervous system from generating, after neuronal death, new neurons and found along the way that there are nerve cells that react with nonfunctional "plastic reactions," by which he meant the growth of dendrites, to injury or grafting. It follows that his brain, if anything, was "essentially fixed."

It's not just that it's hardly possible to conceive of a linear line of progress from these fixed, amoebic, swelling brains to today's plasticity research. It's also that these authors actually used the term *plastic* only very rarely in a small number of their publications, and that where they do, it's in a circumstantial and casual way. They never developed the term conceptually, let alone experimentally.[19] It is thus hard to imagine that the work of Tanzi, Minea, or Wiedersheim mark the historical origin of plasticity research that leads in either a linear or nonlinear way to the present. As in the case of William James, their casual use of the term *plastic* engendered no school of thought or line of research.

The only reason, it seems, that the rewritings of the history of truth by contemporary neuronal researchers mention these nineteenth- and early-twentieth-century authors together is that today, when the brain emerges as plastic, neuronal researchers are looking—exactly as Canguilhem observed more than fifty years ago—for authors whose work could count as origins of the history of truth.[20] In other words, the actual origins of these histories lie in the present, not the past.[21]

The most powerful indicator of the epistemological naïveté of the four origin stories (that is, their confusing term with concept), however, is that they utterly miss the difference between functional synaptic plasticity—which gained momentum precisely because the brain was assumed to be essentially fixed—and the plastic conception of the brain that emerged after the late 1990s and that powerfully undermined fixity and thus the idea that only the synapse is plastic. Virtually all the examples of early plasticity research they present as origins of the plastic brain are presented as precursors to synaptic facilitation, as if functional plasticity were the same thing as the continuous birth of new, yet unspecified and hence literally plastic tissue (on the level of cells, axons, dendrites, spines, synapses).[22] They miss the large-scale conceptual event— the powerful epistemological rupture—that the rise of a genuinely plastic brain has actually been.[23]

In sum, from the point of view of Canguilhem's historical epistemology, there are no nineteenth-century origins of plasticity research—for plasticity research is an event of the late twentieth and early twenty-first century only.

FOUR

Nocturnal

Il s'agit d'une occasion de faire de la science autrement, de montrer son côté nocturne qui n'apparaît jamais dans le discours officiel. [...] Il faut pour cela que l'expérience soit construite autour d'une idée.

ALAIN PROCHIANTZ

In December 2002 I attended a talk on how bleaching techniques enable the identification of molecular movements in the nucleus. On my way back to the lab—the talk was very technical and dry—I ran into Alain, who had introduced the guest speaker. He was full of mockery.

"You see," he greeted me, "this was true science." His voice was loud and his tone aggressive. "It was insignificant, rational, and boring." A frivolous laugh followed.

Over the previous months I had seen Alain several times in a comparable state of furious and challenging mockery, which was quite disturbing in its intensity. I knew that this mockery—this intensity—was the result of his always immediate, almost always passionate reaction to anything he condescendingly referred to as the "scientifically correct"—the comprehension of science as a thoroughly rational, ultimately sober undertaking.[1] But, though I knew what Alain so vividly reacted to, I wasn't sure why he thought of his own work as so very different. Wasn't his work rational? Wasn't it sober? Wasn't it, strictly speaking, scientifically correct?

"Why do you think," I wondered out loud, "that your own work is so radically different?"

He stood still and looked at me with barely hidden anger. If his furious laughter had suggested something like complicity—a shared knowledge that set us apart from the scientifically correct—my question had destroyed it. In that moment it suddenly seemed as if all my understanding of his work—the result of the many, at times intellectually curious and challenging conversations we had over the previous months—had been nothing but an illusion.

Would he answer? Angry, and without a word, he turned around and walked away.

I spent the rest of the day looking for Alain. Perhaps we could talk? I wanted him to know that my question—my ignorance—was genuine. I did not mean to annoy him. I simply was curious and wanted to find out. Why, how, in which sense was his work different? Could he explain to me where he departed from the scientifically correct?

He wasn't in his office. Not this day, not the next one. Eventually, I gave up.

A few days later, though, I was in for a surprise. "I think," he approached me from behind while I was preparing a neuron culture, "that I have not yet answered your question."

"You didn't," I laughed. I remember being grateful. And relieved. And curious to find out what he would have to say. Would he tell me why his work was different? What then followed was one of the most thought-provoking surprises my fieldwork was to generate.

On that day, and for the next several weeks, Alain introduced me to what he called the "nocturnal grounds of scientific work." With this term he referred to all those aspects of science that, as he put it, "cannot be grounded in the bright light of reason, that are essentially nocturnal." At the center of these nocturnal practices was the intimate, passionate, and poetic "work with ideas," which, for him, was the actual ground of all scientific work, conscious or not. Much to his regret, however, the nocturnal engagement with ideas has in contemporary conceptions of science no space of its own. Unrecognized, it remains in the dark, eking out a rudimentary, underdeveloped existence. The reason for this, as he saw it, is that work with ideas cannot be reduced to the scientifically correct. Instead it is grounded in a sensitivity for the beauty of ideas, a willingness to play with them, a pleasure in being overcome and carried away while staying alert to what happens. From the perspective of the nocturnal, scientific work is adventurous, possibly even dangerous (for one may be carried away by an idea and never return). In any case, it makes for extreme experiences, which Alain sometimes described as frenzy, sometimes as flight, but most often as an erotic encounter.

OF ITS OWN KIND

Ideas?

Once plasticity had begun to take shape as my research topic, I spent much of my time documenting how, on the level of experimental practice at the bench, technologies were being invented that enabled—that were constitutive of the possibility for—understanding the adult brain in embryogenetic terms.[2] Could I document the work that would go into the making of a new experimental procedure—of a whole new experimental system, one that would technically generate the possibility of knowing the adult brain as plastic?

When Alain began introducing me to what he called the nocturnal grounds of science, he seemed to challenge the very questions that had guided my research. What is more, he seemed to doubt their validity. At first, I could not say why. After I had listened for a while, however, it seemed to me as if his notion of science was somewhat incommensurable with mine.

I had always assumed—nothing seemed more evident to me—that science is ultimately about the experimental production of truth. Consequently, it was the work that goes into the making an experimental truth possible that I was interested in.[3] Now, what Alain called nocturnal work with ideas suggested an altogether different understanding of science. According to him, science was neither (or not exclusively) about experimentation nor (or not exclusively) about truth, but instead about the work with ideas. Implicit in his lectures was the suggestion—the reproach—that my research questions were naïve. Had I gotten science wrong?[4]

The longer I listened, the more unsettling our conversations became for me—until I gradually began to understand that he was not actually against experimentation. Or truth. The reason that he so vehemently questioned experimentation and truth (or the reason he approached me after my question in the corridor had so annoyed him) was, or so it seemed, a didactic one. He wanted to make his anthropologist sensitive to a whole other comprehension of scientific practice, one that he felt was underappreciated and often not recognized at all, one that he judged to be more important (if in complicated ways) than experimentation. Or truth.

In one of my notebooks I recorded him elaborating on this importance:

> Experiments are wonderful. I love experimentation, love thinking with my hands. I did this for almost thirty years, every day, at the bench. [...] My work led me to recognize, however, that the work with ideas, of ideas, is of at least equal, perhaps even of higher importance. And of an altogether different kind. Experiments are grounded in presuppositions; the truths they allow for are conditioned by ideas. Ideas, you see, condition what is possibly true. To change these ideas, that is, that which is currently considered possible— experiments cannot do that. I know because I tried. The work with ideas, however, can. To recognize ideas, to expose them, to set them in touch with one another, to let them generate new ones—one cannot really foresee how ideas interact—this is a practice of its own kind.

A practice of its own kind, a practice of surprise, one that aims at releasing new possibilities of truth: once I began to understand his argument, my original notion of science began to gradually break open. What if science indeed were less about the production of truth than about the poetic production of new possibilities of truth? What if nocturnal work on the possible, the playful, and poetic engagement with ideas was the unacknowledged ground of all science?

What emerged from these questions was an unexpected, and increasingly exciting, new way of thinking about the story of plastic reason. What if plastic reason was not the result of a technological tinkering that gradually gave rise to a new experimental truth, but rather of the nocturnal fostering of a new possibility of truth? Could I write the history of the work that went into the generation of this new possibility? And could I trace how this new possibility cut across and thereby mutated the established possibilities?

I found myself increasingly carried away by these questions—away from my initial focus on experimentation and truth (though I never completely let go; see chapter 5). And the more I got carried away, the more I had the impression of another world opening up right in front of me, a world yet unheard of, yet unexplored, one that promised to offer a new and surprising understanding of science in general and of plastic reason in particular.[5]

I decided to explore this "other" understanding. What follows is a report of my findings.

ORIGINS

I began by systematically reconstructing the origins. What experience, what reflection—triggered by what—had led Alain to his nocturnal understanding of science?

"That all began with the work on homeoproteins," he explains on one of my tapes that dates to late January 2003. We were having dinner at his house, which was full of photographs of growing embryos, mostly taken by Ariel Ruiz i Altaba, a formerly New York–, now Geneva-based embryologist with whom he had collaborated (one of these photos is reproduced as the frontispiece).

Alain recited the story with which I was already quite familiar—how, in the mid-1980s in New York, he discovered homeoproteins; how he began wondering if they could play a role for single-cell embryogenesis; how Joliot began a PhD project on homeoproteins and the nervous system; and how the two observed that homeoproteins appear to have the capacity to slide between cells.

"In a control experiment we then added Antennapedia to the extracellular milieu of a Petri dish full of mature neurons. The next day, almost all of the homeoproteins were located in the nucleus of the neurons, where they apparently had caused a strong outgrowth of axons and dendrites. At first we thought it was an artifact. A few days later, however," Alain smiled, "this idea occurred to me."

Hadn't he and Joliot found that homeoproteins are also expressed in the adult brain? What was the physiological function of this expression? Could it be that homeoproteins can cross cell boundaries, move through the inner cellular milieu, enter the nucleus, where they attach themselves to the genome and thereby cause the formation of new tissue? Could it be that they do so in the mature as well as in the developing brain? Could it be that the they had found an ongoing, silent embryogenesis that renders the mature nervous system plastic?

"Strictly speaking," I answered, "it could not be."

"It could not be," he replied. "That is exactly right. It absolutely could not be. Beyond the possible." Again he smiled. "And yet there was the beauty of this idea."

In that moment, the story I was so familiar with and the story Alain was telling seemed to part ways. What caught my attention was the way in which he juxtaposed "the possible" with "his idea." The way he told the story that evening, it had a protagonist I had never heard about or noted before—his idea. It was his idea that ran counter to the possible; it upset it, broke it open.

"It was as if suddenly a space opened up," Alain went on, "at once vague and yet clear. I could not just let go what I saw, you understand?"

The first time I had been given an encompassing account of their 1989 experiment was six months earlier, when I was busy reconstructing the history of the lab. "The observation," Joliot had told me at the time, "did not make sense. I thought—well, we all thought—that it was an artifact. Things like that happen all the time. Sometimes the medium is old; at other times the cells were not treated properly. Hence, we were all ready to discard the experiment. Later we found out it wasn't an artifact; it was an observation. And that is how the whole story started."

Alain's story only slightly diverged from Joliot's, but this slight divergence had a maximal effect. Where Joliot had simply moved from artifact to observation, as if this was a smooth and unproblematic transition, Alain's story focused precisely on what had brought about this transformation of a technical accident into a physiological observation. The effect was that he grounded the whole history of his lab's research in the emergence of "his idea" and how it cut across "the possible" (across what, at the time, was considered possible).

While I was trying to capture my emergent nocturnal understanding of plastic reason in one of my notebooks, Alain repeated that he could not let go.

"I had to follow the idea."

I had heard him speak of ideas—of his idea—many times before, but only in this moment did I understand that for him there was a single moment in which his work originated, a moment that marked for him the beginning of an extraordinary adventure—the adventure of attempting to invent a whole new way, an impossible way, of thinking the brain. The adventure, as he later put it, of his life.

The Discovery of the Possible

"I understand that you found yourself intrigued by the beauty of an idea," I began our next exchange. "I also understand that it ran counter to the possible. What I do not understand is, well, the path that led from your having an idea to what seems your systematic way of working with ideas?"

It was an evening in early February 2003. We were sitting in his office on the seventh floor of the ENS science building, overseeing a nightly Paris covered in bird dirt.

"You need to see that we were a small group," Alain began his answer.

I knew from previous conversations that, back in 1989–1990, his lab shrank. Due to the controversial focus of its research, several scientists felt compelled to leave—until only two friends remained, Michel Volovitch and Alain Joliot.

"Given the smallness of our lab," he went on, "the way forward, we thought, was a strict division of labor. We assigned each one of us a single task."

His responsibility, he went on, was to explore his idea and to come up with new ones. Volovitch's task was to add the molecular expertise, and Joliot was to be the *bricoleur* of the team.

"It was in the course of my effort to understand better our challenge, to elaborate it, to give contours to it, that we all learned to appreciate the importance and dynamic of ideas."

"That was too fast," I complained. "Can you explain how this appreciation came about?"

"How? Well, recall that nothing made sense. That homeoproteins—transcription factors—travel from cell to cell. That did not make sense, right? That they cause a morphogenetic outgrowth did not make sense either. A plastic brain? That was not *dans le vrais*. It was impossible, you said last time, right? Well, our task was to create the possibility."

It was not *dans le vrais*, not contained, as a possibility, in what counted as true. I was reminded of an earlier exchange with Alain Trembleau. He had told me in August 2002 that shortly after he entered Alain's lab, he had a conversation with a famous American geneticist, a drosophila expert whom he preferred not to name. Trembleau told him about his new lab's work about the nonautonomous transfer of homeoproteins. Apparently the geneticist laughed out loud and then explained:

> Not only does this make no sense—there is also no need for it. Don't get me wrong, there are important discoveries that at first seem counterintuitive but then you begin to recognize their explanatory power and you see how they add up with what we already knew. But this nonautonomous transfer, it is not just that it does not make sense; it also does not add anything. We understand embryogenesis perfectly well without it. We can explain every step. It has nothing to contribute. We do not need it; the organism does not need it; there is no role for it.

After Trembleau told me this story, I shared it with Alain, who was furious.

"How does this geneticist know? Does this expert know everything? No ignorance? No surprise? No new knowledge? Or only knowledge that goes along with what he already knows? That can be nicely integrated and adds up? Is that science?"

At the time, I could not link Alain's anger to the nocturnal, since I did not yet know about it. Instead I interpreted it as a defense of plasticity against its enemies; though that evening in his office, his response appeared to me in a new light. Perhaps Alain did not defend plasticity, but rather the nocturnal. In that moment I could, for the first time, really, see and appreciate his nocturnal comprehension of science. For Alain science was precisely not the effort to build the house of truth, as if truth production was an ultimately linear, accumulative process. In fact, I had observed on a great many occasions that Alain seemed to despise scientists who spoke in the name of truth—who knew already, who left no space for doubt and, hence, the possibility that things could be different from the way they were currently imagined to be. The challenge of a nocturnal science, as I understood it that evening, was to find the ideas that delimit what counts as true—at a given time, in a given discipline, in a given experiment—and to challenge them, to set them in motion, time and time again, ceaselessly. The challenge was to increase the possibilities of truth, to grow truth by keeping it moving. Now I was more curious than ever to find out when, why, and under what circumstances he had come to appreciate nocturnal work.

"How do you actually create a new possibility?" I wanted to know.

"How? But that is precisely the point. We did not know either. No one knew. All of this was gradual, an insight here, one there; nothing was planned, nothing could be planned, precisely because we did not know. We worked hard, very hard. We felt as if we worked against everybody else. And gradually the work with ideas grew into a practice of its own kind, one that I began to recognize only in retrospect."

I was struck by his answer. Up until this point I had assumed, if implicitly, almost in form of an unexamined presupposition, that his having an idea was equivalent to the emergence of a new possibility of truth and hence with the recognition of the possible. My implicit assumption was that it was this recognition that had led Alain to nocturnal work. I was wrong. Hadn't Alain just told me that in the late 1980s and early 1990s there was no possibility? That they had first had to create it? And hadn't he told me that the recognition of the possible or the work with ideas was an unexpected outcome, rather than the starting point of their work?

No one had ever set out to work with ideas in order to change the possible. There were, strictly speaking, no origins—or only retrospective ones, blurred ones; too many to tell a linear history. I had missed the nocturnal origins of nocturnal work.

We continued talking for several hours. And, gradually, I learned to think of their discovery of the possible as a differentiation process, at the beginning of which was the painful insight that they needed to find a way for thinking the yet unthought of. As a small group, their challenge led them to the division of labor Alain described, and this in turn encouraged Alain, somewhat artificially perhaps, to focus on ideas rather than on molecular biology or technology. Along the way, in conversations with Joliot and Michel aimed at linking his ideas with experiments to be conducted, he and they recognized that his ideas were incompatible with the experiments they all knew. And this then led them, if retrospectively, to the recognition of the possible, the primacy of ideas, and nocturnal work.

When I left Alain's office I understood the outrage—the mockery—with which he often reacted to the scientifically correct. I imagined an encounter with a scientist who acts as if experiments are independent judges of ideas, proving them either wrong or right, as if ideas were neutral machines of discovery. From the perspective of the nocturnal, such a scientist is unbearable. She (he) is impossibly naïve precisely insofar as she (he) is ignorant of the ideational condition of possibility of her (his) experiments and the truths they allow for.

I further imagined that I would try to indicate to this scientist the nocturnal grounds on which he (she) is standing. And then this scientist would critique me, ferociously perhaps. He (she) would style himself (herself) as a guardian of science and truth, a truth threatened by me, and suggest that those who work with ideas (in addition to experimentation) are not proper scientists. This scientist would be more than merely unbearable. How would I react?

How would *you* react?

METHOD

Once I had understood that there were no origins (or too many), I turned to questions of method. What did this nocturnal method for thinking the yet unthought actually consist of? How does one imagine the unimagined? In our conversations—now occurring more often, for briefer periods, as everyday lab life unfolded—Alain described his method in three different ways.

Writing

"How do you actually get in touch with ideas?" I asked Alain in one of our first conversations about method. "I write," he replied.

"You write?" I found it curious that writing should be the medium of nocturnal work.

"I think my answer is only curious to you because you confuse writing with the written. The trap is to take writing as a way toward a text, to determine the meaning and significance of writing from the perspective of a final product." And then he added with a smile, "Having sex is not equivalent to having an orgasm. It may lead to that, if it is good sex, but it does not have to."

If one separates writing from the written—or sex from orgasm—one enters the field of the tentative, explorative. Alain's favorite example of the kind of writing he had in mind was Claude Bernard's *Cahier des Notes,* a posthumous publication that, in the style of a notebook, assembles physiological, philosophical, and epistemological notes.

"From Bernard's *Cahier,*" he told me on another occasion, "I learned to distinguish two types of writing."

In a first and very general sense, writing meant for him simply *prendre de note.* On the level of taking notes, writing is a tool, a technique, possibly a medium for getting ideas. This method of note taking covers a huge terrain: the results of or problems with an experiment, a memo during a phone call, a notice in the course of a dialogue, a short sketch of an idea during a lab meeting, an email to oneself from a conference, an underlined passage in a book recently read, and so forth. Note taking, however, is only one side of Alain's conception of writing, the daytime side.

A second type of writing assumed the form of a meditation on the notes one has written down quickly, in passing, in the course of a day. This meditative work, the actual nocturnal work, happens when one is alone, at night, at home. One assembles the notes, arranges and rearranges them, and begins, by writing, to explore the connections between them. The task is to play with one's ideas, to bring them into dialogue with one another and make them communicate until this communication takes over and gives rise to ideas.

Nocturnal writing is designed to bypass the writer's intentional mind and to create a space in which the unexpected, in the form of ideas, can happen. The task is to write, to lose control, to get carried away while staying alert to ideas that come. After such a flight with ideas, one then reads what one has written, rewrites it, and searches for formulations that capture the distinct quality of an idea until, perhaps, another idea takes over.[6]

A free-floating mind is expected to give rise to disciplined ideas. For this to be possible, Alain identified two indispensable prerequisites. The first is the necessity to *have grown old in experimental work,* and the second is the *dialogue with the dead.*

In the course of my work with Alain, I heard him claim many times that a condition of the possibility of any biologically fruitful work with ideas is that one has worked for a long time at the lab bench. His point of reference, again, was Claude Bernard, who claimed that a physiologist, in order to have valuable intuitions ("*des intuitions juste*") must have grown old in experimental work ("*vieilli dans la pratique expérimentale*"); that he must have been mistaken a thousand times ("*ont été trompés mille fois*"); that he must have felt his way for a long time ("*il faut avoir tâtonné longtemps*").[7] Over the course of our conversations, I gradually learned that what Alain meant was neither that a researcher simply has to search for a long time before she makes an interesting observation nor that she has to have practiced for a long time in order to master the technology, as if biology were primarily a matter of technical work and thus of skill. Rather, he explained, "My point is a correlation between having grown old in experimental work and having valuable intuitions."

Alain was adamant that long-term practical work at the lab bench affects one's intuition, its value, its reliability. What led him to this claim were two powerful "illuminations" (his word). The first was an early career experience dating back to the time when he was still at the Collège de France studying the development of the dopaminergic system in the course of embryogenesis.

"When I was studying the impact of different neuronal populations on one another," he told me, "and then succeeded in inventing pure neuron cultures, I began to understand that technical work is the only means the biologist has available in order to acquire knowledge about living phenomena, even though living phenomena cannot be adequately captured in technical terms."

The conclusion Alain drew from this observation was that the only way to advance his research would be to learn to think of biological questions in technical terms, to learn to convert his ideas about *le vivant* into technical procedures (potentially ones that have yet to be invented).

The second illumination had a gradual and retrospective quality. Over the years, Alain came to recognize that the longer he had immersed himself in technically thinking through a concrete biological phenomenon, the more empirically valuable his ideas became. "What is more," he explained, "they eventually express themselves, automatically, without need for further reflection, as technical possibilities."

Alain drew two closely related conclusions form this observation. First, "experimentally struggling with ones object of inquiry (an organism or an aspect of it) over a long period of time gives rise to a *sens biologique* that expresses itself in valuable intuitions about this object." Second, "[a]pparently, the effort to think of biological problems in terms of technical procedures impacts the way one has ideas. It is as if thinking about and struggling with technical procedures has the side effect of conditioning one's mind in such a way that ideas come immediately in the form of possible, if yet to be invented, experiments."

For successful nocturnal work, the fostering of a *sens biologique* and the conditioning of one's mind are indispensable because they are the only guarantee that one's ideas are not arbitrary. Both have to be achieved to such a degree that even if one is lost in a nocturnal flight, ideas are, no matter how adventurous, informed by a "feeling for the organism" and come in the idiom of technical procedures.[8]

In 1989 (even though this is a retrospective rationalization), when he observed the nonautonomous transfer of homeoproteins, Alain had learned to trust his idea to such a degree that he decided to follow it, against the recommendation of almost everyone else.

Dialogue avec des Mortes

"Writing," Alain said at one point, worried that I would misunderstand his conception of nocturnal work, "is not to be mistaken for autism." He was almost angry. "To write," he explained, "is as well a *façon de converser* [manner of conversation] with others, you understand?"

He insisted that an essential feature of his nocturnal writing is a dialogue with authors of the past who have reflected on questions dear to him, for example, on emergent forms and development. At night, I learned, he sets the notes he has written down during the day in relation to sentences or paragraphs taken from books he has read and worked with. The result, in his words, was a *façon de converser.*

Alain had a veritable obsession for reading. I had first learned about this obsession when we first spent an evening together at his house. "I read everything," he told me that night. The subsequent tour through his library gave me a sense of what he meant. Shelf after shelf, ranging from floor to ceiling, was stuffed with books. Biology authors found themselves next to French historians of science; philosophy books, especially from the eighteenth century, were surrounded by art books and masses of classical literature, primarily French.

Later I learned that some of these books have accompanied Alain for several decades. He has read and reread them again and again over the course of the past thirty years. He has lived with and in them; they have nurtured his intuition, until some, at least, have become exhausted and used up.

"J'ai mon idée des textes" he says about that, "ma façon de les lire. Pas touche. Pollution des œuvres comme on pollue la nature."[9]

By far the biggest part of his nocturnal interlocutors has been the great biological authors of the nineteenth and early twentieth century, that is, from pre–molecular revolution biology. "The old ones," as he explained this preference, "have left us wonderful and very smart books. In reading them, you can learn a lot. You can learn the background story of your own questions and thoughts. It is almost as if you learn how to see."

I heard him insist on many occasions, especially in lab meetings and during his weekly one-on-one discussions with his researchers, that problems contemporary biologists struggle with have been thought about before and that contemporary understandings of biological problems can be fully comprehended only if one understands how they grew out of older ideas and debates. Reading the great biologists of the past, therefore, has for him been a way of becoming aware of the ideas that, often implicitly and barely recognized, inform the way contemporary biologists think about biological problems—for example, the problem of development.

The repeated reading and rereading of dead biologists not only helps him understand past reflections that frame the problems he is struggling with today; it is also constitutive of the form his nocturnal writing takes. From his repeated readings he extracts sentences and ideas that somehow relate to his work and places them in relation to recent experimental results of his lab or notes he has written during the day until, gradually or suddenly, a dialogue emerges. Such a "*dialogue avec des mortes*," which allows him to play with the ideas constitutive of the problems he deals with, is the actual form of his nocturnal journeys and the inexhaustible well from which his ideas and associations spring forth.

AT WORK: ON FRENZY AND METHOD

I turned from method to work: how did Alain's nocturnal encounters actually open new spaces of thought? How, in what concrete ways, did the work with ideas give shape to homeoproteins as plastic forces active throughout life? And how exactly did his nocturnal flights enable him and his colleagues to reimagine the mature brain, against (almost) all currents of neuronal research, in terms of an ongoing, if silent, embryogenesis?[10] Could I reconstruct what the conception of the nonautonomous transfer of homeoproteins as a plastic event owed to the work with ideas?

The unexpected window on Alain's actual nocturnal work turned out to be the reconstruction of his reading list. Whenever he mentioned an author, even if just in passing, I wrote down the reference, looked for the book or article, and started reading. Specifically, I was looking for the passage or passages, or at times even the logic of a larger argument, that he described as having nourished his ideas. I then returned to him (and at times to Volovitch and Joliot) with my discoveries and questions. We talked through my findings until, eventually, I could draw up a map of his nocturnal flights and how they successively opened, on the level of ideas, the possibility of thinking homeoproteins as forces that render the brain plastic, throughout life.

Of course, the map of nocturnal flights I came up with is a (somewhat sober) after-the-fact systematization; it is a catalogue raisonné and hence a mere list. And yet this list is composed of encounters that sparked—and broke open—unexpected spaces of thought. And isn't the generation of such unexpected openings and new possibilities of thinking what nocturnal work is all about?

Among the many interlocutors Alain mentioned, eight assumed a privileged position. I have divided them into two groups. The nocturnal exchanges with the first—composed of Claude Bernard, Hans Spemann and Hilde Mangold, Conrad Waddington, and Alan Turing—gave direct support, in the early 1990s, for considering homeoproteins as plastic (vital) forces active throughout life. His exchanges with the second—made up of D'Arcy Wentworth Thompson, Richard Goldschmidt, and Gavin de Beer—enabled Alain to link his work on homeoprotein expression in the adult to experimental evolutionary biology (which in turn allowed him to link neuronal research, somewhat against the opposition of the then-emerging field of cognitive neuroscience, to more explicitly biological—read: embryological—modes of reasoning).

I briefly turn to each author—not in order to do justice to their works (nocturnal work grounds in decontextualization) but in order to convey something of the excitement, the frenzy, that, together with the almost sober work of thought, was a condition for breaking open the possibility of a plastic brain.

Claude Bernard (1813–1878)

Claude Bernard was for Alain not just any interlocutor. The discussions with the founder of experimental medicine were, especially during the early years of Alain's homeoprotein research, the most important, most form-giving nocturnal encounter he had.

Beginning in the early 1840s, when he was an assistant to François Magendie (one of the founders of physiology) at the Collège de France, Claude Bernard investigated how sugar is taken up, digested, and excreted by animals. In 1855, after he had worked on sugar for more than ten years, and just after he had succeeded Magendie as chair of physiology at the Collège, Bernard made a curious chance discovery. Late one day he killed two rabbits. He carefully washed their livers, but then ran out of time and could analyze the liver of only one animal. The analysis of the second he postponed. When he came back the following day, he found that the second liver contained far more sugar than the one he had analyzed immediately after the death of the rabbits. Could that be? He repeated the experiment:

> By forcibly injecting a current of cold water through the hepatic vessels and passing it through a liver that was still warm, just after an animal's death, I showed that the tissue was completely freed from the sugar which it contained; but next day or a few hours later, if we keep the washed liver at a mild temperature, we again find its tissue charged with a large amount of sugar produced after it was washed.[11]

Could it be that the liver was producing sugar?

When he went public, suggesting just that, Bernard drew considerable criticism. The then-prevailing dual-kingdom conceptualization of nature depicted the animal body as a mechanical incineration plant and the vegetable kingdom as the fuel needed to keep the machine going.[12] For most of Bernard's contemporaries, therefore, sugars present in animals came exclusively from foods and were "destroyed in animal organisms by the phenomena of combustion, i.e., of respiration."[13]

Bernard's sugar-producing rabbit liver was beyond what was then thinkable; it could not be thought of with the prevailing anatomical and chemical concepts. What was he to do?

After some initial hesitation, Bernard seems to have enjoyed both the provocation and the challenge. It's as if he found the conceptual impossibility of his observation attractive, an invitation to elaborate an invitation to

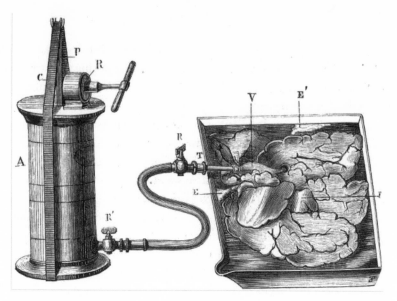

The water pump that Claude Bernard used to wash rabbit livers. From Bernard 1859.

elaborate new concepts, ones that would give contours to the novel physiology of the living that his rabbit liver seemed to imply. The starting point of his conceptual adventure was a departure from the dual-kingdom conception of nature. Certainly, Bernard conceded, the animal body, like all physical matter, is undergoing processes of degeneration and self-destruction. Yet one has to take into account, as his experiments showed, that the animal body is not *merely* physical matter but a *living organism* and as such is capable of furnishing the material and the substances it requires to maintain its form. "*La vie,*" Bernard summarized, "*c'est la mort, la vie, c'est la création.*"

Life is death *and* creation—this was for him the lesson of his sugar-producing liver.

Hidden in this lesson was a powerful conceptual critique of the two disciplines that at the time dominated the sciences of the living—anatomy and chemistry. Anatomy, in the tradition of Xavier Bichat, who famously had described life as the ensemble of forces that resist death, was looking for the trace of disease in dead matter (the body of the deceased). And chemistry—dominated by Lavoisier—understood the animal organism as a combustion machine and was trying to understand the chemical processes that break down (literally burn) the energy provided through nutrition.

Bernard's alternative to anatomy and chemistry, both concerned with death rather than with life, was what he referred to as experimental physiology. With vehemence he argued that a science of living processes had to be grounded in experiments with the living organism, that is, in experiments that could make visible the actual vital—physiological—function of organs.

Claude Bernard's work amounted to a powerful and long-lasting conceptual change. With his sugar-producing liver he biologized the machine view of the animal body predominant since the time of Descartes. He transformed the body into a living organism, and rendered obsolete the hierarchical and teleological division of nature into an animal and vegetable kingdom that had still informed (and was powerfully shaped by) anatomy and chemistry. What is more, he invented physiology as an experimental science of the living. He broke open a new space for thought—and thus for experimentation.

And Alain?

I had noted Bernard's importance for Alain long before I knew about his nocturnal conception of science. Already in our first conversation he proudly told me, "I am a Bernardian." I had also noticed that in many of our exchanges Bernard's name surfaced frequently (if almost always in passing). And I knew that Alain had written a small book about Bernard, *Claude Bernard: La Révolution Physiologique,* published in 1990. But even though I was quite aware that Alain held Bernard in high esteem, it was only in the context of our conversations about things nocturnal that I began to wonder about the direct and immediate relevance the founder of experimental medicine had for Alain's conception of the n-a-t as a lifelong plastic event.

And while I was trying to find concrete traces of Bernard in Alain's work, I suddenly realized that Alain had written his book on Bernard amidst the outrage his work with Joliot had caused. While colleagues attacked him, while friends turned away from him and his coworkers, he had conversed with Bernard.

When I reread the book, it began to dawn on me that Bernard was for Alain a master, that is, someone who had achieved intellectual and ethical superiority and hence could provide guidance, especially in turbulent times. It is only a slight exaggeration to say that Alain modeled his work on Bernard's. For example, there was Bernard's invention of physiology as a science of the living. Alain was adamant that, just as Bernard had biologized the animal body, he was biologizing the brain. In a way, Bernard's sugar-producing liver was equivalent to Alain's lifelong nonautonomous transfer of homeo-proteins—an opportunity to biologize the brain, to render it vital.

This was the challenge Alain had set himself in the late 1980s and early 1990s: Could he vitalize neuroscience, just as Bernard had vitalized physiology?

Then there was Alain's esteem for Bernard the thinker. "Claude Bernard," I noted him saying, "used the implausibility of his observation to rethink the conceptual presuppositions that truth claims make, and then he challenged them." On another occasion he told me, "Bernard actually only conducted one experiment, and then he spent the rest of his life thinking it through. The result was a revolution. He was bringing into existence a whole new, previously unknown world." And at least once I also heard Alain depict Bernard as the prototypical nocturnal thinker, as someone who endeavored to think the yet unthought of. Bernard opened up a novel conceptual space—and this conceptual effort was repeated by Alain. For what was the effort to rethink the brain in plastic terms if not an explicit, if perhaps smaller-scale, attempt at a conceptual revolution?

Alain admired Bernard for his confidence, his courage, and his perseverance. On many occasions I heard him quote a passage from Bernard that he knew by heart: "Quand le fait qu'on rencontre est en opposition avec une théorie régnante il faut accepter le fait et abandonner la théorie, lors même que celle-ci, soutenue par de grands noms, est généralement accepté."

Finally, there were the apparent parallels between Bernard's effort to differentiate physiology as science of the living from anatomy and chemistry—two disciplines that evoked a conception of the organism that was not suited to comprehending a sugar-producing liver—and Alain's angry attacks against molecular biology and against the newly dominant cognitive neuroscience. Both of these approaches, Alain frequently insisted in public (lectures) and nonpublic (lab meetings) settings, conceptualize the brain as essentially fixed and immutable—as a nonliving organ that can be captured in physicochemical terms.[14]

Indeed, Alain was a Bernardian.

In addition to these formal correspondences, I found two passages in Bernard's oeuvre that provided Alain in 1989–1990 with a scaffold for how to make sense of "their artifact." They were something like the anchor point of his work, the ideational condition of the possibility of plasticity. The first is from Bernard's *Cahier des Notes,* the second from the *Principes de médicine expérimentale:*

Il s'agit de prouver que les phénomènes du développement n'existent pas seulement dans l'état embryonnaire, mais qu'ils se poursuivent dans l'état adulte. [...] Prouver en second lieu que les phénomènes de développement sont la cause de tous les phénomènes physiologiques, de toutes les manifestations vitales. Le développement, sa création, est donc toujours le phénomène vital dominateur.[15]

J'admets parfaitement que lorsque la physiologie sera assez avancée, le physiologiste pourra faire des animaux et des végétaux nouveaux comme le chimiste produit des corps qui sont en puissance, mais qui n'existent pas dans l'état naturel des choses. [...] Mais la physiologie devra agir scientifiquement pour opérer toutes ces modifications et se rendre compte de ce qu'elle fait parce qu'elle connaîtra les lois intimes de la formation des corps organiques, comme le chimiste connaît les lois intimes de la formation des corps minéraux. C'est donc dans la loi de la formation des corps organisés qu'agit toute la science biologique expérimentale.[16]

In the first reflection, consistent with his theory that *"la vie, c'est la mort, la vie c'est la création,"* Bernard suggests that developmental—that is, tissue-generating and -forming—processes are the very locus of life itself and that such living processes are not just occurring in the course of development but also in adults. With these claims, Bernard opened for Alain a possibility where before there seemed none: couldn't it be that the transfer of homeoproteins was such a vital process? An instance—perhaps *the* instance—of life itself, in the course of development as much as in the adult? What seemed impossible from the perspective of the classical schema of neuronal research—a silent embryogenesis in the adult—appeared to be, at least from the perspective of nineteenth-century Bernardian physiology, a plausible biological observation.

In the second reflection, Bernard then states that the actual task of a science of the living must be to uncover the laws that stand behind such ongoing developmental processes. Again Alain read Bernard as encouragement: to him, as well as to Michel and Joliot, the suggestion was to think of the transfer of homeoproteins—understood as a living, form-giving (that is, plastic) process—as precisely such a vital "law." Wasn't it their obligation, morally and intellectually, to follow up on their discovery?

In the late 1980s and early 1990s, when Alain's decision to focus on homeoproteins as plastic forces was causing outrage, when his laboratory was actively marginalized, when researchers began to leave the newly founded lab, Bernard's was arguably Alain's most important interlocutor. And his two reflections on physiology as science of the laws of formation were the treasure that upheld the possibility that homeoproteins could transfer between cells and act as plastic forces.

Hans Spemann (1869–1941) and Hilde Mangold (1898–1924)

Hans Spemann was—with Wilhelm Roux (1850–1924), Hans Driesch (1867–1941), and Ross Granville Harrison (1870–1951)—one of the founders of experimental embryology. Whereas earlier embryologists had focused largely on dissection and description, guided by the goal of giving a careful account of the epigenetic formation of the embryo, these three scholars and their students sought to complement description with experimentation. They systematically interfered—a distant echo of Bernard—with growth processes in order to find out the laws of formation. Spemann's perhaps most significant contribution to experimental embryology was his discovery of the inductive logic of embryogenesis—and it was precisely this logic of induction that helped Alain to give further contours to the nonautonomous transfer of homeoproteins.

At the beginning of the twentieth century, Spemann, then working in Rostock, Germany, began studying the embryogenetic formation of the eye in newts (Triton). He was specifically curious to find out whether the formation of the lens (which developed out of the epidermis) was contingent on the formation of the eyecup (which developed out of the medullar plate). More specifically, His idée fix was that the eyecup could have some form-giving—inductive—potency that triggered the formation of the lens.

To answer this question, Spemann ablated the presumptive eyecup rudiment on one side of the embryo with a hot needle and observed that lens formation consistently failed to occur on the operated site. Next, he experimentally removed those parts of the epidermis that give rise to the lenses and replaced them with other, random parts of the epidermis. The eyecup he left intact.

Would lens formation still occur? Would the eyecup induce the formation of lenses in the grafted tissue? If so, lens formation would have to be imagined as an inductive unfolding: the prior formation of one part of the embryo would be the form-giving precondition for the emergence of the successive part, which in itself would not contain the condition of its possibility. And this is precisely what Spemann discovered—the inductive logic of lens formation.

Over the next two decades, Spemann would successively further develop and refine his conception of induction. Around 1919, then, he returned to an experiment he had carried out almost twenty years earlier. In the summer of 1901, then still a *Privatdozent* in Würzburg, he had used an infant hair to constrict newt embryos in the two-cells state. After some initial experimentation, Spemann learned to produce—at will—depending on where he constricted the cells, double-headed embryos with three noses and three eyes or double-tailed embryos. His constriction experiments made Spemann famous. But Spemann suffered from the fact that he could not provide an explanation as to what had caused the deformations his constrictions provoked. If he returned to them now, almost two decades later, it was because it seemed to him that his concept of induction had the potential to provide an answer.

Could it perhaps be, Spemann wondered, that all of embryogenesis—that is, not just the formation of the lens or of this or that organ but literally all of embryogenesis—followed an inductive logic? His idea was that perhaps his constriction experiments had interrupted the communication between the two cells and had thereby caused each one to divide anew (or partly anew), as if it were not already part of a cell cycle. The consequence, then, would be a gastrula that had, depending on where he constricted the cells, two head– or two tail–inducing elements. (A gastrula is the three-layered cell structure that emerges at the end of cell division; it consists of endoderm, ectoderm, and mesoderm—that is, the three cell types out of which the embryo gets built.) The coup of Spemann's speculation was that it implied that the gastrula is composed of parts that have distinctive inductive potential (meaning that one part is inducing the head, another the tail, yet another the eyes, and so on). The project Spemann developed from rethinking his constriction experiments in inductive terms was unheard of: his plan was to map the different inductive potentials of the gastrula.[17]

After some initial experimentation, Spemann was confident that his speculation was correct and his plan feasible. In 1920 he recruited a graduate student, Hilde Mangold, who helped him test his idea. The results they retrieved were as fantastic as Spemann's speculation had been. When they grafted the dorsal lip of one amphibian gastrula to a region of another amphibian gastrula that was known to give rise to body skin, it caused that part to produce instead a new medullar plate (that is, the axis out of which the embryo will be formed). Mangold and Spemann had identified an area in the gastrula that induced a whole new embryo.

Differently put, they had discovered that there is a single Archimedean point, somewhere in the dorsal lip, that induces the entire embryo. With the help of this Archimedean point, one could technically control the production of embryos, possibly even produce new embryos—or part thereof.

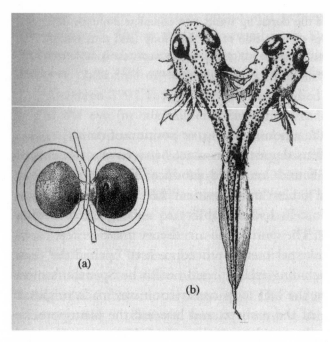

A constricted Triton egg and a two-headed Triton. From Spemann 1936.

When looking for a name for the part of the dorsal lip responsible for the induction, Spemann suggested the term *organizer:* "Ein solches Stück eines Organisationszentrums kann man kurz einen Organisator nennen; er schafft sich in dem indifferenten Material, in dem er liegt oder in welches er verpflanzt wird, ein 'Organisationsfeld' von bestimmter Richtung und Ausdehnung."[18]

Spemann and Mangold made a most important contribution to the space of possibility that Alain, through his conversation with Bernard, had begun to establish. With the two German experimental embryologists, the possibility arose that Bernard's conception of life as ongoing embryogenesis could be linked to small-scale organizing (inductive) forces, understood—here Bernard, Spemann, and Mangold meet—as a condensation of living processes that generate and form new tissue.

What if homeoproteins, given that homeotic genes appear to contain a basic body plan of animal organisms, are a an organizing, inductive, developmental force? One active throughout life? One that induces, for example, the growth of new tissue in the adult human brain?

Conrad Waddington (1905–1975)

A third major contributor to the early years of Alain's nocturnal project was Conrad Hal Waddington, a British developmental biologist. Like many embryologists of the generation that followed Spemann, Waddington was intrigued by the discovery of the organizer but rejected the vitalism implicit in Spemann's work. In the early 1930s, he thus set out to find what he called an "inducer molecule" which he speculated, stood behind induction.[19] In 1933, just a year after a brief stay in Spemann's lab in Freiburg, he seemed to have found what he was looking for. Together with Joseph and Dorothy Needham, two British chemists, he succeeded in producing ether extracts of the newt organizer. These extracts could turn presumptive epidermis into neural tissue.

Waddington was thrilled: had he found the "real" active substance of the organizer? In a 1935 paper he argued just that, and suggested the term *evocator* as the name for the chemical substance he assumed to be the active force behind embryogenesis.[20]After this initial success, however, Waddington's chemical efforts soon proved frustrating. In the course of the 1930s it turned out to be impossible to chemically identify the evocator substance.

In the late 1930s, Waddington then turned away from chemistry and toward genetics, specifically the genetics of Thomas Hunt Morgan.[21] In 1938, he traveled to Columbia University, where he worked with L. Dunn, and in 1939 he stayed for three months at the California Institute of Technology, working with Alfred Sturtevant and Theodosius Dobzhansky. His work in genetics led him to a conceptual coup: the formal equation between organizers and genes.[22] To be more precise, Waddington suggested picturing development as a succession of different branching paths and organizers, with genes as the actual force that decided which direction development would go. Development, he wrote in 1939,

> can best be symbolized as a system of branching paths. The characteristics of each path will depend upon the developmental potencies of the tissue, that is to say, they will be under the control of the genes. We may also expect to find genes which act in a way formally like that of evocators, in that they control the choice of alternatives. Genes of this sort are in fact known.[23]

One of the examples Waddington gives is a gene he calls Aristapedia (first described by Sturtevant in 1923).[24] Normally, he writes in his book *Organisers and Genes* (1947), the antenna of drosophila "consists of a small basal joint, a somewhat swollen second joint, and a third joint which bears the arista, a

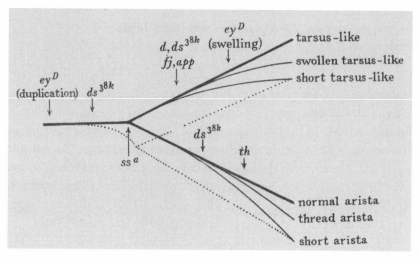

The possibilities of branching that are open to Aristapedia. From Waddington 1947.

tapering chitinous spike having numerous branches." Waddington then goes on to explain that if the Aristapedia gene is mutated, "the arista is transformed into a more or less leg-like organ, consisting of several small joints resembling the tarsal joints, the terminal one of which usually bears two typical tarsal claws; at the same time the third antennal joint is usually less swollen and more elongated than normal." He then concludes: "There is then a branching in the developmental possibilities open to the antennal imaginal bud; it may follow one branch and proceed to develop into an antenna and arista, or the other and develop into a leg-like organ." In other words, there is a formal equivalence between genes and organizers, which allowed Waddington to speak of "evocator genes which shunt development along one or the other of the possible developmental branches."[25]

In Alain's nocturnal work, Waddington occupies a strategically important position. It had been known since 1984 that Aristapedia is a homeobox-containing gene that codes for a homeoprotein with the same name. The possibility thus opened up to think, with Waddington, of homeotic genes as evocator genes, and of homeoproteins as evocator proteins. And this, in turn, opened up the possibility to link contemporary genetics to an older discourse of development as creative processes (Bernard), as organized by small vital (or plastic) forces (Spemann-Mangold), and as an instance of life itself (Bernard and Spemann-Mangold): Waddington allowed Alain to embryologize genetics.

Gradually, homeoproteins gained contour.

Alan Turing (1912–1954)

Our first exchange about Turing left me baffled. Alain told me that for him Alan Turing was "a biologist to whom we owe a profound reflection about the concept of morphogenesis." Turing—the famous decoder of the enigma, thinker of the computer—a biologist?

Alain went on to tell me that "I had conceived of reading Turing as an exercise in critique," and that as an embryologist of the mature nervous system, he had been interested in determining the "insurmountable problems" any effort to understand the brain in terms of computer engineering would run into. "But what I then found was that Turing was not actually trying to understand the brain in terms of the computer. Instead, he was busy understanding computers in terms of brain science."

When I turned to Turing myself, I learned that he had indeed been, for much of his life, a careful reader of brain science—and that his readings were hardly marginal to his work. Turing was intrigued by the possibility that he could construct—literally, not metaphorically—a brain machine. For example, to friends he described his work on "instruction tables" as "building a brain." And he told them that the Turing test, a thought experiment constructed around the question if machines can think, and the Turing machine, which he frequently referred to as a model of a thinking human brain occupied with computation, were for him tools he came up with to facilitate his effort to construct a computer that one couldn't distinguish from a brain busy computing.

The perhaps most surprising finding of my reading adventure, however, was that Turing, in the years after World War II, had systematically worked through articles about how, in the course of embryogenesis, the brain's neuronal structure is formed. The result of his venture into embryology was a "mathematical theory of embryology," which he summarized in his 1952 paper "The Chemical Basis of Morphogenesis." Reciprocally inhibitive chemical substances, he speculates there, diffuse through embryological tissue and thereby build up chemical patterns that in turn trigger the mechanical formation of the embryo.[26]

In an effort to give finer contour to these chemical substances, Turing suggested imagining them as what he called "morphogens, the word being intended to convey the idea of a form producer." He went on: "The evocators of Waddington provide a good example of morphogens. These evocators diffusing into tissue somehow persuade it to develop along different lines from those which would have followed in its absence."[27]

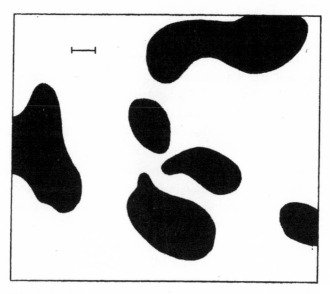

A dappled pattern as it might be produced by a ring of cells organized in the form of a morphogen system. From Turing 1952.

Turing's importance for Alain's nocturnal work was at least twofold. On the one hand, Turing allowed Alain to spin further the line of flight that stretches from Bernard to Spemann-Mangold and Waddington: homeoproteins gain, once again, contour as a plastic force—as an instance of life itself understood as creation, as an organizer, an evocator, a morphogen. On the other hand, Turing extended this line of flight by adding something new and crucial: a way of thinking about the thus far inexplicable nonautonomous transfer. What if homeoproteins were "diffusing form producers," as Turing had it?

In a recent draft of a paper entitled "Are Homeoproteins Morphogens?" Alain and Joliot wrote:

> Homeoproteins are considered as "infectious entities" that invade the neuroepithelium until they encounter a nuclear environment that is unsuitable for their own activation, in part because of the high expression of the antagonist homeoprotein. In fact the protein does not travel far—just one cell—but propagates rapidly by inducing and amplifying its own transcription. All this happens as if the genes themselves were diffusible, a term that evokes the definition of morphogens by Alain Turing.[28]

According to Turing, morphogens diffuse—as do, according to Alain and Joliot, homeoproteins. They leave cells, are extracellular, and then enter their neighboring cells, thereby "infecting" one after the other until a counterhomeoprotein stops their expansion. Perhaps the entire formation of the nervous system, in the embryo as well as in the adult, is grounded in such a not yet known formation process orchestrated by diffusing homeoproteins. Wouldn't the nonautonomous transfer then come into view as a key biological mechanism rather than as an artifact?

WORK ON THE POSSIBLE

Bernard, Spemann and Mangold, Waddington, Turing—these are but a small fraction of the bookshelves of authors with whom Alain converses at night (not to mention the many articles—academic and nonacademic—comments, ephemeral thoughts, and experimental results that also feed into his nocturnal work).[29] But even though they were but a small fraction, this brief overview may suffice to show that and how nocturnal work effectively mutates the possible.

Three basic principles are at play. They partly overlap and yet point in different directions.

First, nocturnality itself. Through writing, Alain is methodologically working his way around his will and intentionality to enable ideas to have a life and dynamic of their own, to have an agency of sorts, which in turn allows them to surprise him.

Second, decontextualization. His readings are devoid of any hermeneutical sensibility. On the contrary, he blissfully ignores context and the intent of authors, which allows for unexpected and hence surprising links between the works he reads and the work going on in his lab.

Third, juxtaposition. When writing, he juxtaposes ideas taken from different, often mutually exclusive contexts and relates them to one another. In the process of writing, these ideas enter, "*comme sous le jeu du hasard*" (as if by chance; his words), into unimagined relations in which, as if independent of the writer, surprising, not yet imagined scenarios are developing themselves.

Together, these three principles—nocturnality, decontextualization, and juxtaposition—allow for the genuine possibility of surprise. They enable the emergence of the unexpected, understood as that which lies beyond the already thought and known, beyond the established configuration of the possible. More technically put, at the core of Alain's nocturnal work with ideas is the methodological mutation of contingencies into surprises—surprises that cut across established pathways of thought to break open new, yet unheard-of spaces of possibility and, at the same time, give shape to these new possibilities.

The more ideas (surprises) Alain comes up with, the more correspondences he recognizes, the tighter the links between the different elements become, the denser the web of ideas gets, the clearer the contours of the space of possibility that he and his colleagues seek to open become.

To provide a sense of what form this thickening took, and in which unexpected direction his nocturnal work on homeoproteins took him I turn to a second set of authors. If Alain's conversations with Bernard, Spemann and Mangold, Waddington, and Turing revolved around the idea of small-scale plastic (vital) forces that shape embryogenesis, then his exchanges with D'Arcy Thompson, Richard Goldschmidt, and Gavin de Beer revolve around the possibility that these plastic forces (aka organizers, inducers, evocators, morphogens, diffusing homeoproteins) could also be active in the adult.

D'Arcy Thompson (1860–1948)

D'Arcy Wentworth Thompson, professor of biology and natural history at the University of Aberdeen, was a curious figure of early-twentieth-century academic life. He translated several Greek works (among them Aristotle's *Historia Animalium*), published glossaries of Greek birds and fishes, trained as a mathematician and physicist, and wrote one very long biology book, *On Growth and Form*, first published in 1917. The book's form and style resembles Buffon's (1707–1788) *Histoire Naturelle* more than the sober journal publications that began to dominate biological authorship in the early twentieth century. But not just the style of the book was untimely. I quote at length to provide a sense of Thompson's Victorian prose:

> The physicist proclaims aloud that the physical phenomena which meet us by the way have their manifestations of form, not less beautiful and scarce less varied which move us to admiration among living things. The waves of the sea, the little ripples of the shore, the sweeping curve of the sandy bay between its headlands, the outline of the hills, the shape of the clouds, all these are so many riddles of form, so many problems of morphology, and all of them the physicist can more or less easily read and adequately solve: solving them by reference to their antecedent phenomena, in the material system of

mechanical forces to which they belong, and to which we interpret them as being due [. . .]. Nor is it otherwise with the material forms of living things. Cell tissues, shell and bone, leaf and flower, are so many portions of matter, and it is in the obedience to the laws of physics that their particles have been moved, molded and conformed [. . .]. Their problems of form are in the first instance mathematical problems, and their problems of growth are essentially physical problems, and the morphologist is, ipso facto, a student of physical science.[30]

For Thompson, an expert in skeletal structures, biology was a branch of morphology and as such a part of physics. *On Growth and Form* was an effort to defend this vision of the science of the living—written against the rise to dominance of genetics in the early decades of the twentieth century.

Thompson distrusted Darwin's conception of evolution, and he distrusted the exclusive focus on heredity it brought about. He doubted the idea that advantageous hereditary mutations could be the only plausible key for understanding evolutionary change. Heredity, he wrote, directly addressing the genetics of his day, was certainly "one of the great factors in biology"—but only one. As another one, which could better account for evolutionary change, he offered the "direct physical and mechanical mode of causation." Consequently, in sharp contrast to Darwinians, he saw his task in studying "the inter-relations of growth and form, and the part which the physical forces play in this complex interaction; and, as part of the same inquiry, to use mathematical methods and mathematical terminology to describe and define the forms of organisms."[31]

Thompson suggested that the emergence of new biological forms was best understood as the result of changes in "developmental growth rates."[32] What brought these changes about, he argued, were physical forces. Transformations, he wrote, occur "where a great change of physical or mechanical conditions has come about, and where accordingly the former physical and physiological constraints are altered or removed."[33] Changes in "climate, rise of sea level," and the like may result in different "growth rates," which result in metamorphoses of the form of given organisms.[34]

The part of *On Growth and Form* that best illustrates Thompson's effort to think through evolution from a general mathematical, physical perspective is the often commented-upon last chapter, "On the Theory of Transformations or the Comparison of Related Forms." There, Thompson compared formal, skeletal differences between species and articulated the idea that evolutionary change is best understood as the result of transformation in the course of an organism's development.[35] The main analytical tool with which he challenged Darwinism was a simple Cartesian coordinate system:

> Let us inscribe in a system of Cartesian co-ordinates the outline of an organism, however complicated, or a part thereof: Such as a fish, a crab, or a mammalian skull. [...] If we submit our rectangular system to deformation on simple and recognized lines, altering, for instance, the direction of the axes [...], then we obtain a new system of co-ordinates, whose deformation from the original type the inscribed figure will precisely follow. In other words, we obtain a new figure which represents the old figure under a more or less homogenous strain, and is a function of the new co-ordinates in precisely the same way as the old figure was of the original coordinates.[36]

Whereas Darwinians explain the rearrangement of physical components as a result of mutation, adaptation, and natural selection, Thompson searched for and found mathematical and mechanical laws of forms and deformations. Even species that superficially look very different could be presented as simple Cartesian transformations of one another: "one form as a definite permutation of another."[37] What were to Darwinians the endless possibilities for mutation were for Thompson "strictly limited, possibilities of permutation and degree [...]. From one form, or ratio of magnitude, to another there is but one straight and direct road of transformation."[38]

Alain encountered Thompson several times. Their first conversation dates back to 1975, when Alain was still in graduate school.

"I was working on the genetics of plant viruses and remained largely indifferent to Thompson's morphological endeavor. For the molecularist I was, a chemist of the living rather than a biologist, D'Arcy was of no apparent interest."

In 1985, during his time in New York, Alain encountered Thompson a second time. Now that he had spent almost a decade dealing with questions of morphogenesis, he valued the author of *On Growth and Form* for his general interest in forms or forms-in-motion. Alain recognized that Thompson fit in a general genealogy of thinkers interested in morphology and that, more specifically, he belonged to the handful of authors who had suggested that the key for understanding evolutionary changes could be found in morphological changes in the course of development.

The third time Alain met Thompson was in the mid-1990s, this time with direct relevance to his effort to formulate a conceptual horizon that would give contour to homeoproteins as plastic forces.

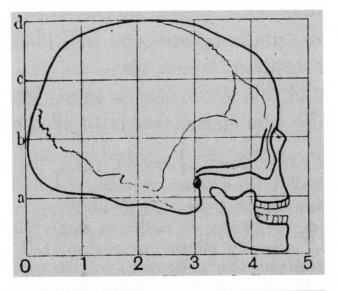

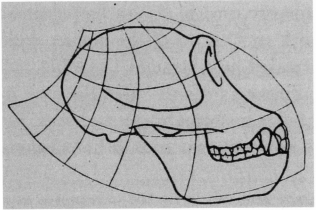

An illustration of permutation from a human to a chimpanzee skull. From Thompson 1917.

"Thompson?" I asked. How, I wondered, could a structuralist—someone who seemed to reduce the living to its skeletal form—be of help for giving contours to homeoproteins as plastic, tissue-generating forces?

Alain's answer to my question of why he suddenly assigned such an important place to Thompson provides a window on his nocturnal method of working by associations. "Thompson," he explained, "considered living organisms as a moldable material, which is under the control of physical forces, for example, surface tension, adhesion, viscosity. In the mid-1990s I had the idea to translate these physical forces into molecular terms."

In short, Alain associated homeoproteins with Thompson's physical forces.

One can see here in nuce how Alain's nocturnal work functions. He literally inscribed his work onto that of Thompson and appropriated it for his own purpose. Through the simple substitution of physical forces through homeoprotein diffusion, Thompson can be linked to Alain's effort to think homeoproteins as plastic forces—forces that shape the *"matière molle,"* as which one might imagine the brain.

But Thompson does not matter to Alain just because he gives contour to homeoproteins as plastic forces. What matters perhaps even more is that by thinking about his work in Thompson's terms, Alain made his work matter to the problems Thompson struggled with, namely evolutionary change. Insofar as Thompson sees the key for understanding evolution in understanding changes in developmental growth rates, or better yet, in understanding the forces that control morphogenetic processes, one can associate homeoproteins and their n-a-t (i.e., exemplary plastic or morphogenetic forces responsible for growth) with evolutionary change. In a word, homeoproteins and their n-a-t (nonautonomous transfer) matter to evolution.

And then there was, as I only discovered after I left Paris, Thompson's own theory of plasticity, which he described in 1917:

> Our bone is not only a living thing, but a highly plastic structure; the little trabeculae are constantly being formed and deformed, demolished and formed anew. Here, for once, it is safe to say that "heredity" need not and cannot be invoked to account for the configuration and arrangement of the trabeculae; for we can see them, at any time of life, in the making, under the direct action and control of forces to which the system is exposed [...]. Herein then lies, so far as we can discern it, a great part at least of the physical causation of what at first sight strikes us as a purely functional adaptation.[39]

When I read this passage to Alain during one of my return trips to Paris, he smiled and said: "I see. You are learning."

Richard Goldschmidt (1878–1958)

The story of Goldschmidt's life is like a window on the profound conceptual incommensurability of, and competition between, early German and American efforts to ground biology in a genetic rationality.

In late 1932, Richard Goldschmidt was a celebrity. He was Germany's first professor of genetics, was working at pre–World War II Germany's most prestigious academic institution, the Kaiser Wilhelm Institute, was the powerful editor of an important journal, the esteemed author of several widely used genetics textbooks, and a leading authority on issues of sex determination, geographic variation, genetics, and zoology. Goldschmidt was "one of the [most] imposing figures of German intellectual life."[40]

Then Hitler came to power. In 1935 Goldschmidt was classified as half-Jew and forced to resign from his position. After a year of uncertainty, he was offered a professorship in zoology at the University of California and left Berlin for Berkeley. Once in California, he did the obvious—he sought to reestablish himself as the important genetic biologist he had been. But in the United States, biology had developed along somewhat different lines than in Germany. Biologists had articulated different questions and had come up with different answers. When Goldschmidt presented his answers and wondered aloud whether his American colleagues had asked the wrong questions, powerful lines of friction emerged. He was on his way to becoming a prewar German biologist in the postwar United States.

The disagreement between Goldschmidt and his new colleagues unfolded along two lines. The first concerned genetics, more specifically the question of what a gene is and what its role for the organism is. Here Goldschmidt's adversaries were Thomas H. Morgan and his followers.[41] The second line of disagreement concerned evolution and evolved around the question of how new species emerge. Goldschmidt's opponents were the authors of the modern synthesis: Theodosius Dobzhansky, Edmond Ford, and Ernst Mayr.

When, in 1939, Goldschmidt was invited to give the Silliman Lecture, he used the opportunity to systematically work out what he thought a proper genetic biology would look like, one that could explain how new species emerge (a year later, he published his lecture as *The Material Basis of Evolution*). The case study he used to make his argument came from his thirty-year-long research on the gypsy moth (*Lymantria dispar*). From the second decade of the twentieth century onward, Goldschmidt had continuously traveled through Asia (mostly Japan) and documented the geographic differences among the variations of the gypsy moth he encountered. The result of his long-term field study, he told his audience, was unambiguous: diversification within species does not lead to the origin of new species. This result ran counter to a core assumption on which Darwin's synthetic theory of evolution was based, namely, that evolutionary change, understood as the result of adaptation, is generally slow, steady, gradual, and continuous, with no apparent break between micro- and macroevolution. In Darwin's own famous dictum: *Natura non facit saltum.*[42]

Goldschmidt did not reject Darwinism altogether. His research taught him that Darwin was right in describing changes within species as gradual and adaptive. However, he insisted that such gradual changes can lead to diversification only within already existent species and cannot account for the emergence of new species. These, he claimed, emerge only in a discontinuous and saltational mode, that is, in a genetic mutation that cannot be explained as adaptive modification. *Natura facit saltum.* Consequently, one had to complement the new synthesis by a saltational theory of macroevolution—a theory of the emergence of new species based on nonadaptive mutations.

The actual genetic experiments that led Goldschmidt to his argument were his inquiries into sex determination. In parallel with his field studies, Goldschmidt had sought to identify the genes responsible in *Lymantria* for sex determination. What he found was that a gene does not produce a unitary trait, as Morgan and his school had it, but some chemical substance, or substances, the ratio of which determine the trait. (That means a trait is not determined by a gene but by an interplay of substances—an interplay that involves the organism and its environment—to which genes give rise.[43]) In the case of sex determination, Goldschmidt called these chemical substances "male and female sex determinants."[44] When he began to alter the expression patterns of these "sex genes" in experiments, he not only succeeded in controlling sex determination. By altering the balance between genetically produced male and female sex determiners in the course of development, he could also produce a series of graded "intersexes" (a term he seems to have invented).[45]

Goldschmidt concluded that the "timing" of gene expression controls developmental and thus morphogenetic processes. It was this discovery that led him to articulate his theory of saltational macromutation:[46] a small-scale genetic mutation that occurs very early in the course of embryogenesis, he speculated, could change the timing pattern of future developmental processes and could thus have a profound impact on the future organic structure of the adult organism.[47] "A single mutational step affecting the right process at the right moment," he wrote in 1940, "can accomplish everything, providing that it is able to set in motion the ever present potentialities of embryonic regulation."[48]

Goldschmidt called the genes that could, if mutated, cause the emergence of a new species "rate genes":

> The mutant gene produces its effect [...] by changing the rates of partial processes of development. These might be rates of growth or differentiation, rates of production of stuffs necessary for differentiation, rates of reactions leading to definite physical or chemical situations at definite times of development, rates of those processes which are responsible for segregating the embryonic potencies at definite times.[49]

Goldschmidt admitted that the vast majority of macromutations could be viewed only as disastrous, what he called "monsters." But, he continued, every once in a while a macromutation might adapt an organism to a new mode of life, generating a "hopeful monster." According to Goldschmidt, macroevolution proceeds by the rare success of these hopeful monsters, not by an accumulation of small changes within populations.[50]

What had attracted Alain to Goldschmidt was, initially, the conceptual mismatch between his work and the dominant schools of thought. The controversy around Goldschmidt was a conceptual event that revolved around the possibility of thinking along lines other than the established ones. There was the promise, somewhere in Goldschmidt's work, that another genetics was possible, a possibility not yet pursued. Alain was also attracted to the poetics of the monster idea, a concept he would frequently evoke in talks and lectures.

However, the more he immersed himself in reading Goldschmidt, the more he became intrigued by his idea of rate genes. Were homeotic genes not a prime example of rate genes? Rate genes produce a series of interacting chemical substances, as do homeotic genes. And wasn't there a correspondence between homeoproteins, rate genes, and Turing's morphogens?

Alain found in Goldschmidt a confirmation of the diffusion idea he had first encountered in Turing: homeoproteins diffuse "until they encounter a nuclear environment that is unsuitable for their own activation, in part because of the high expression of the antagonist homeoprotein."[51]

Alain's association of homeotic genes with rate genes enabled him to consider his work in terms of Goldschmidt's and to make homeoproteins and their n-a-t—insofar as homeoproteins are the active force that actually controls the development of an organism—relevant to matters of evolution.[52] A mutation in homeotic genes, which are known to control the segmentation and the morphogenetic development of the embryo, would change the expression patterns of homeoproteins in the course of development and could thus result in a different pattern of their diffusion by way of nonautonomous transfer. The consequence would be a (potentially powerful) rearrangement of developmental processes—a monster, possibly a hopeful one.

Perhaps the nonautonomous transfer of homeoproteins, and the lifelong cerebral plasticity it allowed for, was the "material basis" of a such a mutation?

If one compares Goldschmidt's work with Thompson's, one can see that the former decisively transforms the conceptual horizon the latter established. Thompson grounded the link between development and evolution in a purely mathematical account of general laws of growth that was explicitly intended to render a focus on genes obsolete by making physical forces the active agents of evolution. Goldschmidt, on the other hand, grounded the link between development and evolution in an explicitly genetic, empirically and experimentally tested account. He geneticizes Thompson's escape from genetics—and thereby affirms Alain's translation of physical forces into molecular ones.

Thanks to Goldschmidt, experimentation with and on homeoproteins and their n-a-t is at one and the same time molecular cell biology, experimental embryology, experimental evolution, neurobiology, and, unifying all of these different aspects, a general Bernardian morphology of living organisms.

One can understand now why Alain called his lab in 1989 *"Laboratoire pour l'évolution et le développement du système nerveux central."*

Gavin de Beer (1899–1972)

Sir Gavin de Beer, a British embryologist, dominated evolutionary theory, at least in the United Kingdom, for more than forty years. This dominance was based on a single book, which he published four times, each time in a slightly different and enlarged version. The first edition, which appeared in 1930, was entitled *Embryology and Evolution;* the later three, published in 1940, 1951, and 1958, were all called *Embryos and Ancestors.*

Like Thompson and Goldschmidt before him, de Beer presumed that the key to understanding the evolutionary emergence of new species is embryology. Unlike his predecessors, though, de Beer actually was an embryologist. Whereas for Thompson embryos were merely shapes, skeletons that gained new forms under physical pressures, and whereas for Goldschmidt they were at best a place of gene expression, for de Beer, embryos actually mattered. They were more than mere conceptual tools, more than just good to think with. They offered, if they were studied in their own terms, the opportunity to understand what actually led to the evolutionary emergence of new species.

There is a second major difference between de Beer and his predecessors. De Beer was not content with being a critical but ultimately marginal voice seeking to keep open the possibility of thinking in ways rejected by mainstream scientists. Instead, he set out to provide a general—and generally accepted—conceptual foundation for "a new coordination of studies in embryology, genetics, and evolution."[53]

His project was to devise a novel foundation for biology.

The frame for de Beer's ambitious project was provided by the problematization of an earlier effort to link embryos and ancestors, Ernst Haeckel's "biogenetic law."[54]

Writing in the late nineteenth century and drawing on his work in comparative embryology, Haeckel had suggested that ontogeny strictly recapitulates the linear stages of phylogeny. For de Beer, more than thirty years of experimental embryology had proven Haeckel wrong, on two counts.[55] First, embryogenesis is not a succession of stages, each stage characterized by the development of an additional feature. Indeed, the construction of an organism is better described as the temporally complex development of single characters. Temporally complex, because the development of each character—for example, teeth and tongue—unfolds along different temporal trajectories at different speeds. While some characters are built over a rather long period of time others emerge quickly.

Second, the successive order in the emergence of characters is not, as the biogenetic law would require it, the same in successive species, with an additional character or feature in each higher species. Development does not obey a strictly linear progression but is instead open to alterations and reversals. While in some animals teeth evolved before the tongue, in others the tongue is formed before the teeth.[56]

For de Beer, phylogeny could not possibly be the driving force behind ontogeny. Rather, a careful reading of embryological literature suggested the opposite: ontogeny was the key to phylogeny. To make this possibility plausible, de Beer asked his readers to picture the embryo as an emergent ensemble of different, developing characters that obey different but interrelated temporal orders and are thus constructed at different developmental speeds.

What, he then wondered, would happen if one of these temporal orders altered its course?

De Beer approached his question by turning to Richard Goldschmidt, specifically to his concept of rate genes. What made Goldschmidt's concept of the gene attractive to de Beer, who had thus far relied exclusively on embryological literature (that is, not on writings by geneticists), was that it allowed him to inscribe genetics onto embryology rather than the other way round. Whereas Morgan and his school had a deterministic understanding of the gene—one gene, one trait—Goldschmidt's physiological conception kept the space for epigenetic changes wide open. For him, traits were the result of a complex interplay that involved genes, organism, and environment.

Citing Goldschmidt's work on sex determination in the gypsy moth, de Beer argued not only that "genes control the structure of the body" (as Morgan had it) but also that they "produce their effects by working at a definite speed."[57] From this genetically grounded conception of embryogenesis as a temporally complex unfolding of different developmental processes, it is but a small step to de Beer's elegant post-Haeckelian coordination of heredity, embryology, and evolution. A change in the developmental speed of characters caused by a genetic mutation would have a profound impact on the structure of the (adult) organism. It could be that while some characters are left untouched by the mutation, thus arriving at maturity in normative time, the development of others is delayed, so that they maintain their developmental stage long after the overall organism has reached maturity. Where such "heterochronic" changes—changes in the temporal orders of the embryo—are of adaptive advantage, the result will be the emergence of new features, possibly of a new species.[58]

For de Beer, heterochronic changes could come in two forms.[59] Gerontomorphic changes—early maturation due to acceleration of developmental speed—decrease what de Beer calls "evolutionary plasticity," that is, the capacity of a species to develop further. Paedomorphic changes—introduction of youthful characters in the adult by retarding the speed of some development processes—increase evolutionary plasticity.[60] Although he assumed that an organism can undergo both gerontomorphic and paedomorphic changes at the same time, he thought one of the two to be generally dominant.[61]

"The most effective mode of paedomorphosis" was for de Beer what he refers to as neoteny—a term he used to refer to heterochronic changes in which sexual maturity has been reached in normative time while other characters of the organism, due to a retardation of developmental speed, are still in a larval or embryonic state.[62] For de Beer, this retardation results in an increase of what he calls—plasticity. For this increase, as he explains, implies that developmental processes are still going on in the adult, that the organism is still plastic, open to future change, and not yet fully differentiated.

Among the examples de Beer gave for neotenic evolutionary change, he presented one as exemplary for a high degree of "plasticity": humans. Drawing on observations first presented by the Dutch biologist Louis Bolk, de Beer explains that "the adult structure of man shows resemblance to those of the embryonic structure of the anthropoid apes."[63] De Beer presents several indications for this "foetalization" of humans (e.g., teeth, hair, fingers), but regards one as central, the human brain. While in apes the sutures of the bones of the skull close around the age of four, in humans they do not close until the age of thirty. As de Beer points out, this example of relative retardation not only is a precondition for the development of the comparatively high brain weight of humans, but also indicates that brain development continues for a very long time after birth. And the closure of the sutures does not necessarily imply the end of developmental processes in the central organ. It could be, de Beer speculates, that "the more or less embryonic condition of the tissues at the young stages can be preserved into the later stages" and that, therefore, "these tissues will still be capable of undergoing a considerable degree of further alteration."[64] If such a "histogenic plasticity" were to exist, it could be that some organs—such as the brain—maintain a lifelong developmental status and thus a lifelong cellular plasticity.

It was important to De Beer to make explicit the implicit biological anthropology that his work on neoteny had given rise to:

> It is worth noting that man, whose phylogeny we have seen to be characterized by paedomorphosis, largely owes his success to the fact that he is not adapted to any particularly restricted mode of life at all. Instead, he is fitted for all sorts of habits, climates, and circumstances. Man himself is generalized, not specialized, and his body has retained a large number of primitive features which other mammals have lost. [. . .] Man is neotenous.[65]

In a word, man is plastic.

How does Alain relate his research to de Beer's? How, and along which lines of flight, does he carry his homeoproteins and their n-a-t into the conceptual horizon of de Beer's work?

The centerpiece of de Beer's conception of embryogenesis, which is also the centerpiece of his theory of heterochrony, is Goldschmidt's conception of rate genes. Rate genes, as we have seen, code for chemical substances whose interaction orchestrates in a temporally complex way the development of an organism and whose mutation is a key for understanding evolutionary change. To the extent that Alain, as in his encounter with Goldschmidt, associates rate genes with homeotic genes, he locates his work at the center of de Beer's and makes it possible to think of homeoproteins and their n-a-t in terms of heterochrony in general and of neoteny in particular.

As far as heterochrony is concerned, the apparent consequence, as in the cases of Goldschmidt and Thompson, is that homeoproteins, understood as active plastic or developmental forces, appear as essential for understanding matters of evolution. As far as neoteny is concerned, however, de Beer's work offers something that neither Thompson nor Goldschmidt nor any other of the previously mentioned authors could provide: a broadly accepted biological narrative that makes plausible why homeoproteins are expressed and diffused in the adult human brain—namely, as a result of a neotenous increase of cerebral plasticity due to mutations of homeotic genes. Perhaps even more significant, it offers an anthropological horizon. For if the evolution of man is due to the neotenous emergence of a fundamental, lifelong plasticity, especially of the brain, and if this plasticity is due to the continued expression of rate genes, aka homeotic genes, then Alain's work on homeoproteins and their n-a-t as an exemplary locus of adult cerebral plasticity has a fundamentally anthropological dimension to it. Indeed, it appears, on an associative scale, as the constitutive element of the human.[66]

WHERE BEFORE THERE WAS NONE

There are two things Thompson, Goldschmidt, and de Beer have in common with Bernard, Spemann, Waddington, and Turing. First, they all assume that central to living processes are plastic (vital) forces that actively build (form) the continuously growing and dying matter of the organism. It is this basic assumption that allows Alain to bring these authors together and to treat them as if they were in a steady conversation, even though they were not.[67] It allows him at one and the same time to inscribe the diffusion of homeoproteins onto theories of evolution, anthropology, and embryology—and to inscribe evolution, anthropology, and embryology onto homeoproteins and the brain.

Second, and perhaps more surprising, neither Bernard nor Goldschmidt, neither Waddington nor Thompson, Turing, Spemann, or de Beer was actually a neuronal researcher. None of the authors, whose works Alain has plundered in order to allow for the possibility of a yet unknown brain actually studied the neuronal organization of the central nervous system.

Can one see here the power of nocturnal work?

"To work with ideas," Alain once told me, "means *se jeté à travers champs.*" In English *se jeté* means "to dare"; *travers champs* means "cross-field." In Alain's rendering, *se jeté à travers champs* means, perhaps, to dare leaving one's own field of study. It means leaving behind one's own little house of truth, and blissfully (perhaps at times also painfully) exposing oneself to other fields, other houses of truth, in order to collect the curiosities one finds. It means, in my philosophical rendering, to dare to know—if knowing means that the growth of knowledge occurs through movement, ceaseless movement.

That authors who have never actually studied the brain can emerge as key to understanding the brain—and that the process of this emergence upends the established order of neuronal knowledge—is perhaps the most powerful way to document how nocturnal work has generated a new possibility for thinking.

Looking back, Alain's nocturnal work was spectacularly effective. In 1989, the internalization of homeoproteins into mature neurons and the subsequent morphogenetic differentiation were considered impossible. It was mere noise, at best an artifact.

A plastic brain? Not *dans le vrais.*

In 2002–2003, at the time of my research, Alain and colleagues had firmly established the possibility that the diffusion of homeoproteins has a physiological function, that it potentially keeps the brain plastic throughout life. Perhaps this breaking open would not have been appreciated, or appreciated in different ways, without the discovery of adult neurogenesis. Yet the opening had been accomplished independently of it due to two and a half decades of nocturnal work.

In 2006, the possibility that this silent embryogenesis is triggered by the nonautonomous transfer of homeoproteins was well enough established for Alain to be elected professor—like Claude Bernard before him—at the Collège de France. And in 2013, a review of Alain's laboratory comfortably spoke of the "shaking of a dogma" and listed the unexpected insights and therapeutic opportunities the work of Alain and colleagues has allowed for.[68]

A bit more than twenty years of nocturnal work with ideas set in motion the century-long conceptualization of the mature nervous system as a fixed and immutable structure. Alain and colleagues have effectively mutated the possible.

QUESTIONS

Why do we have no accounts of nocturnal work on the possible?[69] Why do we have so many studies of experiments—of their social grounds, of their cultural indebtedness, of the unforeseen ways in which technical play generates new knowledge—but hardly any accounts of how scientists work with ideas (as distinguished from experiments) to mutate the possible?

How do scientists get, or get in touch with, ideas? Do they engage with ideas individually or as a collective? How do they deal with the fact that ideas have a life of their own, that they come when it pleases *them,* not the scientists? Do other scientists have a method, or methods, comparable to Alain's?

How do scientists rework the possible? How do they launch new, hitherto nonexisting possibilities? How do they stabilize them? How do they confront the as-of-now impossible?

What different understanding of science (as practice) would an exploration of these questions give rise to? What space of marvel and surprise would it break open? What unexpected insights and possibilities of thought would it generate?

Could one say (excuse the nocturnal provocation) that the many studies of experiments we have document a form of complicity with the scientifically correct?

Vital Concepts

"What does your informant, Alain, owe to the French tradition of historical epistemology?"

I was grateful for the question, posed after I had presented a much earlier version of chapter 4 as a talk. For quite a while I had been wondering about the relevance of Bachelard and Canguilhem for Alain. Wasn't he practicing a kind of epistemology?

I replied that Alain was, in the early 1970s, a student of George Canguilhem. He had taken classes with him and was well aware of his work.

"Couldn't one claim, then," the listener went on, "that what Alain is doing is epistemology? I don't see a difference between what you call nocturnal work and concept work?"

There was the sound of critique in her question. Why do you speak (a bit too pompously) of nocturnal work? Why not just call it the invention of concepts?

"Well," I replied, "I see a difference."

I had been thinking about the relevance of Canguilhem for Alain ever since he told me that he had taken classes with him. Like my attentive listener, I was at first intrigued by the apparent parallels. Wasn't Alain trying to invent a conceptual rupture? Gradually, though, and especially once I learned about nocturnal work, the differences that set the two apart became more interesting for me.

"You are certainly right that there are parallels," I began my response, "though I came to think that the importance of what Alain, not me, calls nocturnal work is precisely that it escapes the work of the epistemologists. I am interested in the alternative space of thought that these escapes seem to indicate."

I listed three lines of escape. The first may appear minimal, but it is just the beginning: epistemology is not usually practiced by scientists or researchers, but rather by philosophically inclined scholars, mostly historians and sociologists. Alain does not fit this picture: he is neither a historian nor a sociologist but a practicing scientist.

The second line of escape makes the relevance of the first more apparent. Most of the epistemological works I am aware of are reconstitutions of the discontinuous histories of concepts. They are after the fact. Alain's nocturnal work, however, was not after the fact. Rather, it was before the fact: he was trying to open a not yet existing conceptual horizon.

The third line follows from the first two. Epistemology as practiced by Bachelard and Canguilhem was in orientation fairly diurnal. One could plausibly argue that this was due to the retrospective quality of their work. Because they worked on things past, Bachelard and Canguilhem could comfortably measure, like technicians on a drafting board, the mutations of spaces of possibility. Alain, however, working amidst uncertainty, couldn't enjoy the comfort of the retrospective gaze.

Provocatively put, Canguilhem and Bachelard were not exactly intellectually creative (or if they were, only in a secondary sense). They merely mapped the already thought (I am aware that this is unfair—but I try to make visible a difference here). Alain, in sharp contrast, faced the challenge of thinking the yet unthought. Whereas they could rely on the ruler of logic to map conceptual ruptures that had taken place long ago, Alain had to find a method for mutating contingency into surprise. There a clean post-fact measurement of the succession of spaces of possibility; here the messy, uncertain challenge of opening up new, yet unknown spaces of possibility.

I don't know whether my listener was happy with my answer—once I had presented her my list, she left and we never met again. Her question, though, kept returning to me. Had I gotten the difference between Canguilhem and Alain right?

At one point, while immersed in reading Canguilhem, I came to think that my response (1) was unfair to Canguilhem and (2) was missing the perhaps most intriguing aspect of the difference between epistemological and nocturnal work.

In an article he first published in 1976, roughly the time when Alain attended his seminars, Canguilhem noted:

> En raison des spécialités scientifiques—physique mathématique et chimie des synthèses calculées—sur le champ desquelles a été initialement élaborée, la méthode historique de récurrence épistémologique ne saurait être tenue pour un passe-partout. Sans doute, d'une spécialité bien travaillée, bien 'pratiquée,' dans l'intelligence des actes générateurs, on peut abstraire des règles de production de connaissances, règles susceptible d'extrapolation prudent. En ce sens la méthode peut être élargie plutôt que généralisée. Mais elle ne saurait être étendue à d'autres objets de l'histoire des sciences sans une ascèse préparatoire à la délimitation de son nouveau champ d'application. Par exemple, avant d'importer dans l'histoire de l'histoire naturelle au XVIIIe siècle les normes et procédures du nouvel esprit scientifique, il conviendrait de se demander à partir de quelle date on peut repérer dans les sciences des êtres vivants quelque fracture conceptuelle de même effet révolutionnaire que la physique relativiste ou la mécanique quantique.[1]

Do different disciplines require different epistemologies? Precisely insofar as they are concerned with different objects, which generate different modes of knowledge production, which give rise to different forms of knowledge? Was the epistemology of Bachelard—that is, the epistemology of the *nouvelle esprit scientifique,* which he arrived at by working on physics and chemistry— applicable to biology? Or was biology, the science of the living, in need of a different kind of epistemology? This is the question Canguilhem was concerned with when he wrote the above passage: what form of epistemology is appropriate to biology?

Canguilhem's answer amounts to a powerful departure from Bachelard. While Canguilhem agrees with his teacher's basic premise—research is about the formation of concepts—he argues that the generation and growth of knowledge in biology requires an epistemology altogether different from Bachelard's.

Bachelard's architectural logic of "ruptures" and "fissures" (the French term is *déchirures*), Canguilhem observes, does not apply to biology, precisely insofar as it is the science of living forms in motion. Not that there were no discontinuities in biology—though these discontinuities were of an altogether different kind. What was needed, therefore, was a different, biology-specific concept of discontinuity. And here Canguilhem turns to his friend, murdered by the Nazis, Jean Cavaillès: "Ce terme de 'fracture'—rapprocher de ceux de rupture ou de déchirure propres à G. Bachelard—est emprunté à Jean Cavaillès: '[. . .] ces fractures d'indépendance successive qui chaque fois détachent sur l'antérieure le profil impérieux de ce qui vient âpres nécessairement et pour dépasser.'"[2]

The formulation echoes one that Canguilhem had written more than twenty years earlier (in 1955): "On peut admettre que la vie déconcerte la logique sans croire pour autant qu'on se tirera mieux avec elle en renonçant à former des concepts, pour rechercher quelque clef égarée."[3]

At the time, these lines were written as a self-defense. Canguilhem felt obliged to make clear that even though he was adamant that biology, science of the living, would never arrive at a stable concept, he was in no way suggesting that one should give up forming concepts.

Twenty years later, Canguilhem was still convinced that research was about the formation of concepts. Likewise he was still convinced that biology would eventually outgrow every concept, would set it in motion, would require new ones. But now he seemed to have found a concept adequate to the growth of knowledge biology allowed for: fracture.

Whereas Bachelard's notion of rupture implied a complete breaking away, the almost independent formation of a new form of knowledge, the fracture concept, as used by Cavaillès, allowed for a different kind of rupture.

Wasn't life about successive fractures of independence, independences— or singularities—that each time they occurred were detaching themselves from the previous fracture, thereby constituting an incommensurability while, at the same time, grounding itself in it?

Canguilhem was struggling with how to reconcile his concept work as epistemologist with the object of biology, with the form of knowledge growth it gave rise to. Fracture was his answer. It follows that Canguilhem was not, as I had assumed in my response to my listener, a mere epistemologist, bureaucratically noting conceptual ruptures as an end in itself. Rather, he was a biological epistemologist of biology—interested in reconciling *le concept* and *le vivant.*

The effect of my new, biological understanding of Canguilhem's epistemology was that it opened up a whole new way of thinking about nocturnal work. It suddenly seemed to me that nocturnal work was Alain's way of struggling with Canguilhem's predicament, that is, with the incommensurability between the concept and the living. Until that point, I had understood nocturnal work in almost technical terms—as a method to mutate the possible. Now the possibility opened up that it was also a kind of concept work.

But was it? What kind of concepts did it give rise to? Here an additional difference between epistemological and nocturnal work arose—a fourth line of escape.

Concept work, from an epistemological perspective—here Canguilhem followed Bachelard—is the rigorous and rational attempt to capture either the logic of a particular way of knowing (if done by an epistemologist) or the logic of an aspect of a particular physiological process (if done by a biologist). In both instances a concept is an instance of logic. Canguilhem held on to this diurnal, constructivist notion of concepts. He was looking for a way to reconcile his epistemology of biology with the living—but he did not reconcile biology and the living. There was, for him, no way for biology to escape the incommensurability of the rigid and rational structural logic of concepts and the partial irrationality of the living. That is precisely what his fracture concept acknowledges.

Concept work, from a nocturnal perspective, had to be an altogether different undertaking. Alain has repeatedly argued in conversations, publications, and lectures that conceptualizations of living phenomena as machines are inadequate.

"They are inadequate," he insisted, "because they are not capable of capturing or coming to terms with life itself, understood"—from his Bernardian (his Bergsonian) perspective—"as ceaseless motion, as intrinsically open, plastic, irreducible to any kind of formula or structure."

Concepts, insofar as they are structured in a definite way, as if the interconnection of ideas resembles a construction plan, are not capable of thinking living phenomena because they mimic a mechanical rationality, which is foreign to *le vivant.*

The challenge was to come up with concepts that would be adequate to the living—concepts that would be as moving, adapting, mutating, surprising as life.

Didn't nocturnal work give rise to precisely such "vital concepts?"

If epistemological concepts are constructs that mimic the construction plan of the phenomenon under investigation, vital concepts are not constructs. For neither is there a *constructeur* nor a construction plan. Instead, they are the result of nocturnal work—the result of the effort to grant ideas a life of their own; to let them interact and generate unexpected offspring; to allow them to grow in unexpected directions, to let them outgrow the established. Vital concepts are a continuously mutating assemblage of ideas. As such, they disclose conceptual horizons that are as open, plastic, moving, growing, mutating as the phenomena they refer to.

Was nocturnal work a method for thinking the living in a way adequate to the living? Was plasticity, as triggered by the nonautonomous transfer of homeoproteins, precisely such a vital concept—a concept, like the plastic brain itself, always new?

Canguilhem—Alain.

Two almost mutually exclusive ways of acknowledging the challenges the living poses for research. For the epistemologist, insofar as he was holding on to a diurnal understanding of concepts, fractures offered the only possibility of acknowledging the concept-defying quality of the living.

Nocturnal work, in contrast, offered an altogether different possibility for reconciling concept work and the living: it generated concepts that were as nonlinear, as unwieldy, as life, as the living.

FIVE

Experimental

The experimenter must be realist.

IAN HACKING

In the Rue d'Ulm, I was a curiosity.

To the scientists, the presence of an anthropologist in their laboratory had something unusual, something enchanting about it. Especially during my first months in Alain's lab, an irresistible attraction seemed to radiate from me. At one point or another most of the scientists felt compelled to give way to their curiosity and to get in touch with me. They wanted to know me, who I was, why I had chosen to work in their lab, what I was hoping to find.

And they wanted me to know them.[1]

Much to my surprise, this aura of the unusual never fully left me. Even after I had been around for several months, had personal relationships with many of the researchers, and had become a familiar part of everyday lab life, they continued to identify me, in addition to the colleague or friend I had become, as the uncommon—an anthropologist in their lab.

Among all the people in Alain's unit, only one seemed indifferent to my presence: Maria-Luz Montesinos, a Spanish postdoc in her early thirties. At first I paid little attention to Maria-Luz's disinterest. After all, why would she care about an anthropologist? The longer I stayed, though, the more her indifference contrasted with the excitement of her colleagues and the more my curiosity was aroused. Was she even aware that an anthropologist had arrived?

Finally, in mid-January 2003, I gave in to my curiosity and approached Alain. Who was Maria-Luz Montesinos? What was she like? Why did she never try to get in touch with me?

"Have you observed her at work?" he asked.

I had not.

"You should. Maria-Luz is perhaps the best experimenter I've ever had in my lab."

"And one can 'see' that?" I joked.

"I don't know if you can see it," he replied dryly. "I can. And I think that by now you should be able to see it too."

And so I began to silently observe Maria-Luz. At first I merely followed her from a distance, though soon I began to arrange my daily work in such a way that we were, at least for a little while, at the same bench or in the same culture room.

Alain was right. There was something unusual, something enchanting, in watching her at work. Her attention was, or so it seemed from the outside, completely captured by her experiments. Something in her technical setups absorbed her, occupying her to a degree that I found curious.

After a week or so of observation, I decided to ask Maria-Luz if she would mind explaining her research to me in an interview. I wanted to find out more about how she related to her work, how she thought about it, why she was so absorbed by it. She agreed, and a week later we sat down and she started to explain.

Maria-Luz was working on Engrailed, a protein responsible, in interplay with a protein from the Wnt1 family, for the formation of the midbrain-hindbrain boundary. Her task was to study the importance of Engrailed's nonautonomous transfer to the emergence of this boundary. Ultimately, she told me, she would produce transgenic mice that would help explain the in vivo function of the nonautonomous transfer for the cellular emergence of the brain.

One of the things that struck me during our conversation was the unusual care with which she explained to me, the nonexpert, the technologies she worked with. She was almost anxious that I would fully understand how—why—she used each tool; how, in which logical way, they built up to her experimental question. At one point, while trying to make me understand what experiments for her are like, she compared the work with the building of windows.

"If well constructed," she said, "experiments are like a kind of window." The way she used the word *window* was almost poetic to me. There was something in her intonation, something in the way she looked at me. In any case, I felt as if she was introducing me to her own personal poetry of experimental work.

One thinks about possible windows, imagines how they would have to be built, in which place. One has a question, one considers the available tools and materials, and then one starts to work. What one will see—if anything at all—depends on where and how and with what material the window is built. The view can be imagined but not anticipated.

I wondered if this "poetics of window making" was the key to her fascination with experimental work. Did she see herself as window maker? Was imagining possible windows what she liked most about her work? Was it the joy of seeing something that she was after, or the technical construction as such? And was window making the reason why she, in contrast to anyone else, had been left untouched by the uncommon, an anthropologist in the lab?

EXPERIMENTAL REALISM

Maria-Luz's poetics of window making provided me with an unexpected opening. At the time of our first conversation (January 23), I had worked at the bench for almost a year. When I arrived in March 2002, Alain had me learn the basics: how to cut off heads, crack or peel off skulls, cut through brains, search for and find different brain regions, and transform these regions into neuron cultures. Half a year and many neuron cultures later, in August 2002, Alain decided that I had mastered the basics well enough and enrolled me in an intensive in vivo class at the Institut Pasteur (the class marked the beginning of my one-year DEA in neuropharmacology). I then spent all of September at the IP, where I learned to experiment on the living brain and to trace, in post-mortem tissue analysis, the effect of these experiments (we focused mainly on the detection of proteins with the help of western blots, Confocal microscopy, and immunocytochemistry). In October 2002, after I had passed the final exam of my experimentation class, I was finally allowed to join the other researchers in Alain's lab in their daily work with homeoproteins. My task was to work with Gianfranco Fazzotta, an Italian postdoc, on the nonautonomous transfer of a homeoprotein called Pax6.[2]

"You will produce a peptide that will bind to Pax6 while it is outside neurons," Alain told me on my return from the IP. "It will neutralize Pax6 and thus stop its expansion. Once you have such an anti-Pax6, you go in vivo and you find out about the physiological function of the nonautonomous transfer."[3]

At first, I was enthusiastic about my daily experimental work with Gianfranco. I was fascinated by the discovery of what I came to call the "pure technicality" of bench work. Every single step involved machines, complicated apparatuses, and strictly followed protocols. Even conversations at the bench, in the hallway, or in lab meetings most often concerned technical matters and took the form of technical reasoning.

Could I uncover what I came to call the experimental, the technical grounds of plastic reason? What experimental technologies would be constitutive of the possibility of knowing the brain as plastic? What would be the material basis of plastic reason? As the lab was busy moving from in vitro to in vivo work, and as my experiments with Gianfranco were one of the key sites of this transition, I imagined that all I would have to do was to carefully map my daily labor at the bench.

Gradually, though, excitement gave way to genuine boredom. Week after week, Gianfranco and I repeated the same technical procedures. First, we had proteins expressed by hybridoma cells, then we checked their expression in western blots, and finally we found ourselves in the Confocal room in order to control whether our proteins transferred from COS cells to neurons and whether our anti-Pax6 had or had not blocked their transfer. Whenever things went wrong—and they often did—our task was to find what exactly had derailed our experiment and why. Once we thought we had an answer, we began anew, only to encounter another unexpected technical problem.

To me, as to Gianfranco, there was nothing particularly inspiring in repeating the exact same technological procedures day after day. Experimentation increasingly appeared to be dominated by technical protocols, a form of technical pedantism largely devoid of any intellectual creativity that would point beyond the merely technical. Wasn't this work on the living?

And then, amidst my growing despair, came Maria-Luz.

Watching her getting absorbed in her experiments, observing the care with which she attended to the technology, listening to her words—evocative words of almost poetic density—was an invitation, an unexpected one, to rethink my disappointment with the experimental, the technical. What captured her so intensely was a promise inherent in her window metaphor— the promise of what I came to call experimental realism.

"A good experiment," Maria-Luz almost confessed to me, "has the potential to open, as a window opens, onto something real, onto a piece of reality not yet seen."

Experimentation, according to her, was the exhilarating possibility of finding a passage through which one could enter an open space, a space no one yet knew of, the contours of which no one could even anticipate. It was the exhilarating prospect—equally aesthetic and intellectual—of being touched by, of being in touch with, a yet-to-be-discovered and thus "pure and pristine reality" (her words).

Thanks to Maria-Luz, I felt as if I was gradually beginning to understand—to get hold of—experimentation, after months of gradual loss of excitement.

Bench work was still all about technical work—about technical rigor, technical protocols, technical pedantism. But now this technical work seemed to point beyond the merely technical. Differently put, at stake in experimentation were no longer technologies as such but the technological venture into and actualization of "the real." The form this "venture into"—this "actualization of"—took was what Maria-Luz taught me to call "variation and repetition" (her words).

One begins with a first question, a question materially arranged in the form of an experimental setup. If the result is negative or if there is no answer, one has given the question the wrong form. The challenge then is to modify the variable one thinks is responsible for the "no" and to repeat the question. This procedure goes on—variation and repetition—until either one has to accept that the question was altogether futile or one receives a positive answer.

"And this answer," she was adamant, "can be, in fact often is, an utter surprise. Something you would never have thought of."

Once one has a positive answer, the challenge is to pose a second question, one that builds on the answer to the first, and then a third, which builds on the answer to the first and the second, and so on, until a series of questions and answers build up to a window that opens onto the phenomena one studies.

Maria-Luz brought back my excitement about experimentation. From the perspective of experimental realism as she outlined it, my bench work was no longer boring or repetitive. Instead I could now think of it as a subtle but exhilarating exchange with the real about the real.

And there was at least one other reason to be excited about experimental realism.

In popular literature (and as well in some scholarly studies of experimental research), one often encounters the assumption that the actual challenge of experimentation is to find the right, the only possible question—as if the real were organized in discrete answers waiting to be discovered. One could call this popular comprehension of research teleological insofar as it assumes an end point—a final, conclusive answer (the intrinsic properties of the thing to be known) that organizes, like a vanishing point, the search for truth. The search might be incremental or full of conceptual and technical ruptures; it might be discontinuous. Yet, once one arrives at the truth, it will be possible to set apart the errors of the past, to tell the history of truth production as the breakthrough to the only possible question.

From the perspective of experimental realism, this teleological conception of research is questionable, probably wrong, and most certainly boring.

It is questionable insofar as the experimental realist knows from experience that there is not just one question. There are always several questions, and more than one possible answer. To be clear, the response one gets depends on the phenomenon one studies; experimental knowledge is not arbitrary. However, the response also depends on the kind of question one is asking—on where and how the window is built. Different questions, different answers.

It is probably wrong because experimental realism can afford to withhold judgment. The challenge is not to come up with an alternative ontology—to explain how the real is organized—but to withdraw from ontological claims and to conduct research, not least for the purpose of opening up the closures the teleologists impose. To experimental realists, claims to having found the only possible question—or the only answer—are thus suspicious and untrustworthy. For how can one know that one has arrived at the endpoint?

And it is most certainly boring because the possibility that the real is neatly organized in discrete entities waiting to be known inscribes experimentation into the grid of the necessary; it takes away from it the possibility of creativity.[4]

It was in my conversations with Maria-Luz that it first dawned on me that what one could call the *perspectivism* that is constitutive of experimental realism—the recognition that the answer one gets depends on the question one poses—is precisely what is exciting about bench work. It is constitutive of the possibility of new discoveries; it is like an invitation to wonder if one could think differently from how one has learned to think; it is an irreducible opening that allows for—that demands—new ways of knowing.[5]

I was grateful to Maria-Luz—grateful that she never sought to get in touch with me. Had it not been for her disinterest in the uncommon—the anthropologist in the lab—I would perhaps never have returned to a project that my discovery of nocturnal work, coupled to the disillusion with bench work, had rendered less and less exciting: understanding the experimental—the technical—grounds of plastic reason.

And I would surely not have returned with so much enthusiasm.

HOW EXPERIMENTS BEGIN

Maria-Luz had taught me that in experimentation, thinking rules, but that thinking in experimentation is a material art.

"You have to learn to think in terms of the technologies you are using," she said. "If thoughts cannot be distilled in a concrete experimental setup—in the form of a question to the organism—they are not real."

Could I learn this material art? Or could I at least learn to recognize traces of thought in the experiments Gianfranco and I were conducting? In such a way that our experimental work would become comprehensible to me as an intellectually and aesthetically exhilarating conversation with the real about the real? As an attempt at window making?

I began asking Gianfranco about each and every technology we were working with. "Hold on, can you explain why we are doing this now? I don't understand. What is the background assumption? What has this to do with the previous work step?"

I hoped that persistent questioning would allow me to get a sense of the thoughts at stake in our technological work. And at first that seemed to work. Most of our conversations focused on western blots, proteins and protein structures, and molecular weights. Gianfranco patiently explained who had invented these technologies, when, in which laboratory, how, and to what ends. And I gradually began to gain a much better sense of what precisely was supposed to happen when we deployed a given tool. Hence, there was an opening.

After a while, though, I began to recognize that Gianfranco spoke about each technology in the abstract. What emerged from his replies were individual, freestanding technologies, each one with its singular history, each one with its distinctive analytical potential. What was absent was a sense of the thoughts—the design—that presumably organized the individual technologies of which Gianfranco spoke into the particular experimental setup we were working with.

What were these thoughts?

No matter how I posed the question, I did not succeed in deducing an answer from Gianfranco's replies. And so I began to harbor doubts again.

Perhaps I had overestimated the importance of thinking, Perhaps misunderstood Maria-Luz. Perhaps she was simply an exception, an outlier.

Construction Work

Things changed only when, late one evening in mid-February, I was working through scribbles from a conversation with Michel Volovitch. Going over my notes, I recognized that he had told me that before Gianfranco's arrival no one in the lab had worked on Pax6. During the day, Michel's remark had not triggered my interest. But now it gripped me.

Why had Alain and the other seniors chosen to work on a new protein? The only answer that I could think of was that the new protein had specific qualities that made it experimentally attractive—more attractive than one of the homeoproteins the lab had worked with previously (such as Antennapedia or Engrailed, the two proteins used to study internalization and secretion). What were these qualities?

While I was wondering about why Alain and Co. had chosen Pax6, it suddenly occurred to me that all of my conversations with Maria-Luz had focused exclusively on bench work. What we never talked about, not even once, was the work that presumedly precedes bench work, that is, the work of constructing experimental projects.

Construction work. The more I thought about it, the more I had the impression as if a whole new world was opening up, one that I wasn't familiar with from my readings in the history of science or in science and technology studies.

Wasn't construction work—the work of coming up with thoughtfully arranged technological questions—the key to the experimental in general? Why, then, do we have so much literature on "how experiments end," but almost none on how they begin, on how construction workers think experimental questions in technical terms, on how they endeavor to bring thought and technology together in such a way that new knowledge becomes possible?

Presumably Alain and some of the other seniors—Joliot, Michel, Brigitte, Trembleau—had regular construction work meetings? Presumably they discussed which kinds of proteins—or which animals, brain regions, technologies—would best allow them to formulate the experimental questions they wanted to ask. Could I gain access to these conversations?

A couple of days later (still mid-February) Alain, Michel, and I met in Alain's office. I was eager to tell them about my conversations with Maria-

Luz, about experimental realism, and about my discovery of construction work. Michel was the first to respond.

"Construction work. Hmm. I think I like the term. I like the idea of being a construction worker."

"I would qualify the term, though," Alain replied. "We construct, but it is not that we simply draw up construction plans and then our experimenters execute a plan. We're biologists, not engineers."

"Alain is right," Michel said. "There is a constant back-and-forth between the surprises of bench work and construction work."

"But if one takes that into account," Alain continued, "you've given a pretty accurate description of our work. It is just important to keep in mind that construction work is often just as messy as bench work. We construct a problem and then follow the experiments, which most often produce some unexpected result. And then our job is to rework this unexpected result into an experimental or biological curiosity that has the potential to move us forward."

"One could even say," Michel added, "that the derailment of our initial constructs—when they do not work and need to be altered—is actually the most exciting intellectual part of experimentation. At least for us."

"It is where knowledge emerges," Alain nodded.

The conversation with the two seniors left me thrilled. When I left Alain's office, I felt as if I had just discovered the intellectual substrate of experimentation, as if I had broken through to the central planning office responsible for conceptual-technical creativity.

If I were to understand the construction work—the thoughts—that gave rise to the Pax6 project, wouldn't that automatically allow me to understand the perspectivism—the thoughts—constitutive of our effort at window making? Wouldn't it allow me to understand our technical work in terms of experimental realism?

I began to work through my field notes and to systematically read through the dozens of papers about Pax6 I had collected over the previous months. Why Pax6? What had made the protein attractive? What kind of conceptual—and technical—considerations had led Alain and the other seniors to favor it over other, already familiar homeoproteins? In addition, I sought to engage the seniors involved in the Pax6 project—Alain, Michel, and Brigitte—in a conversation about why and how they had constructed the experiments Gianfranco and I were conducting. And, gradually, I learned to see traces of thought in the technologies we were working with.

One of the first things my efforts at reconstruction taught me was that I had not paid sufficient attention. I had always assumed that the fact that the lab had shown that the nonautonomous transfer occurs in vitro—and that it had documented the molecular mechanisms that allow for this transfer—implied that it also occurs in vivo. The question merely was, I thought, whether it is of actual physiological significance or not. However, I had moved from the Petri dish to the living animal too fast.[6]

I knew that most of the in vitro experiments conducted in the 1990s had not actually been done with homeoproteins, but with chemically synthesized chains of amino acids that mimicked homeoproteins (or parts thereof). Alain, Joliot, Michel, and Daniele first synthesized a homeoprotein without a homeodomain—the DNA binding part—and found that it does not transfer between cells. Then they began synthesizing, amino acid by amino acid, the three helices that make up the homeodomain (it has two short N-terminal helices and one longer C-terminal helix) until they had established, after ten years of labor, which part of the three helices are necessary for nuclear export, secretion, and internalization.

The result of the in vitro work was thus not—and this is what I had missed—knowledge of homeoproteins, but rather technical knowledge: the capacity to synthesize peptides capable of traveling from COS cells to neurons in a Petri dish. Whether there was anything in this technical knowledge that pointed toward actually occurring physiological processes was precisely the question.

"The mere observation that there are sequences in the homeodomain that are capable of secretion and internalization," Michel explained, "does not at all mean that secretion occurs in the living organism. They could just as well be inactive."

Going in vivo thus presented a huge conceptual challenge. Alain and co. had to find a way to link two different conceptual domains, the technical (synthetic peptides in Petri dishes) and the living (homeoproteins in living organisms). To be more precise, going in vivo amounted to the paradoxical challenge of aligning the living (the yet to be known) with the technical (the largely known).[7] Only if such an alignment were to be achieved could one actually begin an experimental—that is, a technical—conversation with the real about the real (with the living organism about the living organism).

Yet which way would lead from in vitro to in vivo knowledge?

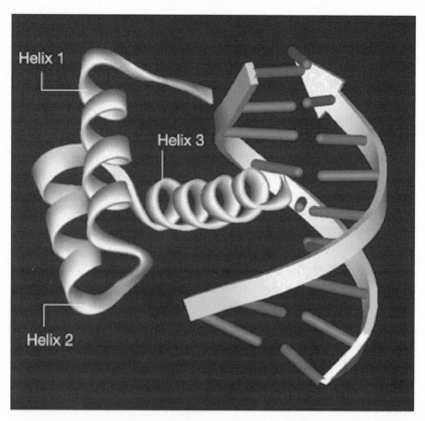

Through rebuilding the homeodomain sequence by sequence, the lab learned which element of the three helices is necessary for the nonautonomous transfer. Helix 3, which is equivalent to the DNA binding site of the homeodomain, is necessary for internalization. The sequence necessary for secretion is integrated in the longer sequence necessary for nuclear export. Both are largely part of the helix 2 but reach out into helix 3. Helix 1 is not relevant for the nonautonomous transfer. From Prochiantz and Joliot 2003.

Constructing Technical Answers in the Form of a Vital Question

In early 2000, Alain thought he had found an answer. Turing, in his 1952 paper "The Chemical Basis of Morphogenesis," had suggested thinking of morphogens as reciprocally inhibitive form producers that diffuse through embryological tissue and thereby build up chemical patterns that then trigger the mechanical formation of the embryo. Alain, in one of his nocturnal flights, had the idea of linking Turing's morphogen concept to one of the findings of the in vitro years: the observation that the actual distance the synthetic peptides they had invented travel in a Petri dish is minimal. They entered only cells in their immediate neighborhood.

Perhaps homeoproteins were, with Turing, diffusing morphogens?

Starting from this nocturnally produced possibility, Alain and co. articulated, in one of their planning meetings, a series of suggestive questions. Are homeoproteins critical for the formation of boundaries between different brain regions during embryogenesis? If so, could it then be that they, through their nonautonomous transfer, are responsible for the emergence of different cell types, each of which is eventually constitutive of a distinct brain region? Could it be that these nonautonomous agents both trigger the generation of new, yet undifferentiated, hence literally plastic cells, and tell these cells what kind of neuron to become, where to migrate, what form to assume, and how and in which direction to expand their axon and their dendrites? And could it be that each homeoprotein thus gradually builds up—or sculpts—a region of the brain until its expansion is inhibited by another homeoprotein, which has built a neighboring region, one made up of different cell types?

In short, are homeoproteins—aka plastic forces, organizers, inducers, evocators—diffusing morphogens? And doesn't the fact that homeoproteins are expressed in the adult brain suggest that the morphogenetic production and maintenance of the brain's cellular composition are a lifelong event?

If taken together, this series of questions amounted to a thoroughly worked-out embryogenetic conception of the brain grounded in the nonautonomous transfer of homeoproteins—one at every point consistent with the technical knowledge gained in the course of the in vitro years.

Call it plastic reason. Call it an in vivo question formulated in in vitro terms.

In Vitro Tool, in Vivo Potential

Constructing the morphogen question in the form of a concrete experimental setup proved difficult. The classical way to test the role of a protein is to produce a knockout mouse, in which the gene that codes for the protein of interest is deleted. Such a deletion can be permanent or temporary. In both cases, the resulting dysfunctions allow one to make claims about the function of the absent protein. But for understanding the nonautonomous transfer of homeoproteins, the knockout technique did not work. Knocking out a homeobox gene would delete the nonautonomous function—but also the cell autonomous function, which most biologists assumed was sufficient for understanding the role of homeoproteins. And even the deletion of the sequence necessary for the secretion or internalization would be futile, as these sequences are found in the homeodomain, that is, the DNA-binding part of the protein. Again, one would not be able to determine whether the observed deformation was the result of the protein's nonautonomous or the autonomous action.

How to produce a cell-autonomous-only mouse—a mouse in which the capacity of homeoproteins to transfer between cells would be turned off while their potential regular cell-autonomous function would be preserved?

"If you work on a problem that falls outside mainstream biology," Michel summarized the lab's predicament in one of our conversations about construction work, "you cannot really rely on the tools mainstream biology provides you with. We had to come up with a new, with our own, technology."

Their "new" technology was made possible by their "old" in vitro work. As they knew which amino acid sequence of helix 3 is necessary for internalization, they came up with the idea of constructing a peptide (a chain of amino acids) that could bind to this sequence while the homeoprotein is outside of cells, neutralize it, and thereby prevent it from entering a neighboring neuron. (This was in fall 2000.)

What Alain called the "beauty" of these minipeptides was twofold. First, they allowed the transfer to be blocked while leaving the cell-autonomous function of the protein untouched. If a change in boundary formation between different brain regions were to occur in the embryo, or in the adult, the lab would not only have established that homeoproteins are plastic forces and that their nonautonomous transfer is a critical plastic event. It would also have established that the brain is plastic, and best thought of in terms of a continuous, silent embryogenesis.

Second, the minipeptides could themselves be used as plastic tools. One could, for example, produce peptides that would merely mutate the sequence necessary for secretion, so that the protein could still be internalized. Or one could produce a peptide that would allow a given homeoprotein to leave but not to enter cells. And one could use both peptides in a single experiment, first turning the transfer off and later recovering it. One could gradually learn to use the plastic forces that organize the brain to sculpt—to resculpt—the nervous tissue.

The minipeptide was an in vitro tool with in vivo potential.

The next step was to find a homeoprotein that would allow the lab to pose the morphogen question experimentally. Alain told me that he and the other seniors had discussed a long list of possible candidates in the course of their regular Saturday-morning construction meetings. What they were looking for were homeoproteins involved in the cellular formation—in interplay with ideally only one other homeoprotein—of distinct brain regions.[8]

After several months of discussion and many preliminary experiments, the Saturday-morning collective eventually chose to focus on Engrailed and Pax6. Engrailed was attractive for several reasons. The lab was already familiar with it (they had used it as a model for understanding secretion); it had a prominent role in the formation of the midbrain-hindbrain frontier (made up of serotonergic and noradrenergic neurons); and it was known to be critical for the survival (and perhaps renewal) of dopaminergic neurons in the adult substantia nigra (the death of dopaminergic neurons in that region causes Parkinson's disease). Perhaps the importance of Engrailed for the substantia nigra lay in the nonautonomous transfer?

"And Pax6," I asked Alain? "Why did you opt for a new protein?"

He replied that there were at least three good reasons. First, Pax6 is critical to the formation of boundaries between the three different areas that make up the embryonic nervous system: the forebrain, the midbrain, and the hindbrain (it had been called a master control gene of embryogenesis).[9] In addition, it is critical to the boundary between the retina (controlled by Pax6) and the astrocytes and oligodendrocytes of the optic nerve (Pax2).[10] Second, the protein that seemed to inhibit the expansion of Pax6 was Engrailed. And third, Pax6 was active not just in the embryo but also in the adult. Around the year 2000 a German researcher named Magdalena Götz (who visited Alain's lab while Gianfranco and I were conducting our experiments) had reported that the presence of Pax6 is critical for the maintenance of adult cerebral tissue in the olfactory bulb and the hippocampus, that is, in the two major sites of neurogenesis in the adult brain.[11]

"Are you suggesting that Pax6 nonautonomous transfer is regulating adult neurogenesis?" I asked Alain.

"You are moving too fast. But let's say that there is a chance that one could one day use the minipeptide you and Gianfranco are working toward to explore this," he smiled.

Eventually, Alain and the Saturday-morning collective worked out two Pax6 experiments, both of which were focused on the embryonic formation of the brain. (The plan was to first establish the new conception of embryogenesis and to then show that it is relevant for understanding the adult.) The first experiment was Brigitte's. Her task was to study the interaction of Pax6 and Engrailed in the formation of the diencephalon-mesencephalon boundary by way of constructing an anti-Engrailed minipeptide. The second, focused on the formation of the eyecup and the stalk, was Gianfranco's (and mine) and concerned not only Pax6 but also Pax2.

Pax2 has a paired DNA binding domain but no homeodomain. In contrast to Pax6, it lacks helices 2 and 3—the helices necessary for homeoprotein export and import. Our task was to add the sequence necessary for internalization and secretion to Pax2, to knock it into a mouse, and to then examine the cup-stalk border. It was expected that the domain of Pax6 expression would be reduced and that the stalk would take over part of the optic cup.[12] In addition, the plan was to develop an anti-Pax6 peptide that would block the passage outside the cell by binding to the protein. As the size of the eyecup is linked to the amount of cells that express Pax6, one would expect, that a blockage of Pax6 decreases the number of cells that synthesize Pax6 and thus the number of cells in the eyecup, and hence reduces the size of the eyecup. In addition, one might assume that the stalk-cup border would be malformed and that the stalk would take over parts of the eyecup.

Logic of Plasticity

As a consequence of my emerging understanding of the construction logic of the Pax6 experiment, the technologies that Gianfranco and I worked with began to gain intellectual contours. Thought and technology began to come together. It was especially the work with Alain that was responsible for this new comprehension.

He had replied to my many questions almost exclusively in passing—between door and hallway, while waiting at the printer, over a brief coffee, in the elevator. And yet his scattered comments added up and provided guidance.

Four tentative conclusions framed my nascent understanding of the logic of experimentation. First, the aim of experimentation is the production of unprecedented knowledge. As the new might, conceptually speaking, escape the already known, a major challenge of experimentation is to not constrain the possibility of new knowledge. The way to achieve this is to make derailment—and the reinterpretation of the noise derailment gives rise to—a key methodological element of experimental knowledge production.

Second, experimentation unfolds along two related, though different, scales. On the one hand, there is construction work, the task of which is to create the *possibility* of unprecedented knowledge. The challenge is to abstract from the available technologies possibilities of constituting the organism or organ in technical terms, of using the logic inscribed in the tool available to think the logic of the living so that, in the abstract, an experimental engagement of the organ(ism) in a technical conversation becomes possible. On the other hand, there is bench work, the task of which is to *produce* unprecedented knowledge by involving the living (the real) in a technical (and surprising) conversation about the living (the real). The challenge Gianfranco and I faced was thus to use the fragments of thought Alain and co. had tentatively provided us and to begin exploring their actual productivity.

Third, there was an emergent sense that the outcomes of experimentation, at least in biology, are *vital technologies*. Vital technologies, because knowledge about living organisms is contingent on and captured by technologies. It is as if knowledge of living organisms is ultimately a technically actualized possibility of knowledge. I found this most curious, for it seemed to imply that experiments do not actually discover. Rather, they pose a question—open up a possibility—and then (if successful) actualize it.

And fourth and perhaps most important, I could now see the perspectivism constitutive of our work. The minipeptide we struggled to produce (in itself a way of engaging the living technically) was designed to allow for the possibility of engaging the brain in a conversation about whether or not unexpected embryogenetic processes—the nonautonomous transfer of homeoproteins—render it plastic. If Gianfranco and I were to succeed in blocking the transfer, and if there were a transformation of the boundary between stalk and eyecup (Pax6 and Pax2), or between diencephalon and mesencephalon (Pax6 and Engrailed), homeoproteins would come into view as diffusing morphogens. And our vital technology would have opened, and actualized, the possibility that the brain is plastic.

I was eager to return to the bench. Now that I understood the technologies that Gianfranco and I used as fragments of thought that coded for the possibility that diffusing plastic forces sculpt the brain, could I make sense of our day-to-day endeavor in terms of experimental realism?

At least as curious was I about something else: experimental knowledge. In the aftermath of my recognition that experiments do not so much *discover* as *actualize* the possibility of knowing that they themselves open up, I began to wonder what experimental knowledge actually is. If experiments do not discover, then what is actually experimentally known? And what, strictly speaking, does experimental knowledge consist of?

There was only one problem. Just when I learned to articulate these questions—just at the time experimentation was opening up—my time at the bench with Gianfranco ended. One of the requirements of my DEA in neuropharmacology was that students join another lab from mid-February 2003 to mid-April 2003 (I was working with Joliot's group). Where was I to go from here?

I returned to my notebooks. During my months with Gianfranco I had assembled a large, convoluted set of scribbles—observations, ideas, marginalia, technical descriptions, reading impressions, relational troubles. Most of them revolved around how my interlocutors spoke about experimental "variables." Before I knew about experimental realism—about construction work—the importance my lab mates seemed to assign to "variables" had seemed to me as a possibly useful tool for understanding experimentation.

Would the field notes in which I documented their talk and my own reflections about variables allow me to understand how, on the level of thought and technology, Gianfranco and I actualized the possibility of knowledge Alain and the other seniors had constructed around Pax6? Even though I had written these notes before I knew about experimental realism? And would they speak to my nascent curiosity about experimental knowledge?

What follows is a reconstruction, from my scribbles, of the five scenes that initially triggered my curiosity about variables and that framed my comprehension of experimentation at a time when I had not yet discovered experimental realism.

During the first two weeks I spent with Gianfranco, he was still busy coming to terms with the neurobiology of homeoprotein transfer. He often made jokes about the work and described himself as a "convert."

"Before I arrived, I strongly doubted that such a transfer occurs," he grinned. "And now I am firmly convinced."

Perhaps to erase the last doubt, Gianfranco decided to conduct some preliminary experiments. He wanted to see for himself if Pax6 could really travel between cells and cause an intense morphogenetic outgrowth, even in already mature neurons. Hence, we transfected COS cells—modified monkey cells that express extraordinarily high amounts of the protein with which they're infected—with Pax6 DNA, and then cocultured them with neurons in order to see if Pax6 proteins would transfer from the former to the latter. When they did, Gianfranco was genuinely surprised. He repeated the experiment several times. The result was always the same.

"This is really amazing," he told me. "I would never have thought that this is possible. Cells are usually autonomous, you know."

Then, in late October, we began to work on the anti-Pax6 that Brigitte had constructed before Gianfranco had arrived. (Alain had asked her to begin working on the Pax6 project and then to help Gianfranco to carry it further). From that point on, our daily work almost always followed the same pattern: We ran western blots to test our anti-Pax6.

A western blot is a method for detecting proteins by mass (according to their molecular weight, measured in daltons). The procedure went as follows: Every day Gianfranco and I made a (polyacrylamide) gel with several contiguous "wells," or vertical columns. In each of these wells we injected different, chemically treated proteins. On top of each well we added color (ink). The first well is usually reserved for a marker, a commercially available mixture of proteins having defined molecular weights (measured in kilodaltons). Next to the marker we usually injected first Pax6 soluble and then Pax6 insoluble fraction, which we had produced from the mesencephalon of embryonic mice (dissection and production of cell culture were done once a week). Finally, we had one well with a negative control, usually Engrailed. Once we had loaded the wells, we electrically charged the gel; and the proteins, because of their electrical charge, started migrating down their well-column—a process called electrophoresis. Because of the staining, the migration of the proteins leaves bands in the gel. How far a protein travels depends on its molecular weight. Heavy proteins travel less far than light ones. Once the electrophoresis was completed, we transferred the gel, by way of a transblotting machine, onto a paper membrane. Next, we treated the membrane with antibodies. In a first step we added a primary antibody to the membrane. This primary antibody was specific to the protein we were looking for, in our case, the anti-Pax6 peptide produced by Brigitte. After a certain amount of time (which could range from thirty minutes to twenty-four hours or more) we thoroughly washed the membrane to make sure that antibodies that did not bind to the anti-Pax6 were cleared away. Then we added a secondary antibody that is specific to the primary antibody and that is usually linked to a reporter enzyme, such as horseradish peroxidase. The reaction between primary and secondary antibody causes a luminescence reaction. In the final step of the western blot we placed a sensitive sheet of photographic film against the membrane, and the exposure to the light from the reaction created an image of the antibodies bound to the blot. The result is an image of bands in vertical columns. As we knew the dalton size of the protein we were looking for, we could compare its bands with the bands of the marker of the first well, and we could tell whether or not "our" protein is expressed—and whether the antibody did or did not recognize the protein.

If things had worked out as planned, our anti-Pax6 would have recognized Pax6 but not Engrailed. And, ideally, we would have gotten the same result no matter how often we conducted the experiment. This, however, was never the case. Either there was no reaction at all, or our antibody recognized both Pax6 and Engrailed. Why was entirely mysterious to us.

The blot we did on November 5 was particularly bewildering. The day started early (roughly 8 A.M.). We had recalculated for the nth time the structure and length of the antibody, centrifuged the bacterial cells that expressed it, used the supernatant (soluble fraction), and tested it as our primary antibody in a western blot. When, around 2 P.M., we exposed the membrane to a filmstrip, the result was devastating. We could see hardly anything. The blot was dirtier than ever before. When I asked Gianfranco why this was the case, he introduced a phrase that was to become our constant companion.

"We go and check the variables," he said. And after a brief pause he added, "And the best way to check variables is to ask an experienced experimenter."

Then he walked straight to our bench neighbor, Bernadette Allinquat, a woman in her fifties who worked with her own small group, within Alain's lab, on Alzheimer's disease. Bernadette listened, asked questions, and then indeed listed a number of "variables" we should check.

How did you produce the antibody? Are the cells old? How old? And the medium? When did you renew it? Is the primer used for anti-Pax6 bad? Where did you get it from? Is the Pax6 good? Did you test it beforehand? What second antibody did you use? How long did you wash the membrane? After she listened to Gianfranco's responses, she offered advice. Wash the membrane overnight, not just for a few hours. Also put it overnight in the cold room, at four degrees Celsius. This inhibits the growth of fungi. And use another, more clarifying secondary antibody.

We followed Bernadette's advice and started a new western blot. At 8 P.M. I put the membrane in the cold room where it would be washed overnight. When we arrived the next morning, we added a secondary antibody and then exposed the membrane to a photographic film. The picture we got was indeed much clearer. What we saw, however, was as discouraging as our previous results. Despite our recalculation of the antibody and despite having followed Bernadette's advice, the anti-Pax6 still reacted to both Pax6 and Engrailed.

Gianfranco was angry. I was curious. What's next, I asked? What does one do if one has checked the variables and the experiment still doesn't work? Annoyed, he explained that there are many more variables to be checked. Back at the desk he began to compare the structure of the third alpha-helix of Engrailed and Pax6.

"They coincide to 37 percent," he said, and then, realizing that this did not mean anything to me, added, "this is reasonably high."

"You mean this is the reason why anti-Pax6 reacts to Engrailed?" I asked.

"It could be."

"And now? What are we doing next?"

"Well, we repeat the whole thing again. You can go and start a gel. I'll take care of the protein."

"Do it again?" I asked. We had already done it again. What was the point of yet another repetition? What would we look for this time? When I asked Gianfranco, he replied that we have to talk to Alain and ask him "how to play around" with things.

"Play around?" I asked. "With what?"

"As I said, we talk to Alain. And then we change this and that variable, until we get an idea what the problem is. We'll have to repeat things often."

December 7: Epistemological Variables

Once or twice a week Alain visited us at the bench and asked how things were going. Usually he was extraordinarily supportive and gave advice. It sometimes happened, however, especially on Monday mornings, that he stopped by to ask Gianfranco why he hadn't been in the lab on the weekend. Angrily, he then explained that Gianfranco was not for leisure in Paris but for work.

Gianfranco and I found these predictable Monday-morning attacks amusing. After all, nobody in the lab, aside from a few grad students, worked on weekends, certainly not on Sundays. So when Alain approached us on a Monday morning in early December, we were prepared to listen to his standard complaints about Gianfranco's work ethic. Counter to what we expected, however, Alain was friendly, asked how things were, and then explained that he wanted Gianfranco to take part in a meeting with him, Trembleau, Michel, and Joliot. These are regular meetings, he explained, in the course of which we discuss current work. We would meet on Saturday morning at 10:30 in the lab meeting room. I could come as well.

When Gianfranco and I arrived on Saturday morning, not only the four seniors were present but also Brigitte and Laure Sonnier, a graduate student of Brigitte who worked on the n-a-t of Engrailed in mice. After some general chatting and coffee drinking, Alain began the meeting by briefly summarizing the work of Laure and Gianfranco and by raising questions about how the two projects should be continued. From that point onward, there was an open exchange of ideas, suggestions, and doubts.

I was struck by the asymmetry of the meeting. In his opening remarks, Alain addressed neither Laure nor Gianfranco nor me. And the ensuing conversation took place exclusively among the four senior males, with Brigitte making a brief comment every now and then. Without any explicit statement, it was clear to all that Gianfranco, Laure, and I were subordinates. Juniors were not meant to talk except when asked.

Their conversations evolved around what Michel described as "our three models, mouse, chick, and Homo sapiens," and about how one could work on one and draw conclusions about the others, based on the work with Engrailed and Pax6.

Could one transfer experimental results from mice to chickens or Homo sapiens? Are the peptides they develop applicable to all three models? Would they need different peptides?

For the most part, they spoke about Engrailed, which Volovitch frequently described as "*notre meilleure cheval*"—the best horse in the stable. Everybody agreed with him, and there was a consensus that Laure, who had developed an anti-Engrailed peptide, should soon conduct in vivo experiments on both mice and chicken. Gianfranco's Pax6 work was rarely mentioned.

While listening to Alain, Joliot, Michel, and Trembleau discuss the various possibilities, I found two things remarkable. The first was the sheer intensity of the meeting. In sharp contrast to the lab meetings, there was little laughter. The exchange was serious, at times even tense. The second was that their exchange, which was solely concerned with technical procedures and how they could be modified, took place in the conjunctive. It was a constant "but . . . if . . . and . . . consider instead . . . what about . . . but on the other hand . . . one could also say . . . have you thought about . . ."

Weren't they conducting a kind of epistemological work, I wondered?

Just when I had scribbled "epistemological work" in my notebook, I heard Trembleau say "If we take this variable into account, then. . . ." I was electrified. Wasn't Trembleau talking about epistemological variables? Was this the purpose of our meeting? A discussion of the epistemological grounds, and variables, of the experiments Laure, Gianfranco, Brigitte, and I were conducting in the lab?

Just as Gianfranco and I checked technical variables, I noted for myself, so the seniors check epistemological variables. Perhaps they had invited Gianfranco and Laure so that they could listen and learn about some of these epistemological variables?

December 9–11 (2002): Relational Variables

In mid-December Gianfranco and I were still trying to figure out why Brigitte's anti-Pax6 did not work. Alain had asked us to first make sure that neither our Pax6 nor our Engrailed or the secondary antibody we used was the problematic variable. Once these possibilities were excluded, he asked Gianfranco to go over Brigitte's notes, recalculate her construction of the anti-Pax6, and check the western blots to ensure the anti-Pax6 we had was indeed an anti-Pax6. In the course of this work Gianfranco discovered, by chance, the variable responsible for the fact that anti-Pax6 was not functioning properly.

We began December 9, a Monday, with the production of new anti-Pax6 peptides. We ran a PCR with Brigitte's primer and the cDNA she had produced, and then inserted the DNA sequence coding for the minipeptide into bacteria.[13] To access the peptide produced by the bacterial cells, we later transferred the cells from dish to test tube and centrifuged them. The centrifuge smashes the cell walls and separates pellet (insoluble fraction) from the supernatant (soluble fraction) in which the peptide should be found in high concentration.

For no apparent reason Gianfranco decided to run the blot not only with the supernatant but also with the pellet. And that made a difference. The blot showed that anti-Pax6 was expressed but not secreted: we found it in the pellet but not in the supernatant. Thus far, though, we had worked exclusively with the supernatant.

We got the results of the western blot late in the evening. Alain had already left, so we had to wait till the next morning to share the good news with him. He was overjoyed and immediately engaged Gianfranco in a discussion about why the protein was not secreted. Although nobody used the term, I thought that we were again checking variables.

They agreed that the problem was either that Brigitte had misconstructed the antibody or that the bacterial cells were old or otherwise bad. Alain suggested two procedures. First, we should calculate the exact weight that anti-Pax6 should have and then compare it with the weight we measured in the blot. He suspected that perhaps Brigitte had constructed the antibody a bit too short so that the leader peptide, which is critical for the secretion of the anti-Pax6 (2.420 daltons), was not part of the cDNA and hence the peptide stayed aggregated in the pellets.

I was amazed by the standardized references and the calculation procedure. Pax6 consists of 750 base pairs. Divided by three—the genetic sequence is made up of trinucleic units called codons, each coding for one amino acid—this makes 250 amino acids (aa). One aa has 110 daltons. The C-terminal of Pax6 has 87 base pairs, hence 27 aa, hence 30.470 daltons. If Alain were right—that is, if the leader peptide, which weighs 2.420 daltons, is not part of the cDNA—then the band we got on the western blot should have been below 30.000. The band we got, however, was at 35.000 daltons. The peptide was not smaller, as Alain had speculated, but larger. Why?

Alain's second suggestion was that we chemically treat the bacterial cells so that the peptide is no longer aggregated, but secreted, and thus found in the supernatant. Before centrifuging the bacterial cells, we treated them with PMDI (polymeric methylene diphenyl diisocyanate), lysine, and other substances. And it worked. We found anti-Pax6 in the supernatant. The band was weak but clearly visible.

The good news spread quickly and was met with great enthusiasm. To my surprise, the actual molecular weight, which was still around 35.000 daltons, was no longer of concern. Everybody agreed that the weight was of no interest as long as the peptide would work, that is, as long as it would recognize Pax6. Our task now was to increase the amount of anti-Pax6 in the supernatant and to then test whether it would recognize Pax6 in western blots and, if that was the case, whether it would block the transfer of Pax6 in vitro. After that we could begin with in vivo work.

The next day, Wednesday, December 11, I arrived late in the afternoon. (On Wednesdays I attended lecture classes for my DEA.) When I saw Gianfranco, I immediately knew that something had gone wrong. He was in a rage. Brigitte had approached him that morning, he said, and explained that she had tagged anti-Pax6 with Myc and not, as we assumed, with HA.

HA (short for anti-human hemagglutinin) and Myc (a transcription factor, a member of the Myc-protein family) are so-called epitopes. Epitopes are part of an antigen against which the immune system builds antibodies. In molecular biology such epitopes, which are commercially available, are frequently incorporated into recombinant proteins. If one tags, for example, the anti-Pax6 peptide with an HA, one can use an anti-HA as the secondary antibody to detect the protein on a western blot membrane. This is precisely what Gianfranco and I did. We had used an anti-HA, assuming that Brigitte had tagged her anti-Pax6 with an HA tag. That she had in fact used a Myc tag meant that the results we received the day before were useless. The bottom line was that we had to repeat the experiments we had done the previous two days.

To me the story seemed regrettable but of no major consequence. Gianfranco disagreed with that assessment. He took Brigitte's mistake personally. Why did Brigitte not tell me, he asked? She stood next to us whenever we talked about our experiments. We always talked about the HA tags, so why didn't she say that she had used a Myc tag?

The relation between Gianfranco and Brigitte had been delicate from the start. To me, it seemed as if Brigitte was sad—*envious* is perhaps too strong a word—because Gianfranco had taken over "her" project. And then there was Gianfranco's suggestion, made shortly after he arrived in the lab, that the lab meetings be held in English. As Gianfranco knew that Brigitte didn't speak English, she was hurt by his suggestion. Both were furious and yelled at each other. The result was an embarrassing silence. They did not talk to each other for almost two weeks. And once this changed again, their encounters always reminded me of joking relationships.[14] Most often they teased each other with mildly ironic critiques—Gianfranco would call Brigitte "so French," and Brigitte Gianfranco "polyglot" or "cosmopolitan"—thereby avoiding major confrontation.

Be that as it may, Brigitte was the one who approached Gianfranco and told him about her mistake. She felt terribly sorry and apologized over and over again. I never had any reason to doubt Brigitte's good intentions. What had happened was simply unfortunate. Yet Gianfranco disagreed.

"For weeks," he told me bitterly, "we have been checking all kinds of variables. We took all variables into account but not this one. Fine, now we know."

I was surprised that Gianfranco simply declared Brigitte to be one of the variables of our work, as if she was some sort of technical procedure. When I asked him whether he had recognized that he had just extended the variable concept to his social relations, he replied that social trust and reliability is as much an element of experimental work as a western blot.

December 17: Cultural Variables

Just two days after the incident with Brigitte, on Friday, December 17, Gianfranco was again enraged. We had spent the rest of Wednesday doing another western blot, this time with the required anti-Myc antibody. The result, fortunately, was the same. We found anti-Pax6 in the pellet and also, if to a lesser degree, in the supernatant. Alain was satisfied and Gianfranco became calm again. Together they agreed that it was prudent to first test whether the anti-Pax6 we had would recognize Pax6 in a western blot. Alain wanted to make sure that we did not waste time replacing the bacterial cells and constructing a new plasmid if the anti-Pax6 didn't work. The next day, Thursday, we ran the experiments and the result of the blot was positive. Anti-Pax6 recognized Pax6. We were enthusiastic. Three months after Gianfranco had arrived, the antibody seemed to work. We immediately walked over to Alain's office and presented the results to him. To my surprise, his reaction was reserved. In a sober tone he explained that we had made a mistake. Both our Pax6 and our anti-Pax6 had a Myc-tag. Since we had used an anti-Myc as the secondary antibody, we could not be sure that the reaction we saw on the film strip was caused by our anti-Pax6; it could have been caused by the anti-Myc reacting to Pax6. Alain asked us to replace the Myc-tag in the anti-Pax6 with an HA tag and to do the experiments again. This was fairly easy to achieve, but Gianfranco had no time to do so. It was Thursday evening, and he would leave the next day for Italy, where he would stay until January 5. Alain briefly pondered whether I could do the experiments, but then shook his head and decided that we would have to wait until January.

On Friday, December 17, Gianfranco visited the lab just briefly. He cleaned up the bench, put his lab notes in order, stored the cell cultures in the cold room, and completed all other errands. Not long after he arrived, Michel stopped by and told Gianfranco that he had asked Laure to replace the Myc-tag with an HA tag and to run a western blot on his behalf. Michel smiled. Gianfranco blushed. He nodded but didn't say a word. Righter after Volovitch left, however, he freaked out. In an angry tone he repeatedly explained to me that the Pax6 project was his, his alone. Who is Volovitch, he asked? What is he doing here? He does not even have a proper research group! Why does he tell me what to do? Who does he think he is? I am happy if he is interested in my work, but I work with you and Brigitte and not with him. He's not my director; Alain is my director. Gianfranco closed by saying in the most pejorative of tones that this lab was the weirdest place he had ever seen in his career. He added: "It is so French here. You should really visit other labs."

After lunch break, shortly before Gianfranco took a cab to the airport, we had a final meeting with Alain. Gianfranco explained what he would do once he was back in January—reconstruct the antibody, make a new plasmid, insert bacteria, and so forth. Alain, in a rather unfriendly tone, explained that the work Gianfranco suggested was well thought through but of no relevance. I could not help but think that he was trying to provoke Gianfranco.

"I don't give a shit about the bacterial cells," Alain said. "All you are supposed to do is block the intercellular transfer; this is what I need. Once we have the right cDNA, we inject it in the mouse and go in vivo."

Alain wanted Gianfranco to stay focused on what was to him essential, to clarify the relevance of the nonautonomous transfer of Pax6 for the formation of the eyecup and the midbrain-hindbrain frontier.

When Alain turned to his computer screen, signaling that the conversation had just ended, Gianfranco began talking about Michel. In carefully chosen words, so as to avoid any provocation, he explained that he thought that the Pax6 project was his project, not Michel's. Could he, Alain, talk to Michel?

Without turning away from his computer screen—he was reading his emails—Alain explained in neutral, almost sterile terms that Gianfranco was wrong. "First of all, it is not your project but my project. Second, this lab is very different from other labs you might know. In my lab there is a strong collaboration between people. I think that this is good, and in any case I like it better. Michel Volovitch," Alain went on, "is involved in almost all projects because he is our MCB [molecular cell biology] expert. Whenever we have an MCB problem, we give it to Michel. Without Michel's help Brigitte could not have constructed the anti-Pax6 you work with now. So he already worked on Pax6 before you arrived. And, by the way, Michel had first asked Brigitte to do the experiments, but she was worried that you might take it personally and so she suggested that he ask Laure."

Gianfranco didn't say a word. But his face expressed deep frustration.

"The problem," Alain continued, still starring at his screen, "will broaden. Alain Trembleau will teach you how to inject in nuclei. Then you will have to analyze embryos, and this is fairly difficult, especially the midbrain-hindbrain frontier."

"I think that collaboration is great," Gianfranco tried a modest response. "And I understand and respect the traditions of your lab, but I really would like to do the experiments myself and not have Volovitch decide that Laure should continue my work while I am away, you know?"

"Look, if you work on my project, in my lab, you have to agree, okay?"

When we were about to leave his office, Alain turned away from his computer and asked me to stay. After Gianfranco left, he offered coffee and explained that his lab, with its strong collaborative orientation, is very different from most other labs.

"Why is this so?" I wanted to know.

"Well, this is in part due to the peculiar circumstances of our project, but in part it is due to the fact that we're in France, I guess. Also, Michel, Joliot, and Trembleau are friends. We discuss things together and work together. I like it better that way. You should visit different labs to understand what I mean."

I found it striking that Alain had made the same suggestion as Gianfranco had. Both seemed to agree that the lab was, in its collaborative orientation and its emphasis on a common project, a "French lab." Evidently, this is to say, both agreed that there were profound, to a certain degree, "cultural" differences in the way experimental work was organized and conducted. Of course, what for Alain had positive connotations had negative ones for Gianfranco. For him it was precisely the Frenchness, especially the focus on the French language, which prevented the lab from being a cosmopolitan consortium of sorts, with postdocs and visiting scholars from all over the world.

January 22: Experimental Systems

When Gianfranco returned to the lab on January 7, he quickly learned that Laure had done the experiments and that the results were positive. Anti-Pax6 recognized Pax6 in western blots. As if to prove to himself—and to the others—that the Pax6 project was his, he repeated the experiments several times. Like Laure, he found that anti-Pax6 recognized Pax6.

In mid-January, we began to test whether anti-Pax6 would block the transfer of Pax6 in vitro. For us, this meant that the times when we ran several western blots per day ended. From now on our days were dominated by immunocytochemistry.

Immunocytochemistry refers to the chemical detection of proteins in cells in culture with the help of specific antibodies that have been labeled with a fluorescent dye. The antibody binds to the protein one seeks to detect, and the fluorescent dye allows one to spot, with the help of a laser or Confocal microscope, the location of the protein in question (*Confocal* is short for Confocal laser scanning microscopy).

In practice, immunocytochemistry looked as follows: Once a week Gianfranco and I produced neuron cultures. We cut open pregnant mice, dissected the brains of the embryos, roughly ten to fourteen at a time, isolated their developing midbrain, chopped it up, and grew the neurons in a milieu made up of calf serum. The rest of the week we then used the cultured neurons in always the same experimental procedure. First, we transfected COS cells with Pax6 DNA tagged with HA. Next we cocultured the transfected COS cells with neurons from our cell culture, knowing that Pax6 would transfer from the former to the latter. To prevent this transfer, we added our anti-Pax6, which, if things worked well, would bind to Pax6 outside the cell. Then we left the Petri dish untouched, at times for only half an hour and other times for twenty-four hours. Finally, we transferred the mixture of COS cells, neurons, and anti-Pax6 onto a cover slip, treated it with an anti-HA labeled with fluorescent dye, and then checked it under the Confocal microscope for the location of Pax6. Ideally, the Pax6 would be found exclusively outside the neurons. It would have made its way out of the COS cells but, due to the anti-Pax6, not into the neurons. However, we could never achieve this result. No matter how often we repeated the experiment, Pax6 was not expressed by our COS cells or only to a small degree. It was found in the COS cells but nowhere else.

Our first reaction was to check whether something was wrong with the antibody we had tagged onto our Pax6. Different antibodies, Gianfranco told me, are suited for different kinds of things. We tried a whole cascade of them, but to not avail. Next we tested whether it would make a difference to add our anti-Pax6 later. Perhaps our anti-Pax6 prevented Pax6 from being secreted? But that didn't make a difference, either. Then we stored the mixture at different temperatures, again without any success.

Finally we focused on the COS cells. Perhaps they were the problem. Gianfranco ordered a new line of COS cells, and we transfected them with Pax6 and then cocultured them with our midbrain neurons—but without our anti-Pax6. And indeed we found that Pax6 had literally flooded the neurons. At that point it seemed as if we had identified the problem. But when we then tested the anti-Pax6 to see if it would block the transfer, the result was the same as before. The COS cells did not express Pax6.

The situation was frustrating. Again we found ourselves discussing and checking variables. To me, experimental work had gained a labyrinth-like quality. You try different directions until you find one that takes you further than the others. This, however, does not mean that you have found the exit; it just means that you have found a path to walk a bit farther. In experimentation, one solves a problem only to encounter yet another one. Nobody really knows how long this will go on, or when one will find an exit—or if at all.

Gianfranco decided to talk to Bernadette. She suggested only things we had already tested. Next Gianfranco asked Brigitte. I found that step curious, given his frequent expressions of ambivalence about her. But, then, Brigitte, in contrast to Bernadette, had several years' worth of experience with homeoprotein biology. Brigitte, in a way, was an expert. She seemed to very much appreciate that Gianfranco asked her for help and indeed she offered several suggestions. In her work she had recognized that if one treats the cells in a certain way, the proteins transfer better. Also, she suggested that the amount of DNA with which we transfected the COS cells was perhaps insufficient. We should increase the amount of DNA and coculture neurons and COS cells for forty-eight instead of twenty-four hours.

We spent the next two days following Brigitte's suggestions. The result of our experiments, however, was the same. Pax6 was not expressed by the COS cells. Finally, Gianfranco decided to ask Alain, whom he had tried to avoid since his return from Italy. Alain told Gianfranco that he thought we should discuss the problem with Michel, as he was the expert on such questions. Michel, however, was away until the following day.

While Gianfranco, Michel, and Alain met, on January 21, I passed my midterm exam. When I returned and asked Gianfranco what they had suggested we do, he shrugged and said that both thought that we probably made a mistake somewhere in our handling of the cell culture, the transfection, or the use of the Confocal. In addition, he added, they decided that we should present our work in the lab meeting.

To me, the path that led us from Bernadette to Brigitte to Alain to Michel and finally to the lab meeting was illuminating. Our effort to solve an experimental problem led us through a hierarchy of competence and decision making that was nowhere clearly articulated but that silently structured the lab and organized its work processes, from bench neighbor to lab head, to expert, and finally to the united effort of the whole lab.

In the lab meeting, which took place the next morning, the seniors agreed that Gianfranco did great work but that, as Volovitch explained, "he was perhaps not yet familiar with the experimental system" the lab worked with. After more discussion, Alain decided that Gianfranco should work with someone who knew the chemistry and the biology of the transfer well and who was familiar with using the Confocal. His decision fell on Michel Tassetto, a graduate student of Joliot who had spent years working with the Confocal to make visible the nonautonomous transfer in vitro.

After the lab meeting I walked straight to Michel Volovitch's office. I wanted to know what exactly he meant by the term "experimental system."[15] Why was knowing the "experimental system" central to blocking the transfer of Pax6 in vitro? And what kind of experimental system did the lab work with? Could he explain to me what this system consisted of?

In the conversation that unfolded, Michel made a distinction between "technology" and "experimental system." He emphasized that Gianfranco had good technical skills and that the way he handled the technologies was elegant but that nonetheless there might be a problem in the way he had composed the medium or the way he transfected the COS cells or the way he used the Confocal. "After all," he concluded, "Gianfranco just arrived in the lab and is not yet familiar with our work."

"I am not sure I understand what you mean," I replied. "What has this to do with an experimental system?"

"None of the procedures we work with," Volovitch explained, "is [self-] evident. Neither the cell medium nor the use of the western blot nor the Confocal microscope. Instead they are the result of several years of experimentation in which we tried to determine the circumstances of the transfer."

"And what's the experimental system?" I asked.

"The experimental system we work with is made up of the experiences and results of our previous work. And of the assumptions that are built into these results."

"And the results—are these the technologies you work with?"

"Look, Penetratin was once an experimental object; now it is a technology.

"So previous experiences and results are the building blocks of the system?"

"That's perhaps a bit too generalizing but you could say so, yes."

"And each of these building blocks might be a variable Gianfranco has to test now?"

"Well, not all of them *are* variables but they can *become* variables. You have to understand that experimental results are always tentative. That's the way our work is. A result we get today might tomorrow appear in a different light. It might even be that you encounter a problem that requires you to return to what you thought was a solid result, that you have to redo the experiments that produced it, that you need to change this or that aspect of the experiments, or your interpretation of it. That's good, actually, for this allows for surprise and progress."

"So surprise is the form through which an experimental system grows?"

"To a certain degree, yes. Anyway, for now we're not dealing with such problems. We think that Gianfranco merely needs some assistance. And Michel Tassetto—here I agree with Alain—is an excellent choice for helping Gianfranco. He knows the procedures and assumptions we work with. I hope he will not take this personally, which, as you know, he tends to do."

Gianfranco had himself become a variable that needed to be checked. He knew the procedures, but there was the worry that he could not yet, to use Alain's words, "think with them."

On January 27 Michel Tassetto began spending his days with Gianfranco and me. For one week we worked together and redid all the experiments we had conducted for the past two or three weeks. The results, however, remained the same. The COS cells did not express Pax6. Gianfranco felt affirmed and was happy. He, it seemed clear, was not the problem and hence not the one to be blamed. Finally, in March, after another month of work, it was discovered that Michel Volovitch's vector, that is, the DNA inserted in bacterial plasmid to produce Pax6, was bad.

Anthropology of the Concrete

Would these anecdotes allow me to make sense, in retrospect, of the work Gianfranco and I carried out, in terms of experimental realism? Would they allow me to reconstruct how—on the level of thought, through technical work—we sought to enroll the brain into a conversation about its plastic becoming?

After I finished a first reading of my notes, my answer was a clear "no." At first sight, what made them interesting was that they made no qualitative distinction between relational and cultural variables on the one hand and technical and epistemological variables on the other, as if relational variables were as central to experimentation as epistemological ones. However, since I had written those notes, I had gotten to know experimentation better, with the consequence that I had come to distrust the very concept of symmetry found in early social studies of scientific knowledge. Wasn't the idea of symmetry contingent on the refusal to learn how exactly experiments produce knowledge? Couldn't one maintain the idea of symmetry only if one ignored the art of thinking in technical terms about biological processes?

In the aftermath of my encounter with Maria-Luz, though, it was precisely this art that interested me. It was just that my convoluted field notes had little to say about this art. They conveyed a good sense of the actual technical work Gianfranco and I carried out, but not of the thoughts that organized and were at stake in our technical work.

Differently put, the above-five anecdotes reflected a concept of the experimental as the merely technical—as work with technologies; as checking technical variables; as, in its advanced state, thinking through the epistemological presupposition that organizes a given technology, that organizes the assumptions about what would happen when a particular technology was used.

But then, upon a second reading, it suddenly seemed to me as if I was wrong, as if the five anecdotes actually did provide an answer, if an unexpected one, to the question of how Gianfranco and I enrolled the brain in a thoughtful, technical conversation about plasticity. The critical turning point came while I was working through my conversation with Michel Volovitch. At the time the conversation took place, in late January 2002, Michel's elaborations were exciting to me because they seemed to elevate my work with Gianfranco beyond the merely technical. Wasn't Michel suggesting that we were not, after all, mere technicians, that we were actually conducting epistemological work, even if we did not know it? I had understood Michel to be making a technical point—that every experimental technology was also an epistemological variable insofar as it stood in for *technical* presuppositions about what actually happened when it was deployed. This technical understanding of Michel's elaboration was consistent with the understanding of the experimental as the merely technical that had emerged from my work with Gianfranco.

"Even epistemology," I noted for myself, "is concerned with technologies, that is, the merely technical."

Since my conversation with Michel, however, my encounter with Maria-Luz and my discovery of construction work had radically changed my understanding of the experimental. Where before I had seen "mere" technologies, I had now learned to see "vital" technologies, that is, tentative—perspectivist—configurations of thought, technology, and living processes.

And it was this substitution of mere technologies by vital technologies that gave a new meaning to Michel's concept of an experimental system—a meaning that opened the possibility of understanding how precisely Gianfranco and I sought to produce new knowledge, a meaning that allowed for a powerful reinterpretation of the relational troubles and variables my field notes reported.

HOW EXPERIMENTS PRODUCE KNOWLEDGE

Had Michel not suggested that an experimental system is composed of thoughtfully arranged vital technologies, each one of which is the result of a previous experiment (his example was Penetratin)? Usually, or so I understood him now, the epistemological quality of an experimental system is dormant. As long as the system produces the expected results, the vital technologies it is composed of are taken for granted. But in the course of an experiment it may happen that the experimental system, or some element of it, becomes problematic and is questioned. The consequence then is that one or several of the vital technologies it is made up of will be transformed back into an experimental inquiry.

The encountering of a problem, thus, has the potential to mutate a given into a question, and working through this question requires one to transform a vital technology back into the experimental setup that initially produced it, so that one can go back and check each variable—thought, technology, living process—of that setup until one has found the one that needs to be altered in order to move forward. As no one knows in advance which variable will need to be adjusted—and as (almost) each variable is itself potentially a vital technology that can be decomposed in the experiment that initially produced it—the process can be long and complicated and full of tension and conflict.

What emerged from my reading of Michel's explanation of experimental systems from the perspective of construction work was a sense that producing experimental knowledge (often) meant moving forward by moving backward—insofar as the new knowledge (vital technology) one is working toward is contingent on already established knowledge (vital technologies), and insofar as the derailment of a given experimental setup may require one to critically rethink that older knowledge (those older vital technologies).

Wasn't the work that Gianfranco and I carried out a prime example of such a moving forward by moving backward?

In October 2001 we began working with the fragments of thought Alain and Michel had provided us. Each one of these thought fragments was a product of the experiments carried out since 1989, when Alain and Joliot first thought that perhaps homeoproteins could transfer between cells and cause a powerful morphogenetic outgrowth. Soon, though, our experiments got derailed, and Gianfranco and I found ourselves checking many of the vital technologies our experimental setup was composed of—vital technologies that were now part of the experimental system that once produced them. The cell medium; the amount of protein with which we transfected the COS cells; the coculturing of COS cells and neurons; how long we washed the membrane; at which temperature we washed them: None of these vital technologies, as Michel put it, was evident. Each was a specific outcome of many years of experimentation, of the effort to study the conditions of the nonautonomous transfer of homeoproteins in vitro. Next we checked Brigitte's construction of the anti-Pax6, which was contingent on the knowledge produced during the in vitro years, specifically on the many experiments that had determined which part of the three helices that homeoproteins consist of was necessary for internalization (as internalization was to be blocked).

Each one of our work steps implied transforming older experimental results—stabilized into vital technologies—into variables to be checked and, if necessary, adjusted, so that we could move our experiment forward, as well as the whole experimental system on which our experiment was contingent. In short, Gianfranco and I consistently moved forward by moving backward.

This, then, is how we sought to produce unprecedented knowledge—by exposing the fragments of thought we were provided, by letting them be derailed by the living processes we were studying, and by using this derailment as an opportunity to rework the nuances of the experiments that had given rise to the vital technologies upon which our fragments of thought were contingent. Eventually, if successful, our work would have aligned thought, technology, and living processes in such a way that the plastic becoming of the nervous system would be experimentally known (in the form of a vital technology contingent upon the experimental system that produced it). An experimental system, thus, is itself a giant vital technology, a particular, perspectivist actualization of the living.

If experiments are efforts to open windows, then experimental systems are something akin to a (perspectivist) glass house.

Retrospective

Once I had come to terms with the way Gianfranco and I sought to experimentally engage the brain (the real) in a conversation about plasticity (the real), my time with Gianfranco, and the relational troubles I had documented in my field notes, appeared to me in a new light.

First, I began to wonder whether or not Gianfranco was actually aware of the particular notion of what an experimental technology is, which was constitutive of the lab in which he had arrived. Was he? At the very least, it seemed that Gianfranco's notion of technology was radically different from that of his new seniors.

When Gianfranco began working in Alain's lab, he had just completed his PhD in developmental molecular biology at University College, London. He viewed the technologies constitutive of molecular biology as in themselves neutral, as just instruments—tools—that produced more or less objective knowledge about the molecular organization of living organisms. Alain's lab, however, had come to distrust this "neutral" understanding of technologies as mere tools. In the aftermath of their 1989 observation, Alain, Joliot, and

Michel had to learn that technologies were less neutral tools of or for discovery, but encoded "philosophies of life."

As Joliot once put it, they had to learn that tools do not so much discover as "produce" biological truths, and that most commercially available tools were tailored to "reproduce" and "refine" the already known, that is, the dominant genomic and cell-autonomous conception of the living.

The challenge of experimentation, for Alain and the other senior researchers, therefore, was to find new technologies that would make possible another, different knowledge of the biological processes that gave rise to the brain. Differently put, a large part of their job, insofar as they were working toward a plastic conception of the brain, was to problematize the technologies that Gianfranco took for granted and to either readjust them or come up with alternative ones.

If this were true, then wouldn't it explain why my work with Gianfranco led me to think that experimentation is merely technical work That it is somewhat devoid of intellectual, biological creativity? That it is mere technological groping in the dark? All Gianfranco saw, all he could show me, were technologies, not materially arranged fragments of thought, testing grounds for an alternative philosophy of life.

Second, it seemed to me as if my new notion of what an experimental system is was putting what I had called cultural variables into perspective. What I had hoped to capture with the term *culture* in the days before I met Maria-Luz were Gianfranco's problems in adjusting to the new environment. I thought that his animosities toward other researchers made plain that a thoroughly international discipline like molecular (neuro)biology, organized by global, nonlocal standards and norms, is, in the way it is practiced, subject to local variation.[16]

Gianfranco, who had been introduced to lab life in London and Heidelberg, was struck by, and suffered from, the "Frenchness" of the lab, by which he meant its focus on the French language as much as the insistence on relational forms of experimental inquiry. He longed for a more cosmopolitan and individualistic organization of science, one independent of place, where everyone spoke English, where everyone had his or her proper project, where people from all over the world got together and exchanged experiences. Alain and co., for their part, identified Gianfranco's idea of a cosmopolitan science as thoroughly Anglo-Saxon, just as Gianfranco identified theirs as thoroughly French.

Now, however, I wondered whether behind these conflicts stood not culture, but the specific experimental system the lab had elaborated since 1989.

Wasn't it more appropriate to say that what provoked the conflicts was an experimental system that was new and unknown to Gianfranco, one that defined itself precisely by putting into question the experimental system, its implicit understanding of the living organism, that Gianfranco was trained in?

And third, I began to wonder whether my understanding of experimentation wasn't also changing what I had called "relational variables." Initially, the phrase was little more than a gesture toward the importance of trust in experimental work. Gianfranco's ongoing disputes with and ambivalence about Brigitte (or about Volovitch or several other members of the lab), the fact that he declared her to be one of the variables we have to take into account in our work, and the fact that he himself was ultimately identified as a moral variable that had to be checked by Michel Tassetto—these stories seemed to point to the significance of trust and moral reliability for the collaborative undertaking that experimentation inevitably is.[17]

But now I wondered. Perhaps what trust means depends on the relational form experimental life takes in a given lab. That Gianfranco insisted on being an individual, that he was adamant that Pax6 was his experiment and no one else's, did not fit well with the ethics of relationalism constitutive of Alain's lab and its experimental system. Gianfranco became morally suspicious, not trustworthy.

What Is Experimentally Known?

The question that remained was: What does experimental knowledge consist of? What kind of thing do experiments get to know if they do not so much *discover* reality as *actualize the possibility* of knowledge they themselves open up?

My work with Gianfranco on Pax6 and my interpretation of this work in terms of experimental realism eventually led me to think that the first step to answering this question is the appreciation that it is not actually humans who produce experimental knowledge, but the technological procedures and machines that humans work with.

In experimentation, knowledge is not gained through the human senses, a curious eye, or the insights of an inquiring mind. Instead, it is produced by machines and technical procedures.[18]

To be sure, humans, are the ones who build machines, negotiate or establish norms, and make interpretations of results. It is humans who perform nocturnal work, who discuss what experiments to conduct, who look at data and have associations, who feel electrified, and so forth. However, the actual *Erkenntnisprozess* (process of producing knowledge) is thoroughly dehumanized and desubjectified. Not the human mind but machines are the media of producing knowledge.

This appreciation of the techno or technocentric rather than anthropocentric quality of experimental knowledge production is critical because it makes clear that—and to what radical degree—the experimental sciences actually escape the Cartesian epistemology and its clear-cut distinction between subjects and objects that is commonly held to be constitutive of modernity in general and of modern knowledge in particular: The process of gaining experimental knowledge has little to do with an individual Cartesian subject (or its various manifestations, from Hume to Husserl and Popper), who has an idea and then goes and tests it in order to see what is evident. Between the intentional subject and the object to be known, experimental science puts procedural work with machines—not as a passive device designed to enhance the subject's discriminatory capacities, but as the actual knowledge-producing act.

Strictly speaking, therefore, experimental knowledge is not gained. Instead it is produced, by machines and machinelike procedures. And what they produce depends—as we have seen—less (or at least not primarily) on the phenomena to be known than on the space of possibility a particular experimental system can create (hence, the inappropriateness of the term *discovery,* which suggests a discrete object that has been uncovered by the human).[19]

What, then, is experimentally known? What kinds of things are the object of experimental knowledge?

Here are three, still somewhat tentative suggestions.

The first is that experimentally known things are necessarily and inevitably emergent things. They are known and come into existence gradually, through the work with vital technologies that bring into view certain aspects of a process or thing and thereby give it form. This emergent quality inevitably implies that experimental things are intrinsically open or fluid in their contours. As what defines them is an emergent list of assumptions one can experimentally control, every new feature has the potential to change what the experimental things are.[20]

The second tentative suggestion is that experimentally constituted things are inevitably bound up with the thoughts that organize them (the technology constitutive of them). That is, they are irreducibly partial. Had one worked with a different kind of experimental system, had one begun a different conversation, based on different questions, one would have produced different answers and results, and hence the thing itself would have appeared in a different light and have different contours (a different space of possibilities makes the thing in question appear in a different epistemic perspective). Of course, this does not mean that experimental results are arbitrary and depend exclusively on the questions one is asking or on the tools one uses. It means, however, that the questions and tools provide the framework within which the response can be interpreted.

The third suggestion, finally, gestures toward what could be described as the *romantic quality* of experimentally known things, that is, their potential inexhaustibility. As they are constituted by vital technologies and not discovered, the project of fully knowing them appears to be, at least in principle, without end. There is always the possibility of asking yet another question. Of course, when answers get repetitive, one stops posing questions. But then, one is never quite sure whether an experimental system is exhausted or one just needs to find a new, unexpected question that can tap the system's yet unexplored and surprising potential.

After all, they are almost living things.

HOW EXPERIMENTS END

I left Paris in May 2003.[21] A few weeks later, in late July, Gianfranco reported that he succeeded in blocking the transfer of Pax6 in vitro—and then he left as well.

"At that point," Alain later explained to me, "I returned the project to Brigitte. That seemed only fair. After all, it was Brigitte who had initially begun the Pax6 experiments."

When I returned next time, in May 2005, I found that the Pax6 experiment had significantly changed. Brigitte told me that when she repeated the final experiments Gianfranco had conducted, she found, counter to what Gianfranco had told, that the anti-Pax6 did not block the transfer in vitro. "I had to begin the Pax6 experiment from scratch," she laughed. "And that," Alain later added, "was simply too much work for her alone. I thus asked her to drop the mesencephalon-diencephalon project."

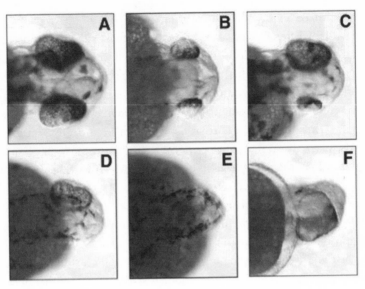

A monster of hope: Brigitte's one-eyed fish. From Lesaffre et al. 2007.

In mid-2004, after Brigitte had constructed a new, functioning anti-Pax6 and she finally succeeded in blocking the transfer in vitro and was about to begin in vivo work, Alain decided on two further changes. First, he suggested dropping the construction of Pax2+3. "Despite thorough efforts," he explained his decision, "the project had made little progress since Gianfranco's departure. It seemed therefore better to let go and to let Brigitte concentrate on the in vivo project." The second change concerned the animal Brigitte would work with. "Instead of working with mice," Alain went on, "as initially planned, we thought it would be better to work with zebra fish."

"Why zebra fish?" I asked Alain, a bit surprised.

"Well, it is a far simpler organism," he replied. "And eye formation has been well studied in zebra fish."

By the summer of 2004, then, a project that had originally been constructed as a multifaceted conversation with the real about the real—with Pax6 about its role in the embryogenetic formation of the nervous system—had become a single dialogue about the role of Pax6 nonautonomous transfer in the formation of the eyecup.[22] In fall 2004, Brigitte finally began with in vivo work. When I visited the lab half a year later, she had assembled quite astonishing results: where she had blocked the transfer, there were no—or only rudimentary—eyes to be found.

When I first saw Brigitte's pictures, I was struck by how beautifully these monsters produced a logic of plasticity. The pictures of her one-eyed fishes were powerful pictorial evidence for the plasticity of the organism. They showed Pax6 as a plastic force, its nonautonomous transfer as a plastic event, and the brain as a plastic organ. Brigitte had succeeded in enrolling the brain in a logic of plasticity—a logic that allows conceiving of homeoproteins as diffusing morphogens that first produce a plastic tissue and then sculpt it.[23]

AND THE ADULT?

For Alain, Joliot, Michel, Trembleau, and Brigitte, these results were profoundly satisfying. Almost two decades after the first observation of the nonautonomous transfer, in 1989 at the Collège de France, they had established that the n-a-t was not just a curious, though pharmacologically valuable, artifact, but they had also shown that it has an important in vivo function: homeoproteins are plastic forces and their nonautonomous transfer is a decisive plastic event that shapes the nervous tissue.

Given the success of Brigitte's work on Pax6, I was curious to see how the lab would go ahead and apply the minipeptide technology to the adult brain. What experimental setup would they come up with? What animal, what protein would they choose for their work? Who would conduct the project?

When I returned to Paris in summer 2006, however, I quickly learned that no one was thinking about Pax6 anymore. Once the in vivo role of Pax6 had been established, Alain and the Saturday-morning collective had begun to construct other, to them more exciting projects. Simply put, if one were interested in the adult, other proteins and other brain regions offered more interesting, more compelling venues.[24] Alain and the other seniors had begun to construct new projects—about the role of Emx2 for adult olfactory neurons; about the significance of HOP (homeodomain-only protein) for adult neurogenesis in the hippocampus; about the relevance of Otx2 for the control of critical periods.[25]

This is how experiments end. They engender new, unexpected questions, which lead to the construction of unanticipated experimental problems— new possible windows—which continue the variation and repetition and thereby advance the experimental system, this massive endeavor to engage the real in a conversation about the real.

Plastic Anatomies of the Living

Looking at Brigitte's one-eyed fish, I could not help but think about plastic anatomy. Plastic anatomy—I had stumbled over the phrase while researching the history of the term *plasticity;* it refers to the emergence, in the mid-eighteenth century, of sculptures of human and animal bodies in wax, specifically in the medical schools at Bologna and Florence.[1] The purpose of these plastic anatomies, which could be found in medical schools across Europe, was anatomical instruction; it was an opportunity for medical students to learn about the anatomy of the human body without actual dissection.

Weren't Brigitte's fish plastic anatomies of sorts?

I began to read through books and articles about plastic anatomy, wondering if I could find lines, broken or linear, that would lead from the eighteenth-century wax models to Brigitte's cyclopic fish. And gradually, more by chance than by design, I discovered what I came to think of as the untold history of *plastic anatomies of the living,* that is, the history of the transition of tools and techniques from sculpting organisms in wax to sculpting the living organism itself.

A beginning was made by the young Wilhelm His, specifically in his 1868 *Untersuchungen über de erste Anlage des Wirbelthieres: Die erste Entwicklung des Hühnchens im Ei,* a careful analytical description of the early formation of the chick embryo. According to most historians of embryology, His's *Untersuchungen* was an event in the history of science because it attempted a purely mechanical explanation of embryogenesis.[2] Until His, most embryologists had been vitalists. They explained embryogenetic growth in terms of vital forces that gave shape to the embryo and that could not be assessed in terms of science. His radically departed from the vitalism of his colleagues and predecessors, opening the possibility of a modern, empirical and experimental—rather than idealistic and vitalist—embryology.

When I read His (I vaguely remembered from readings that he had modeled embryos in wax), I could certainly see this insistence on the mechanical rather than the vital.[3] But what stood out much more was the seeming continuity of his conception of embryogenesis with that of his vitalist precursors. Despite his insistence on the laws of mechanics, His was actually holding on to nearly every aspect of the plastic comprehension of embryogenesis that the vitalists had come up with. For him, just as for them, the embryo was a growing plastic tissue that was gradually sculpted into form. But whereas the vitalists had argued that the sculpting was done by vital forces, His thought that he could explain the sculpting in terms of the mechanical pressures produced by growth and expansion. Could it be, he wondered, that the different parts of the plastic germ layers gradually grew larger—and that they thereby not only built up the embryo's tissue but also exerted pressure on it, a physical force that—like a sculptor—molded the tissue until the embryo assumed form?

His's major contribution was to mechanize the vitalist conception of embryogenesis. And, even if it may sound surprising, what made this mechanization of the vital possible were his attempts at plastic modeling.

Around 1866, His built a new kind of microtome, a section cutter that enabled him to serially cut embryos into extremely thin slices. From these slices, he sought to reconstruct the embryo's inner composition. And once he had cut his way through a whole series of embryos at different embryogenetic stages, he arranged them in a linear series and reconstructed from them the embryo's gradual spatial emergence.

Just a year after he had begun working with his microtome, in 1867, His wrote to Adolf Ziegler, a physician who had been modeling anatomical wax models of organs in the tradition of eighteenth-century plastic anatomy. Ziegler had made a name for himself in medical schools where his models were used to instruct the students. What His was interested in, though, was not anatomical instruction but anatomical research. He had suffered from the limits his slides imposed on him. It was rather challenging to abstract from them a sense of the embryo's spatial growth. His hope was that Ziegler's plastic anatomies could help. And they did—if in an unexpected way.

Once Ziegler sent His the first embryos in wax, and once His began aligning them with his thin slices of embryonic tissue, he made the, for him, flabbergasting discovery that he could understand the embryo itself as a kind of plastic anatomy: just as the sculptor formed wax, the growth of tissue shaped and sculpted the embryo into form—it added plastic material and at the same time exerted a physical pressure on it.

His had accidentally discovered the plasticity of the living.

The effect of His's eureka moment was an indistinguishability between embryos in wax and embryos themselves, between the methods of plastic anatomy and the methods of embryology. And it was this insight into the mechanical sculpting of the embryo itself that opened up the possibility of His's mechanic embrace of the vitalists' conception of an embryo's irreducible plasticity.[4]

In the late 1860s, His's conception of embryology as a kind of plastic art was at best an event of local relevance. And it might well be that this would have never changed, that His's appropriation of plastic anatomy to embryological ends—he spoke of his models as *plastische Anschauungen* or, later, as *plastische Synthesen*—would have remained a personal idiosyncrasy of no further relevance, were it not for Ernst Haeckel.

In 1866, two years before His published his *Untersuchungen,* Haeckel, professor at the University of Jena, began to argue that the best way to understand embryogenesis was in terms of evolution. Haeckel was adamant that embryogenesis was the mere recapitulation of the evolutionary stages that gave rise to a given animal. His (like Gavin de Beer later) thoroughly disagreed with Haeckel's "biogenetic law," a phrase Haeckel began to use in 1870. He lamented that Haeckel was blind to what he, His, who had spent so many years studying growth processes, had come to understand as the key to embryogenesis—its logic of plasticity.[5]

Haeckel, who quickly emerged as a celebrity among physicians as well as the educated public, seems to have cared little. He went ahead and published a long series of popular science books and articles in which he argued that the way to understand the embryo was not through some imagined plasticity but through the proper study of evolution. He was adamant that the best thing embryologists could do to understand embryogenesis was to become evolutionary biologists.

When Haeckel, in 1874, published *Anthropogenie oder die Entwicklungsgeschichte des Menschen,* a popular science book that explained human embryogenesis in terms of the biogenetic law, His had enough. He reached out to the public with his own popular science book, *Unsere Körperform und das Problem ihrer physiologischen Entstehung.*[6] Carefully he explained to his readers the logic of plasticity that organizes embryogenesis and also the importance of plastic modeling for understanding how the embryo is formed. He measured Haeckel's pictures of human embryos and showed where and why the evolutionary stages that Haeckel insisted on were untenable. And, after every proof of error, His insisted that seriously advancing the medical sciences required not another theory of embryogenesis, but an embryology for embryology's sake, one capable of studying and understanding the plastic processes that shape the embryo mechanically. His's way forward was a plastic anatomy of human becoming.

After he had published his rebuttal, His set to work. He knew that a popular science book would not suffice to convince his colleagues that Haeckel was wrong. He needed empirical proof. So he embarked on the largest systematic study of human embryogenesis that had ever been undertaken. For almost a decade, he cut his way through human embryos of various embryogenetic stages and reconstructed from them the plastic processes that gradually formed the human—by arranging the slices produced with his microtome in linear sequences and by plastic modeling. Again His was assisted by Adolf Ziegler. After Adolf's health declined, his son Friedrich, who had been trained as a plastic artist, worked alongside His. The culmination of His's work was his three-volume atlas *Anatomie menschlicher Embryonen* (Anatomy of Human

Embryos), which was published between 1880 and 1885 and could be purchased with models from the Zieglers.

Most histories of embryology describe His's *Anatomie* as the beginning of our modern understanding of human embryonic development. In this historical reading, the importance of His's work was that it was the first to offer a systematic, methodologically rigorous overview of human embryogenesis.[7] From the perspective of the story I seek to tell here—the story of the plastic anatomy of the living—this focus on methodological rigor is grossly insufficient. First, it conveys a conception of science that hardly does justice to the plastic art His practiced. Second, it fails to bring into view that what His actually hoped to impart with his *Anatomie* was not so much technical acuity as the appreciation of the plasticity of the embryo. And third, it completely misses the form-giving consequence that His's plastic conception of embryogenesis had on subsequent generations of embryologists. When one reads the work of His's successors, it becomes apparent that what they took from him was hardly his mechanical conception of embryogenesis—which they criticized—but rather his insistence on the embryo's plasticity. Wilhelm His established for a whole generation of embryologists—from Roux and Driesch to Spemann, Harrison, von Dürken, de Beer, and many others—that the embryo is plastic and the challenge of embryology is to understand the processes that shape its plastic matter into form.

I emphasize the significance of plastic anatomy for His and his successors in order to illuminate what is usually lost from sight: it was His's embryological appropriation of plastic anatomy that was constitutive of the possibility of the experimental search for the laws that his successors took on. More than that, they largely understood their experiments as a continuation of His's plastic art by other means. And the consequence of this continuity was a most marvelous event: the discovery—reminiscent of Claude Bernard's *loi de formation*—of the possibility to model the embryo itself as if it were of wax.

After His, Wilhelm Roux and Hans Driesch worked out two mutually exclusive understandings of embryogenesis. Roux, who ablated one of the cells of the blastula, observed that the whole embryo then died. After repeating the experiment several times, he suggested that the fertilized egg obviously contains all of the information necessary for the embryo to emerge, and that if one damages any of the cells that subsequently emerge from it, the embryo misses a vital part and is aborted. When Driesch repeated Roux's experiments, he made a different observation. After he separated blastula cells from one another, the embryo didn't die. Instead he got several, smaller embryos. Consequently, Driesch concluded that each cell of the blastula contains all the information necessary for embryogenesis to occur.

Around 1901, Hans Spemann set out to solve this conflict by constricting the two-cell blastula of the Triton. Would he receive two embryos or no embryo at all? Spemann found that when he tightly constricted the two cells, he could produce two embryos. But much more interestingly, he also found that, depending on where he constricted the blastula, it would eventually have either two heads or several eyes or noses.

Looking at Spemann's two-headed and two-tailed embryos, I could not help but think that they must have been the first successful attempt to apply His's experimental adaptation of plastic anatomy to the living organism. Spemann's two-headed or two-tailed amphibian embryos were the first *plastic anatomies of the living.*

If the plastic art was still rudimentary at the turn of the twentieth century, the work that led Spemann from his constriction experiments to his work on lens formation in frogs, and from there to his discovery of the inductive logic of embryogenesis in the early 1920s, was something like its continuous refinement. And in 1924, when Spemann, together with his graduate student Hilde Mangold, learned to induce entire embryos in indifferent embryonic tissue, he achieved mastery: he learned to control the plastic forces that themselves organize embryogenesis.[8]

If His's work marks the very moment at which plastic anatomy ceased to be a tool of instruction and emerged as an experimental, knowledge-producing method, then Spemann's constriction experiments of the 1890s mark the transition from modeling embryos in wax to modeling the embryo itself.

From Spemann's plastic anatomies of the living, it is but a small step to Brigitte's one-eyed fish. Couldn't one say that her Cyclopes were the latest achievement of a line of thinking and experimenting—of thoughtful experimentation—that could be traced back to Wilhelm His's adaptation of eighteenth-century plastic anatomy? And couldn't one say that the significance of the work of Alain—of Brigitte—was that it sought to extend the plastic anatomy of the living from the embryo to the adult?

SIX

Ethical

Science is meaningless because it gives no answer to our question, the only question important for us: What shall we do? How shall we live?

MAX WEBER

A few weeks before I left Paris, three minor (if taken by themselves) events occurred in quick succession and thereby accidentally accumulated to a question that none of them could have generated alone—a question that first challenged and eventually changed my understanding of the stakes of plastic reason. The first of these events occurred late one Friday evening in April 2003, in the laboratory of Philippe Ascher.

At the time of our conversation Philippe, one of the best-known French electrophysiologists, was in his early seventies.[1] We initially had gotten to know each other because he was on the committee that interviewed me when I applied for my DEA. Philippe was a strong supporter of the idea that an anthropologist would study French brain research and invited me to visit him in his lab. When we met for our first conversation, I learned why Philippe was so enthusiastic about my work: he told me that his secret passion was the history of science in general and of the French neuronal sciences in particular. To him I was like-minded, someone with whom he could discuss the stories that had shaped his field. And Philippe's repertoire of stories was impressive, to say the least. He had been one of the last students of the Institut Marey, the once famous center of French electrophysiology, founded in 1947 by Alfred Fessard, who had worked with both Sherrington and Adrian and who succeeded in institutionalizing the electrical study of the synaptic, chemical brain. Philippe knew personally many of the people who had shaped the French neuronal sciences. Most of them were either, his teachers or his friends. Philippe had much to tell, and I was eager to listen. That evening in April, he had invited me so that we could talk about the battles fought in the late 1970s between the electrophysiologists of the Institut Marey, led by the senior Fessard, and the molecular neurobiologists of the Institut Pasteur, led by the young Jean Pierre Changeux.[2]

At one point in our conversation Philippe made the following remark: "The nervous machine"—he was pointing to his head—"is organized in fixed and immutable neural circuits. We've known [. . .] since the 1940s that these neural circuits are governed by chemical molecules and electronic signals. The arrival of molecular biology didn't add any basic insights. It did not revolutionize our conception of the brain. It was a new tool, that's all."

Philippe's claim caught my attention because it seemed to me to deny the significance of the work of Alain.

"You just said the brain is organized in immutable circuits," I interrupted him. "What, then, is the place of Alain's lab in the history of the neuronal science? You know that he claims that the brain is profoundly plastic and that he thinks the challenge neuronal researchers face today is to think the nervous system from the perspective of this plasticity."

Philippe nodded, serious.

"Look," he replied in a sober tone, "I like Alain, but his work, you know, it is speculation. From the perspective of electrophysiology his claims don't make sense. There simply is no space for plasticity in the adult."

After a pause, he turned the question back on me.

"Where would plastic changes occur in an adult brain?"

I smiled.

"But the adult brain," he said, apparently taking my smile as an expression of doubt, "is already wired. It is already wired. It really is!"

The scene held something of a snapshot. Philippe, who had untamed gray hair, was dressed in black, and wore huge black glasses was surrounded by black walls and shelves from which colorful power cords hung above his head and over his shoulders. The unplanned effect was that his body seemed to fade into the black wall—and that he appeared as a mere head, a head accentuated by his huge glasses and his grey hair, a head directly wired to the machines that surrounded him. For a mere second, Philippe, while insisting that the brain is already wired, looked himself like a wired electrical machine.

Perhaps the scene was unremarkable. Yet I noted it anyway, because it seemed to speak to the curiosity I had once so carefully fostered but that had somehow evaporated after I abandoned biotechnology in favor of neurobiology, the curiosity about the relation between life and science. Hadn't Philippe just provided me with an example of how the latter might intersect with the former?

Just a few days later—I had already forgotten about life and science again—I was sitting in the coffee corner of Alain's lab, chatting with Laure Sonnier about her research. Laure, a graduate student of Brigitte, was working on the significance homeoproteins for the birth and survival of new dopaminergic neurons in the substantia nigra. At one point in our conversation we were joined by Christo Goridis, director of a neurochemistry lab located on the same floor as Alain's.

"Neurogenesis exists," he explained after he had listened to our exchange for a while. "It exists in the olfactory bulbs. Fine. But does it have a function as well in the hippocampus? Does it occur in the cortex? Far from clear, even doubtable. In any case, neurogenesis is a minor phenomenon. It might be interesting from a pharmacological perspective, as in Laure's work, but not from a scientific perspective. It will not change the way we think about the brain."

He was staring at us, holding on to his coffee and cigarette. Christo was tall, very thin, and always seemed a bit tense—an impression that his intense way of smoking enforced. His three-day-old beard lent him a sharp, angular look.

"Alain," he raised his voice and head, "he believes in plasticity!"

He took his glasses off, forcefully rubbed his eyes, and then—apparently performing a lecture—continued to instruct us.

"The character of a person is basically formed around age twenty-five. Afterwards this doesn't change anymore. There's no escape!"

With almost exaggeratingly long steps he began walking up and down the little corridor, puffing on his cigarette.

"Whether we like it or not," he went on, "we are machines."

He looked at us, provocatively.

"I know that many people don't like that idea" he went on. "They waste their time and energy to show that man isn't a machine. Only, man *is* a machine. We are machines. In the adult, the neuronal circuits are fixed. They are—and hence we are—regulated by chemical processes. There is no plasticity, the brain is a chemical machine."

I wanted to affirm that people don't like to think of themselves as machines, but before I could finish my sentence, Christo interrupted me with a gesture bordering on the grotesque. He raised his brows and shoulders and looked at me with an intensity that made me feel embarrassed.

"At least when people are sick," I wanted to make my apparently silly comment forgotten, "they like to be machines."

Christo laughed, cranky. "And why? Because machines can be repaired! However," he added with a somber voice while tapping on his head, "this machine is highly complex and we're far away from repairing it."

He stubbed out his cigarette decisively and walked away with his too long steps to continue his experiment or whatever he had been working on.

I was struck by the intensity of Christo's performance—and suddenly felt reminded of my encounter with Philippe a few days earlier. Wasn't Christo's lecture another example of how life and science might interact? Christo's insistence to Laure and me that the brain is a chemical machine had something so intensely machinelike that it was almost frightening. His whole appearance—his sharp, angular look, the mechanical way in which he was smoking, his very long steps, the tenseness with which he spoke and lifted his shoulders and rubbed his eyes—was, in that moment, for me, one of a nervous machine.

Like Philippe, I thought, Christo had performed a statement about the brain, a bodily performances enacted to counter the claim that the brain is plastic.

Walking back to my lab space, I wondered if I could remember a similar encounter with Alain, one that had left me with the impression that he had *met en scène* his plastic conception of the brain. I could not think of any telling incident. Also, I wasn't sure what to look for. What would a bodily enactment of plasticity look like?

The next day I got to the lab early, as I had several experiments to prepare before Gianfranco arrived. Alain must have been waiting for me, for as soon as he saw me walking through the door, he jumped from his chair, ran out of his office, and threw himself in front of me.

"I am not coherent," he shouted. "I don't need a psychoanalysis!"

I was so baffled by his aggressiveness and intensity that at first I couldn't react.

"I am not coherent!" he aggressively repeated. "I don't need a psychoanalysis!"

Why was he so furious?

I tried to calm him down but I could not appease him. As if caught in a loop, he repeatedly shouted that he was not coherent and did not need a psychoanalysis. Eventually, I succeeded in maneuvering him into his office, all the while uttering that I understood, that I was not a psychoanalyst, that of course he was not coherent. In his office, he refused to sit down and stared at me with a challenging posture. I stared back. What had made him work himself up into this rage? The only answer I could think of in that moment was that he was worried that I, the anthropologist, would transform him into what he did not want to be—a coherent person. I explained that I had no idea how he could possibly arrive at the assumption that I would try to make him coherent or to psychoanalyze him.

"I am an anthropologist of your lab," I said, "not of you."

His answer was a strange laugh—something between hysterical and artificial, perhaps with a mild shot of relief.

"I am not coherent, anyway," he added. "So it would be a waste of time." He sat down and began to read his emails. "Isabelle," he said without looking at me, "has very good data. Engrailed seems to have an in vivo function in the guidance of adult retinal axons."

When I left Alain's office, I was thrilled. Wasn't his outrage the exemplary enactment of a plastic conception of the brain that I had been looking for but couldn't find? The enactment of a brain that is neither a fixed chemical machine nor an already wired computer, but instead a living organ characterized by ceaseless cellular becoming?

"Today, the once hegemonic idea that the brain is a stable organ, fully and irreversibly achieved by the end of puberty, is dead," I had heard Alain explain during a lecture he gave at the Cité de Science in La Villette a few months earlier. "In truth, the brain is undergoing a constant renewal. There is nothing that is stable. And therefore it would, from a strictly neurobiological perspective, be wrong to say that we are coherent beings. There is no coherent ego—we are always in the process of becoming."

There is no coherent ego. As in the case of Philippe and Christo, Alain's conception of the brain was not an abstract conceptualization but a physically lived statement about it. Only this time that lived conception wasn't enacted to reject plasticity, but instead to reject what Alain called the *régime fixiste*.

LIFE AND SCIENCE

I was immensely excited by these three events—by the way in which they spoke to and reinforced each other—if only for nostalgic reasons. "Just at the time when I am about to leave France," I scribbled in my notebook, "the relationship that had initially brought me to Paris returned, unexpectedly, out of nowhere, the relationship between life and science."

At least since the 1830s European philosophers have insisted that science—constitutive of modernity—has no relevance for life. Science, they argued, is meaningless because scientific knowledge—rational, sober, objective, value free—is useless for mastering the turbulences that trouble life. Also, it does not provide any answers to the questions that frame a life. Why am I here? Where do I come from? How should I live?[3]

Specifically in nineteenth- and early-twentieth-century Germany the idea consolidated that science cannot provide any guidance for what ever since Greek antiquity has been called *the ethical*—the challenge of relating to oneself, of actively living one's life, of transforming oneself into an object of thought, amidst the irreducible openness that frames life.[4]

I had spent years reading about how life and science became mutually exclusive categories—and began to wonder what would happen when living organisms (humans) produce scientific knowledge about living organisms. Wouldn't humans then be at stake in the research they carry out? And wouldn't that provide them with an ethical vocabulary for how to think—for how to relate to—oneself?

If I was thrilled about my encounters with Philippe, Christo, and Alain, then it was because they spoke precisely to these questions, if from a neuronal rather than, as I had initially envisioned, from a biotechnological perspective. Here were three examples that showed that science—brain science—was not at all meaningless for the ethical challenge of living a life. On the contrary, Philippe, Christo, and Alain were ethically at stake in their science. More than that, all of them were seriously convinced that it was their brain that is constitutive of their humanity, their individuality. Conducting brain research was for each of them a form of work on the self. It was only consequential, therefore, that they used neuronal concepts as ethical tools, as means to transform themselves into an object of thought, to set themselves in relation to themselves, in order to actively live their life in accordance with truth.

"Philippe, Christo, and Alain" my notebook entry concludes, "are all three *neurologically human*."

I enjoyed this reminiscence of the past for a few days and then was ready to let go. As my stay came to a close, time had become precious to me. There were many people I hoped to meet, many conversations I wanted to at least begin so that I could perhaps continue them at a later time. But then a chance discovery pushed my research in an unanticipated direction.

When I was going over the three encounters one last time, I suddenly recognized that they showed not only that science was not meaningless for living a life, but also that different neuronal conceptions of the brain allowed for different ways of living a life and being neurologically human: Philippe, a wired machine; Christo, a chemically regulated machine; and Alain, a plastic organ in process of ceaseless cellular becoming.

The longer I thought about these three different neuronal lives, the more it seemed to me as if I could deduce from them an analytical grid: weren't these episodes suggesting an analytical distinction between, on the one hand, the particular *ethical space* a given neuronal conception of the brain provides for being human (the space of possibilities within which a given conception of the brain—fixity or plasticity—requires one to be human) and, on the other, the always unique *ethical equipment* for living a life it provides to all those who live their life, deliberately or not, as brains (that is, the knowledge, concepts, and metaphors the given conception of the brain offers for making sense of oneself as a brain; here, electrophysiology/wires, neurochemistry/transmitters, and plasticity/movement)?[5]

I was electrified. Not only by the distinction between ethical spaces and equipment as such, but also by the unexpected question this distinction gave rise to: could it be that the emergence of plastic reason was actually an ethical event, insofar as it overthrew the ethical spaces and equipment the neuronal sciences, or at least electrophysiology and neurochemistry, had provided before?

Until that moment my fieldwork had led me to think of plastic reason as a sweeping conceptual event (a conceptual event made possible by nocturnal work, one that had relational refractions and that was only real insofar as it was grounded in experiments). Plasticity, I thought, has been breaking open an unexpected, unruly, not yet conceptually stabilized possibility for thinking and knowing the brain—the human—differently from how it was thought and known thus far.[6] And it was my task, I thought, to study the breaking open of this unruly space.

Now, my encounters with Philippe, Christo, and Alain suggested that I had perhaps missed a significant aspect of the story of plastic reason. Or, at the very least, that an analysis very different from the ones I had already conducted was possible—an ethical analysis.

Could I study the contested emergence of a plastic conception of the brain from an ethical perspective—just as I had studied it before from a relational, conceptual, nocturnal, and experimental vantage?

At stake in this question, or so it seemed to me, was the possibility of a kind of *genealogy of morals* of neuronal knowledge, a history of the neurological human, constituted by the temporal succession (however blurred) of the ethical spaces and equipment that the neuronal sciences had provided over time to all those who lived their lives as brains.[7] At stake as well was the possibility that perhaps plasticity was not so much rejected for conceptual as for ethical reasons.

Could it be that the work on homeoproteins and their nonautonomous transfer caused such resistance, deep anger, and fierce polemics not because it undermined the conceptual horizon that had long structured neuronal knowledge production, but because it threatened to powerfully mutate what it means to be neurologically human? Could it be that it was Alain's plastic way of being—of living a scientific life—which aroused his colleagues' decisive disapproval of plasticity?

What follows is an effort to rethink the emergence of plastic reason in terms of ethical spaces and equipments.

THE NEUROLOGICAL HUMAN, ca. 1891 TO ca. 2002

I returned to the library in the basement of the ENS, though this time not to trace the history of the idea that "synapse is liberty" (as Jean Pierre Bourgeois had it), but rather to research the untold history of the neurological human. What venues for living a life, for being neurologically human, have the neuronal sciences opened up since 1891, when Wilhelm Waldeyer introduced the term *neuron*?[8]

My plan was to read the works that make up the history of neuronal research and to systematically reconstruct (at least some of) the ethical spaces and equipments the neuronal sciences provided from roughly the 1890s to the early 2000s. And my hope was that such a chronological map would allow me to understand whether—and if so, in which concrete ways—the elaboration of a homeoprotein-induced silent embryogenesis in Alain's lab amounted to a radical mutation of (all) earlier figures of the neurological human.[9]

I began my genealogy of morals by turning to Ramón y Cajal, whose histology, strictly speaking, marks the emergence of the neurological human. From Ramón y Cajal I then went to German cytoarchitecture, and from there to the emergence of neuronal electrophysiology. Next I worked through cybernetic theories of the brain and the effort to think the central nervous system in terms of a formal logic of computing. Finally, I moved on to the emergence of neurochemistry, of molecular neurobiology, and of plasticity. For each one of these different neuronal conceptions of the brain I asked three questions.

What is a neuron? How were neurons conceptualized? How were neurons thought to come together and constitute the brain/the human?

Instance of Growth (1890s)

What, for Santiago Ramón y Cajal, was a neuron?

When Ramón y Cajal began to experiment on the brain, little was known about its cellular composition. Was there any sense of order? The central nervous system seemed too complex, too convoluted an organ for anyone to hope that any coherent logic of construction could be discovered.

When I read Ramón y Cajal's oeuvre a second time, I could not help but think that his brilliance was that he approached the challenging complexity of the brain in genealogical terms. Ramón y Cajal's coup was that he deduced from the works of His and Forel a speculation that Golgi's silver-staining method made empirically accessible: if His and Forel were right, that is, if nerve cells are individual, contiguous units, then couldn't one use Golgi's silver-staining method and study how the brain gets built, nerve cell by nerve cell?

What Ramón y Cajal then found when he set out to transform the development of the nervous system into a linear series of ink-pen drawings was that neurons must be thought of as instances of a free, experience-dependent growth—a growth he was among the first to refer to as "arborization."

For Cajal a neuron was a tree. The brain, however, was a forest.[10] All the trees of this forest were generated and put in place during embryogenesis, but the spectacular growth of their branches (axons and dendrites) really took off only after birth. The branches grew and grew until they had used up all the space they had available for their spectacular arborization (i.e., once adulthood was reached). Then, for the rest of its life, the forest was an "essentially" unchanging structure. Some of the branches would eventually dry out and die, which for Ramón y Cajal was an explanation of old age senility and loss of memory.

And the neurological human?

The figure of the neurological human as it emerged from the work of Ramón y Cajal—from his scientific publications, his recommendations to young scientists, his autobiography—was that of an exquisite forest. And the

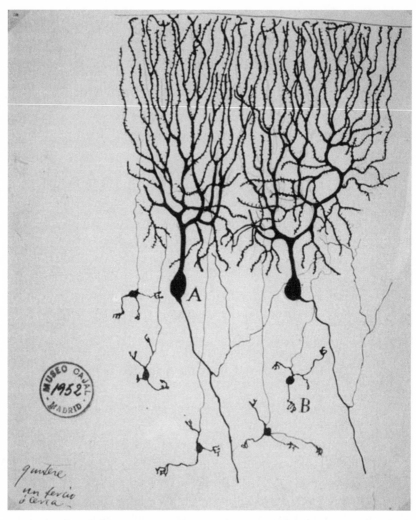

Santiago Ramón y Cajal invented the first neuronal depiction of the human. When the Spanish histologist looked at humans, he saw trees like these. Courtesy of the Instituto Cajal.

challenge of living a life in accordance with neuronal reason was to understand oneself as composed of neuronal trees. To understand oneself, to understand one's humanity, to live true to human nature, meant for Ramón y Cajal, as much as for those who surrounded him (specifically Pío del Río-Hortega and Fernando de Castro), to think of oneself in terms of growing branches. Consequently, the key term of Ramón y Cajal's ethical equipment was "cultivation."

"The cerebral cortex," he wrote in 1894, "is similar to a garden with innumerable trees, the pyramidal cells, which can multiply their branches thanks to intelligent cultivation." And the form this cultivation ideally took—Ramón y Cajal was adamant about this—was the histological work on the brain, with the consequence that his neuronal studies and his work on the self coincided. "My work caused me pleasure," he writes in his autobiography, "a delightful intoxication, on irresistible enchantment. Indeed, leaving aside the egocentric flattery, the garden of neurology offers the investigator captivating spectacles and incomparable artistic emotions."[11]

However, given Ramón y Cajal's concept of "essential fixity," the possibilities for actually cultivating one's forest were rather small. They were small because the ethical space his cerebral forestry allowed for was open only to the growing brain. Self-cultivation was possible almost exclusively to the growing brain. Once adulthood was reached, the forest was already fully grown (almost).[12] In Ramón y Cajal's 1913 formulation: "Once development was ended, the fonts of growth and regeneration of the axons and dendrites dried up irrevocably. In the adult centers, the nerve paths are something fixed and immutable: everything may die, nothing may be regenerated."[13]

Form as Function (ca. 1900)

Only a few years after Ramón y Cajal published the first volumes of his *Textura del Sistema Nervisio* (1897), a somewhat different figure of the neurological human emerged in the work of the German cytoarchitects.[14] The reference here is mainly to the work of Oscar (1870–1959) and Cecile Vogt (1875–1962), Korbinian Brodmann (1869–1918), and Constantin von Economo (1876–1931).

For the cytoarchitects, who ruled the neuronal study of the brain in German-speaking countries from roughly 1900 to the 1930s, a neuron was in principle what it had been for Ramón y Cajal—the individual, freestanding functional unit of the brain. However, where the Spaniard and his students saw the free, experience-dependent growth of neurons as the actual key to understanding the brain, the cytoarchitects had little interest in the concept of growth. What mattered to the Vogts, Brodmann, and von Economo—and their many lesser-known contemporaries, for example, Max Borcherdt and Max Lewandowsky—was not the free arborization of the fine structure, but the morphological classification of the different kinds of neurons out of which the cerebral cathedral was constructed.[15]

For the cytoarchitects a neuron was thus an organic building block. And the task of the cytoarchitect was to discover the architectural logic—the construction plan—that organized the brain, organ of the human.

The main analytical tool available to cytoarchitects was the section cutter. After they had removed a brain from the skull, they froze it, cut it in extremely thin slices, and then stained them, usually with a method invented by the German pathologist Franz Nissl (Nissl staining). From such stained brain slices, they reconstructed the always singular, cell-architectural composition of a brain and its different histological areas. The majority of these reconstructions took one of two forms. On the one hand, there were carefully crafted topographical maps. The aim here was to distinguish different brain areas from one another, exclusively by looking at form, pattern of arborization, and density of cells. The results were often stunningly beautiful brain maps, of which Brodmann's map of the cortex remains the most famous.

From 1901 to 1909, Brodmann, working at the neurobiological laboratory at the University of Berlin, had endeavored to come up with, in his words, "a topographic analysis of the human cortex with respect to its cellular construction." His ambition was to uncover the "laws of construction of the cortex," to identify the "organizational principle" that underlay "the construction plan of the cortex cerebri." After eight years of cutting, staining, and drawing, Brodman had identified fifty-four distinct cortical areas, which he grouped into eleven histological regions.

On the other hand, the cytoarchitects used their inquiries into the brain's construction logic to find means to correlate form and function. Carefully they compared the brains of different human beings according to their construction logic and then sought to discover links between character traits and the size and density of particular brain areas. Oscar Vogt's analysis of Lenin's brain is, if not the most significant then certainly the best-known exploration of the neuro-architectural basis of the human. Shortly before Lenin's death in 1924, Vogt was consulted for his medical advice and then, after Lenin had died, Vogt asked to study the cerebral basis of his intellectual capacities. According to Vogt, Lenin's exceptional intellect was the consequence of the high density of unusually large pyramidal cells—he referred to them as associative cells—in the cortex.

What figure of the neurological human emerged from the works of the early-twentieth-century cytoarchitects? What ethical space, what ethical equipment, did the writings of the Vogts or of Brodmann provide to all those researchers, patients, and laypeople who lived their lives under the spell of the brain?

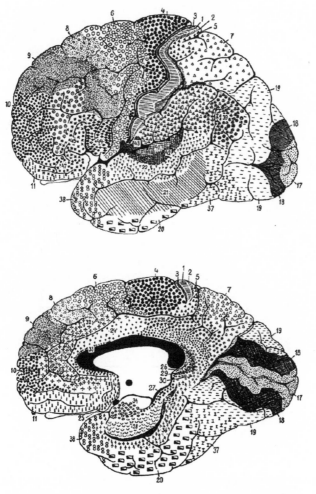

Brodmann's map of cortical areas. Each area was composed of one distinctive morphological type of neuron. For Brodmann and his colleagues, such maps were the neuronal equivalent of the human and could capture, if focused on individual variations, the neuronal basis of an individual's traits, capacities, and potential. From Brodmann 1909.

I came away from readings in cytoarchitecture with a sense that the ethical space opened by the study of the cellular construction logic of the brain was exquisitely minimal, perhaps even more so than it had been for Ramón y Cajal and his students. For whereas the Spanish foresters had allowed for at least some growth, and hence for some possibility of self-cultivation, the German cartographers of cerebral architectures viewed the brain as fully

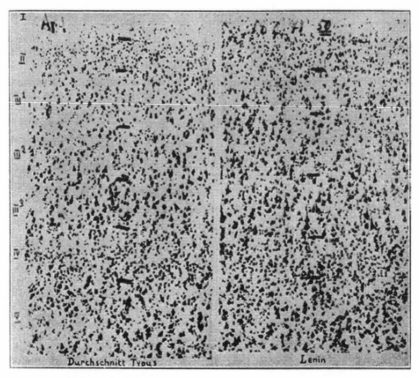

The cytoarchitects invented a new kind of neuronal depiction of the human. Here, Oskar Vogt's comparison of an average brain (*left*) with Lenin's cortex. According to Vogt, Lenin's intelligence was the result of an above-average density of well-branched pyramidal cells (visible in the form of black spots). From Kahn 1929.

constructed. Once adulthood was achieved, the building was complete and it was impossible to add new architectural elements.

The ethical equipment that emerged from cytoarchitecture, however, differed markedly from the one provided by Ramón y Cajal's human forestry. For the cytoarchitects the challenge was no longer to think of oneself as the direct result of the particular growth of trees and branches, which could be trimmed, straightened, and hedged. Rather, the challenge was to understand oneself as architectural form. To live true to nature required thinking of oneself in terms of cell density, form, morphology, composition, and also volume. To be neurologically human, at least in one province of neuronal reason in the early twentieth century, meant to be an organic, architectural structure.

What the German cytoarchitects shared with Spanish forestry was an organic understanding of the brain. For the cytoarchitects, the brain had to be understood as a *Gebilde* (construct or formation), as organized by a *Bildungsplan* or *Bildungsgesetz* (construction plan or law of formation). The key concept, made popular by Johan Gottfried Herder in the late eighteenth century, was *Bildung,* a term which means both "organic formation" and "construction." And for the Spanish epigeneticists, the brain was the result of naturally occurring growth.

At the turn of the twentieth century, a radically different kind of neuronal brain began to flourish in physiology labs in London and Cambridge. At stake in Britain was neither growth nor *Bildung*—histology had never really arrived in a country dominated by physiologists—but instead the technical prospect of inventing tools fine enough to allow for the study of how nervous impulses, electricity, flow from one set of neurons to another. What thrilled the young Keith Lucas, Charles Sherrington, and Edgar Adrian was not organic growth but the possibility of getting to know the brain as an electrical machine.

How and along which paths does nerve information travel? Where and how are nerve impulses coordinated? And how does this coordination allow the organism to adapt to the environment?

Sherrington's answer to these questions was the "synapsis," that is, the electrical reaction that he speculated would occur in the gap between dendrites and axons, at least in the cerebellum, and that would somehow integrate and coordinate the electrical stimuli that the periphery sent to the center (and vice versa).[16] Lucas and Adrian, working in Cambridge, had little interest in the speculative concept of the synapse. What interested them, rather, was their finding that the flow of information from one area of the nervous system to another—they had focused on the relations between the retina and optic nerve—was highly patterned.[17] And their hope was that they could correlate the logic of these patterns to different brain functions.

In the still-young conceptual history of the neuron, its electrification was a sweeping event. If for cytoarchitects a neuron had been a structural building block and for the histologists an instance of free growth, for the electrophysiologists a neuron had become an electrical information-processing unit in systematic relation with other such units. And whereas the histologists and cytoarchitects viewed the brain as an organically grown—or built—

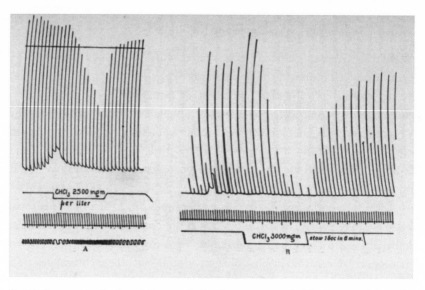

A radically new visualization of the neurological human emerged with electrophysiology. For electrophysiologists, graphs like this one, taken from Sherrington (1906), were the true representation of the human. To live a life in accordance with neuronal reason now meant to learn to think of oneself in terms of wiring, electrical flow, and transmission of information.

structure, the electrophysiologists understood the brain as an exquisitely complex switchboard.

For Sherrington, Lucas, and Adrian, as for their many students, postdocs, and other followers, humans were neither forests nor architectural constructions but simply electrically wired machines.

Along with the shift from the organic to the electrical came a whole, previously unknown ethical equipment. The challenge of living a life in accordance with neuronal reason, of being neurologically human, entailed thinking of oneself with concepts borrowed from the nascent sciences of electrical engineering and telecommunication studies: wires, charges, information processing, electrodes, telegraph, switchboards, reaction. To be neurologically human in early-twentieth-century Britain was to live one's life as an electrical machine.

Yet, however thoroughly electrophysiology changed what it meant to be neurologically human, it hardly changed the ethical space available to those who lived their lives as brains. Neuronal reason had mutated, radically so, and along with it the ethical equipment. However, for Sherrington and Adrian, just as for Ramón y Cajal or the Vogts, the mature central nervous system was a fixed and immutable structure. If anything, the electrical machine was even more structurally rigid than the brain of its organic predecessors.

As Philippe Ascher put it in our conversation in his laboratory, "There simply is not space for plastic changes in the adult. [...] The brain is already wired." Of course, much changed in electrophysiology from the early days of Sherrington and Adrian to the days of Philippe Ascher. A large series of new tools and concepts were invented—from the capillary electrometer (1870s) to mini-electrodes (1950s) and patch clamps (1970s), from the conception of the synapsis as an electrical reaction (1890s) to the end-plate potential (1930s) and long-term potentiation (1970s). Each of these tools and concepts further contributed to and slightly changed the ethical equipment provided to neurological humans. And yet each of these technical and conceptual innovations stayed within the framework established by the original application of electrophysiology to the neuronal brain.

For electrophysiologists, the brain, and along with it the human, remained, from the late 1890s to the late 1990s, an immutable electrical machine made up of already wired neurons.

Computers (ca. 1940s)

The next mutation of the neurological human occurred in the 1940s and was prompted by the emergence of cybernetics in the United States and Britain.

The effort to conceive of the brain in terms of mathematical computation emerged somewhat rapidly. If in the mid-1930s it was still unknown, by the mid-1950s almost all of the major works (and machines) that prepared the ground for analyzing the brain as a computation machine were published (built).

A beginning was made in 1937. That year, Alan Turing, then a young mathematician at Cambridge, published a paper, "On Computable Numbers," in which he sought to challenge an argument the Austrian mathematician Kurt Gödel (1906–1978) had presented in 1931—that systems, or machines, were capable of only the most trivial versions of arithmetic computation. Young Turing felt provoked by Gödel's delimitation of mechanical computation and worked out a sketch for a machine, later known as the Turing machine, that in principle could solve any mathematical problem, no matter how complex.[18]

In the early 1940s, two researchers at the University of Chicago—Waren McCulloch (1898–1969), a neurophysiologist who had worked for years on the functional (electrical) activity of the cerebral cortex of chimpanzees, and Walter Pitts (1923–1969), a young logician who had worked with Rudolf von Carnap—wondered whether they could find a way to formalize cellular transmission to such a degree that they could apply Turing's theory of computation to the neuronal brain as it had emerged since the 1890s. In 1943, after a year of discussion, the two published the first explicit computational conception of the central nervous system, "The Logical Calculus of Ideas Imminent in Nervous Activity."

Once Turing had established the possibility of a machine capable of solving complex mathematical problems, and after McCulloch and Pitts had established the formal possibility of applying models of computing machines to the neuronal brain, W. Grey Walter (1910–1977), Ross Ashby (1903–1972), and John von Neumann (1903–1957) sought to integrate the brain with what by then was increasingly called "the computer."[19]

In 1948, the year Norbert Wiener coined the term *cybernetics,* Grey Walter, an American-born, British-educated neurophysiologist, built the first electronic autonomous robots—he named them "Elmar" and "Elsie"—and advertised them with the claim that they, their technical make up, could serve to explain the "secret organization of living organisms."[20] The same year, Ross Ashby, a British psychiatrist, presented what he called the Homeostat, the first automated computing engine capable of adapting itself to the environment. And after Ashby published his *Designs for a Brain* (1952), an effort to think of the brain in terms of mechanistic design, Walter began to build CORA, an automaton organized around a Pavlovian reflex circuit that allowed the machine to be conditioned.[21] Finally in 1951, John von Neumann, a Hungarian-born mathematician and physicist at Los Alamos, presented a paper in which he worked out the possibility of understanding cells as self-regulating automata—subsequently called von Neumann automata—an idea that he later, in his 1957 *The Brain and the Computer,* systematized and expanded.[22]

What conception of the neuronal brain—of neurons—was made possible by the emergence of computational brain science? From a cybernetic perspective, a neuron was neither about free arborization nor was it an organic form element. Rather, it was a formalized unit of logical operation. On the one hand, this formal and algorithmic understanding of neurons was not all that different from the electrophysiological conception of a neuron as an information-processing electrical unit. Both looked at the brain as an electrical machine of sorts, and both largely disdained the organicism of their histological predecessors. On the other hand, cybernetics pushed in a direction very different from the application of mini-electrodes to single neurons. Not that McCulloch, Pitts, Grey, Ashby, or von Neumann lacked interest in actual mini-electron recordings of the action potential of neurons. But most of the cyberneticists were logicians, not electrophysiologists. What excited them was less the invention of a new recording devices than the formal possibility to think of the brain as a self-regulating automaton, that is, as an algorithmic machine, a computer. What excited them, as well, was the possibility of thinking of machines as brains.

And the neurological human?

With the emergence of cybernetics, a whole new ethical repertoire of sense making emerged. With respect to the cybernetic brain, the challenge for those living their lives in accordance with neuronal reason became to think of themselves with the help of a language directly derived from the theory of closed signaling systems: input, output, feedback loops, and signaling were the major ethical concepts. To be human now was to be a large, self-replicating machine organized as an algorithmic exclusion chart: if this, then not that. The idea of control had replaced the idea of cultivation as the main venue of work on the self, as the major form of ethical practice.

However, even though the cybernetic researchers so clearly broke with the organic brains that had flourished in Spain and Germany around 1900, the computational brain they elaborated was still, if silently, organized by an observation first made by the organicists: that the adult human brain is fixed and immutable. Cybernetics was contingent on the presupposition that the brain was a closed system. The ethical consequence of this contingency was that the ethical space provided by cybernetics, just like the space provided by electrophysiology, hardly differed from the one provided by the histologists (whether foresters or architects). It was still the exquisitely minimal space that first emerged with Ramón y Cajal.[23]

Neurochemical Machines (ca. 1950s)

In the immediate aftermath of cybernetics, the most radical mutation in the early history of neuronal reason occurred—the rise of neurochemistry.

After neurons had been instances of growth, trees, architectural building blocks, forms, and information-processing units, the works of Wilhelm Feldberg, Alfred Fessard, Stephen Kuffler, Bernhard Katz, and John Eccles

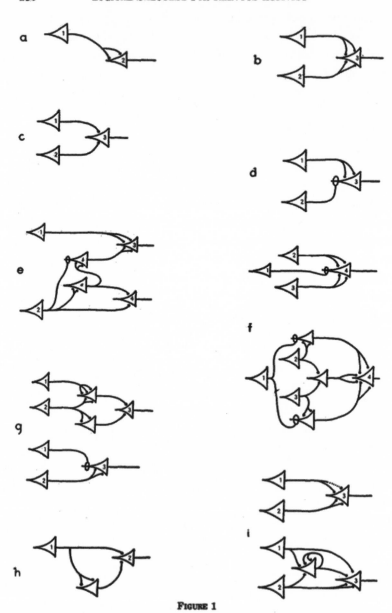

FIGURE 1

With the emergence of cybernetics, a whole new, previously unknown visual—and ethical—vocabulary for representing the true neuronal grounds of the human emerged. With the works of Turing, McCulloch, Pitts, Grey, and von Neumann, the human became an automaton, an algorithm executed by neurons. From McCulloch and Pitts 1943.

made them into chemical factories for the production of neurotransmitter substances to be released or taken up by synapses. The brain became a chemical, synaptic machine.

The international—global—emergence of neurochemistry after World War II brought about a most far-reaching conceptual and experimental reconfiguration of the neuronal sciences. The chemical inquiry into the brain not only changed what a neuron is but also brought about previously unthought-of ways for understanding the functional makeup of the brain. For example, if, up until the mid-twentieth century, morphological studies were the only way to map the cellular organization of the brain, Eccles's 1954 observation that most neurons produce but one single neurotransmitter allowed for a whole new, chemical understanding of brain topography.[24] In the aftermath of Eccles, chemists around the world began to classify neurons according to the one transmitter substance they produced—GABAergic neurons, cholinergic neurons, serotonergic neurons, dopaminergic neurons, and so on—and to discover that the distinctive morphological cell types histologists had described corresponded to distinctive chemical types: there were whole neurotransmitter-specific regions of the brain, just as there were large-scale neurotransmitter-specific networks that linked various brain areas together. It was the discovery of the chemical topography of the brain that soon then allowed links to be uncovered between specific chemical areas and mental and chemical processes, specifically between dopamine and excitement, and norepinephrine and depression.[25]

With the emerging dominance of neurochemistry, the human was enrolled in a whole new rationality, with the effect that a previously unknown ethical equipment for thinking of oneself—for living one's life—emerged. The language of wires and computers was quickly replaced with concepts such as catecholamines, inhibitors, epinephrine, receptors, dopamine, reuptake, serotonin, and acetylcholine. To be neurologically human, now, was to understand oneself as a chemical, synaptic machine. And for hundreds of millions of humans it meant understanding themselves in terms of a chemical imbalance that left them depressed, schizophrenic, or manic—and, hence, in need of chemical adjustment. To be neurologically human, beginning in the mid-1950s, meant to be a neurochemical self.[26]

And the ethical space available for those neurochemical selves?

Even though neurochemistry provided a previously unknown vocabulary for relating to oneself, primarily with respect to mood and behavior, the space within which it was possible to live one's life as brain was still the

What neurochemists saw when they looked at the human was a chemical composition. With the rise in the 1950s of neurochemistry, the human became accessible by—and thus was simultaneously transformed into—a set of chemical diagrams like this one, taken from Schildkraut's 1965 paper on affective disorders. To be happy or sad, to be angry or in love was now reducible to a chemical composition.

minimalist space it had been before. The neurochemical selves that emerged after the 1950s were as immutable as their electrical and anatomical predecessors. Fixity, here too, defined the limits of the possible (the human).

Genetics (1980s)

The last (major) reconfiguration of the neurological human before the emergence of plasticity was brought about by the application, at the turn from the

1970s to the 1980s, of the tools of molecular neurobiology to the study of the brain. That came as a surprise for me. During my fieldwork I had frequently heard, primarily from chemists and electrophysiologists, but from Alain and Michel Volovitch as well, that the arrival of molecular cell biology in the neuronal sciences did not significantly change the understanding of the brain that had emerged with neurochemistry.[27] As Philippe put it (and Alain might have agreed), "The arrival of molecular biology didn't add any basic insights. It did not revolutionize our conception of the brain." However, when I began working systematically through the first articles that analyzed neurons or neuron-to-neuron communication in terms of genes—the earliest papers came from the labs of Jean Pierre Changeux (Pasteur Institute), Francis Crick (Salk Institute), and Eric Kandel (Columbia)—I found that these papers actually did "revolutionize our understanding of the brain." Perhaps the revolution was subtle—but its effect was nonetheless powerful and far-reaching; it thoroughly changed the conceptual understanding of what a neurons is.

The argument of many of the neuronal researchers who had belittled the significance of molecular biology was that the study of the brain in genetic terms was "only" an event on the level of tools. As Alain put it, "Molecular biology was a methodological, not a conceptual advance."

On the one hand, this emphasis of the methodological was fair. Up until the late 1970s, the predominant ways to analyze the brain came from either chemistry or electrophysiology. The former enabled researchers to determine which transmitter substance a given neuron metabolized, and the latter to record the electrical impulses triggered by the release or uptake of transmitter substances. Exquisite knowledge was produced with the help of these methods. The chemical topography of the brain was mapped; relationships between neurochemicals and affective disorders were established; the intensity with which synapses communicate were successfully correlated to a panoply of behaviors, notably memory formation.

With the arrival of genetics, however, a whole new, much finer-grained analytical possibility for understanding the neuronal brain opened up—the analysis of the molecular processes that presumably coordinate the production, release, and uptake of neurotransmitters. More than that, simply by tagging and then following a given molecule, one could now trace concrete synaptic circuits in ways formerly thought impossible. And one could, for each molecular movement of the brain, identify the genes that actually code for these molecules. Molecular neurobiology was thus a major methodological opening.

On the other hand, however, the reduction of recombinant DNA technologies to a mere method concealed the powerful conceptual innovation that this method actually transported. For the effect of the works of Crick and Changeux and of their many successors was that they enlisted the neuron in the genetic rationality that had been assembled since the early twentieth century.

With the rise of molecular studies of the brain, neurons became what they had never been before: one kind of biological cells among many other biological cells, each endowed with a genome, made up of protein-coding genes that would organize the organism, each to be understood in the terms of molecular cell biology. And synaptic communication became what it had never been before as well: one variant of biological cell-to-cell communication by way of the release or uptake of signaling molecules, the production of which was controlled by—what else?—genes.

Of course, one could still look at neurons as information-transmitting units, as a computation event, or as a metabolic factory. And of course mini-electrodes didn't disappear from labs. However, underneath these processes—transmission, computation, metabolism—neuronal researchers now discovered what had emerged since the 1950s as the universal language of life: DNA, RNA, proteins. And the consequence was that mini-electrodes were increasingly marginalized, or at least decentered, by the arrival of a whole new technical armamentarium that was constitutive of the molecular vision of life: blotting and PCR and sequencing machines, centrifuges, bioassays, refrigerators, cell culture rooms, antibodies and anti-antibodies, pipits, calf-medium, and so forth.

The effect of the molecularization of the neuron on the neurological human is perhaps best described as *continuity across change*: *continuity,* because the basic conception of the brain as composed of neurotransmitter-specific neurons that are organized through chemistry and function-specific synaptic circuits was little altered by the arrival of the machines and apparatuses of molecular biology; and *across change,* because the genetic analysis of neurons significantly altered the understanding of the actual cell biological events (rather than merely chemical or electrical happenings) that constitute transmitter production and "synaptic signaling" (as it was now called).

Humans thus continued for much of the 1980s and 1990s to be neurochemical selves. However, the ethical equipment available for neurological humans changed significantly. Whereas until the early 1980s the challenge was to think of oneself in terms of available amounts of neurotransmitters, living true to human nature now required understanding that the production of neurotransmitters was organized by transcriptional and translational processes in neurons. The concepts available for sense making were no longer, at least no longer exclusively, composed of a chemical vocabulary that revolved around secretion, inhibition, or metabolism but were instead made up of a biological language of DNA, amino acids, SNPs, transcription factors, splicing, RNA, signaling molecules, modulation, and many other terms.

What didn't change, however, yet again, was the ethical space available for adapting to neuronal reason. Again the opportunity for work on the self was limited to the narrow confines of a fixed brain.

Plasticity

And plasticity? What was a neuron for Alain or Michel or Brigitte?

It may sound curious but I think that a neuron was in Alain's lab what it had been for the histologists of the late nineteenth and early twentieth century, an instance of free, experience-dependent growth (and a matter of form). That said, there was one far-reaching difference between Alain, Joliot, Michel, Brigitte, and Trembleau on the one hand and their nineteenth-century predecessors on the other. For the histologists the growth of new neurons was (ever since Richard Altmann's 1881 privately printed article) restricted to embryogenesis and the growth of the fine structure (ever since Ramón y Cajal's 1897 *Textura*) to the period of development. For Alain and his colleagues, however, neuronal growth, whether of new neurons or of the fine structure, occurred throughout life. On the seventh floor of the Rue d'Ulm, neither the neuronal composition of the brain nor the form of a neuron ever stood still: the brain was never actually fully developed (or accomplished). A neuron, beginning at some point around 1990, became an instance of ceaseless movement, at least in one Parisian lab.[28]

The effects of the mutation of neuronal reason in terms of movement and growth—once it left the confines of Alain's lab and intermingled with adult neurogenesis research (around the year 2000)—were perhaps the most radical and far-reaching in the one-hundred-year history of the neurological human. Just how radical and far-reaching becomes visible when one arranges in chronological order the different figures of the neurological human that have existed in the history of the neuronal sciences. Two observations stand out. The first one is the frequency with which quite radically new ethical sets of equipment were made available to neurological humans.[29] Arguably, it

glu gln ser glu gly gln asn pro glu thr glu ser his ser arg arg lys arg ser
gag cag tcg gaa gga caa aat cct gaa acg gaa agc cac tca agg aga aaa cgg tct

val leu thr pro ser leu ser ser leu gly glu ser leu glu ser gly ile se rlys arg
gtc cta acg cct tcg ctt tcg agt ctt ggt gag ctc gag tca ctc gag tct gga atc tct aaa cga

```
1    2    3    4    5    6    7    8    9   10   11   12   13   14   15   16   17   18   19   20
ile  ser  ile  asn  gln  asp  leu  lys  ala  ile  thr  asp  met  leu  leu  thr  glu  gln  ile  arg
atc  tcc  atc  aac  cag  gac  ttg  aag  gct  atc  aca  gac  atg  ctg  ctt  aca  gag  caa  atc  cga

21   22   23   24   25   26   27   28   29   30   31   32   33   34   35   36
glu  arg  gln  arg  tyr  leu  ala  asp  leu  arg  gln  arg  leu  leu  glu  leu  lys  gly  lys  arg  ser
gaa  agg  caa  agg  tat  ctc  gct  gac  tta  cgc  caa  cgt  ctc  ttg  gaa  aag  ggc  aag  cgg  agt
```

ser gly val ser leu leu thr ser asn lys gly arg gly asn cys *** ***
tct ggc gtc agt ctg ctc acct cc aac aaa ggc aga ggg aac tgc tgaaagcgataagca

acctcttgaactaatgaaacagtctgtaa

The machines and apparatuses of molecular cell biology opened a new chapter in the history of the neuronal depiction of the human. For geneticists, the human brain and its function are reducible to a linear series of nucleotide sequences. Rows and columns of letters like these are thus the direct equivalent of the human. From Scheller et al. 1982.

makes quite a difference if one actively thinks of oneself—if one actively seeks to live one's life—in terms of the architectural logic of neuroanatomy, the engineering logic of electrophysiologists, the chemical (or pharmacological) logic of neurochemists, the cybernetic logic of communication scientists, the genetic logic of neurobiologists, or the plastic logic brought about by Alain's lab. Each of these approaches offers a different kind of ethical equipment for living a (neurological) life: different words, concepts, metaphors, and images for making sense of one's existence.[30]

The second striking observation is the relative continuity of the ethical space available to neurological humans. No matter how sweeping the mutations in the ethical equipment available to neurological humans, the differences were quite negligible—until the emergence of plastic reason. They were negligible because the ethical spaces these various conceptions provided were essentially identical. No matter how one thought about or experimented on the brain, it was always imagined as a fixed and immutable anatomy or machine.

The significance of the emergence of plastic reason has been that it radically broke with this continuity by mutating, for the first time, not just the ethical equipment but also the ethical space available for those who live their lives as brains.

Plastic reason mutated the ethical space in that where the nonautonomous transfer of homeoproteins triggers plastic changes in the adult—whether by the proliferation, differentiation, and migration of new neurons, or the appearance and disappearance of synapses, or the continuous sprouting of axons and dendrites—there is no more need to conceptualize the human, no more need to find means to conceptualize the human, from the perspective of fixed and immutable circuits, chemical or electrical. On the contrary, with the advent of plasticity the challenge is to conceptualize the human—to live a life—from the vantage point of a brain believed to continuously change, to undergo ceaseless morphogenetic transformations. It is almost a one-to-one inversion: Where once fixity reigned, now plasticity rules. Where once the basic feature of the neurological human was immutability, it is now openness, its openness toward the future, its capacity for ongoing adaptation.

And plastic reason mutated the ethical equipment in that once the neurological human ceases to be "essentially fixed," it also ceases to be an immutable structure, an electrical switchboard, a chemical machine, or an information-processing computer. And with this cessation a large part of the ethical repertoire assembled over the course of the twentieth century has been marginalized. The language of wires, switchboards, computers, programs, neurotransmitters and receptors—once so central for thinking of the human, for making sense of oneself and of one's experiences—no longer applies to a brain characterized by an ongoing silent embryogenesis. It is replaced by talk about growth, differentiation, proliferation, flexibility, morphogenesis, adaptation, individuation, and the like.[31] For the first time in more than a century of neuronal research a radically novel, plastic figure of the neurological human emerged.

Was this sweeping mutation the key to understanding the conflicts that surrounded the work of Alain's lab?

A BATTLE ABOUT THE HUMAN

During my final month in Paris, July 2003, I picked up a new habit that was to stay with me for years: I began to systematically collect and read biographies, biosketches, obituaries, autobiographies, and autobiographic sketches of neuronal researchers. One effect of accumulating masses of life reflections in neuronal terms was that at one point I recognized that the relative continuity of the ethical challenge of living a life within the fairly narrow confines the fixed neuronal brain allowed for had led, already in the early twentieth century, to an ethos that I gradually came to think of as *the heroic*.

The heroic, because twentieth-century neuronal conceptions of the brain required, at least from all those living their lives as brains, a "heroic" act: to submit their lives, their physical existence, their mental particularities to the narrow space that the different comprehensions of the brain as fixed allowed for. *Heroic* this act was not, as a romantic take would suggest, because life in all of its perplexity, irrationality, and intensity had to be subordinated to science as such: the sober, neutral, rational—but rather because science, the anti-romantic, de-illusionary, realistic practice that it has been for most of the authors I read (and talked to) required heroically facing the scientific truth that we are fixed and immutable machines.[32]

In Christo's exemplary words: "Whether we like it or not, we are machines. I know that many people don't like that idea; they waste their time and energy to show that man isn't a machine. Only, man *is* a machine. We are machines. There is no escape!" Or, as Philippe put it, "The brain is already wired; it really is!"

The more I read, the more it seemed as if the heroic effort to live a sober life within the narrow confines the neuronal sciences provided for being human had been, throughout the twentieth century, the precondition of becoming, and remaining, a good and successful neuronal researcher. The heroic—think of Philippe's and Christo's efforts to contain the possibility of the plastic— was an ethical practice based on which neuronal researchers judged each other; it was a code of conduct that helped them evaluate themselves, their colleagues, and, especially, their juniors, whether they were histologists, electrophysiologists, logicians, chemists, or geneticists. The heroic was the normative ethos of the discipline: show me how you live, and I will tell you if you have the potential to be—to become—a good neuronal researcher.

All those who didn't submit to this heroic ethos—who made claims about the nervous system incommensurable with a vision of the brain as fixed— were looked at as unscientific or, when things became more intense, as irrationals, metaphysicians or enemies of science. Those who claimed that new neurons are added to the adult brain—Joseph Altman in the 1960s, Michael Kaplan in the 1970s, Fernando Nottebohm in the 1980s, Elizabeth Gould and Fred Gage in the 1990s—are a case in point. They were, just like Alain, isolated, ridiculed, and confined to the margins.[33]

If one looks at the emergence of plastic reason from the vantage of the heroic, the intense turbulences that surrounded Alain's claim for plasticity appear in a new light: as the fallout from a most intense battle about the human—what it is, how it should be lived. What I mean by this is that what made Alain—his work, his way of being, his performance of the neuronal sciences—so outrageous was perhaps not only, perhaps not even primarily, that his insistence on a homeoprotein-induced plasticity was conceptually irreconcilable with the fixed and immutable cellular structure the brain had been for so long. Certainly, the emergence of plastic reason was a conceptual scandal; however, my readings in the ethical history of the neuronal sciences led me to think that a much more significant reason for the outrage provoked by Alain was that his work amounted to a sincere claim that the neuronal understanding of the human on which the heroic was based was, well, wrong—that it was a relic, an artifact from a time when we did not yet really understand the brain. For the heroic only made sense as long as the brain was an immutable structure.

Perhaps one has to pause for a moment to appreciate the full scale of the provocation that plasticity has posed. When Alain claimed that the brain is plastic—when he aggressively began to live the plastic—he not only performed a new neurological human but also confronted his colleagues with the claim that they were living an unscientific image of the human.

They may have been ethically inclined—but they failed to live in accordance with reason.

My new habit of collecting and reading neuronal sketches of the self had gradually mutated my understanding of the stakes of plastic reason. At stake in the battles that surrounded Alain's lab, or so it seemed to me then and now (2015), were hardly scientific, conceptual disagreements alone. At stake, rather, was the ethical question how one should relate to oneself, how one should live life truthfully.

At stake was the human.

My encounters with Philippe, with Christo, and with Alain were windows onto this lived debate.[34]

I wonder if one couldn't rethink other controversies in ethical terms?

Humility

"I have time right now," Alain approached me from behind. "Would you like to talk?" I remember being surprised. Why did he want to talk to me?

It was a Tuesday morning in early May 2003. During the previous months that I had spent in his lab, Alain had never approached me with a similar offer. It was almost always the other way round—I wanted to talk and asked him if he would have time.

I looked at Gianfranco, with whom I had been chatting. He nodded, suggesting that we continue our conversation later.

"Sure," I replied, grabbed my pen and notebook, and followed Alain to his office.

"I know you have to write about your work here," he eventually began.

From previous conversations I knew that he was worried about what I would write about his lab.

"You should write whatever you want," he went on. "This is none of my business."

I smiled.

"I just want to give you one piece of advice." He looked at the floor, hiding his face, and paused. "I don't want to appear as if I am right."

Only now Alain turned to me, revealing a despair I had never before seen in him. "Please don't write as if I am right," he repeated. "I might have gotten everything wrong, from day one onward."

I admired Alain. I found myself impressed by his extraordinary wit and intellect, by his apparent courage, by the heat of his passion and the devastation of his anger. Never would it have occurred to me that, all along, he had been haunted by doubts and despair—until that day in early May 2003.

Only a few weeks earlier, in April, experiments were for the first time suggesting that homeoproteins did indeed transfer in various brain regions, throughout life. That Alain introduced me to his doubts in the moment of a possible triumph was not only moving; it was also a way of initiating me to the ethos with which he practiced and understood science. Indeed, it could still be that there was no homeoprotein-induced plasticity, neither during development nor in adulthood. But even if homeoproteins were the plastic forces Alain envisioned them to be (which seemed likely in spring 2003), it would be inappropriate to present the story of his lab's work as a triumph, for that would suggest that he and his friends—Joliot, Michel, Brigitte, Trembleau—had gotten it right. But who could tell? Those working in the lab since the early 1990s had learned to distrust scientists (among others) who claim to be right and speak in the name of the truth.

"I am not a man of truth," Alain once informed a baffled audience at the end of a talk, "but a man of doubt."[1]

"Of doubt," he later told me, "because doubt assures movement."

For Alain, the task of science was not to build the house of truth, brick by brick, adding discovery upon discovery. The story of his research gradually taught him to think of science differently: as the challenge of keeping the horizon open, of appreciating the accidental that unexpectedly opens possibilities for thinking that have never before occurred to oneself, possibilities that perhaps derail how one has thought thus far. Science as doubt was not about the production of truth—or at least not exclusively. Rather, it was about the production and maintenance of humility, a grateful appreciation of one's ignorance.

Of course there are many in the sciences who appreciate ignorance. But more often than not, ignorance is celebrated as an invitation to keep on building the house of truth: there is *still* much to discover. If I were to abstract from what I learned during my stay in Alain's lab, I would say that this is a naïve ignorance, an ignorance without doubt (and the sense of humility that follows from it): for it is the doubt vis-à-vis all truth claims, especially one's own, that opens up the possibility of novelty, of being surprised, of learning new things. And it is the constant overflowing of the already thought and known, made possible by doubt (and discovery), that makes ignorance a continuous, not a temporary condition of science.

Indeed, the story of plastic reason hasn't been about the triumph of truth but about the triumph of doubt—and of the surplus of possibilities of truth that doubt has given rise to, a surplus no one can ever exhaust. My aim has been to capture something of this surplus—as well as its effects.

SEVEN

Letting Go

I left Paris for the first time in summer 2003. In 2005 I briefly returned to conduct a few follow-up interviews and to ask some clarifying questions. It was good being back. I enjoyed seeing my old friends and learning how their research had continued. My next return, however, in 2006, was very disconcerting.

It may sound naïve, but while I was writing a first version of *Plastic Reason,* the story of the lab and its research had gradually sedimented into a story with a clear beginning (the 1989 observation) and a clear end (the turn to physiology and Alain's election to the Collège de France). But what I found upon my return was that while "my" story had an end, the story of the lab had continued.

The overarching questions that had structured the work of the lab from its inception in 1989 to 2004–2005 when the first papers on the function of the nonautonomous transfer were published, was, Do homeoproteins transfer between cells? Is this transfer an important embryological process, one that organizes the cellular emergence of the brain, one that renders the adult brain plastic? My research had followed the emergence of these questions and the efforts to answer them. And once they were answered, my story had come to an end. What I now found myself confronted with, however, was that the answers that concluded my story were merely the beginnings of a new episode in a story much larger than my research.

Also, the people who had advanced the lab's experimental system when I conducted my fieldwork—postdocs such as Gianfranco and Maria-Luz, PhD students such as Laure, Isabelle, Stéphane, and Michel Tassetto—were no longer there. The friends with whom I had shared my time, who had taught me what relationalism means, had all left. They had finished their research, secured postdocs or research positions elsewhere, and had been replaced by a new cohort of graduate students I didn't know (and who didn't know me). Even though the seniors were still all there, the lab was no longer the same. It was relationally differently composed and hence a somewhat different place.

When I left Paris after my visit in 2006, I had for the first time a vague sense that the field was beginning to outgrow the story I had been part of and could tell. This sense of parting ways—of outgrowth—was intensified when I returned to Paris again three years later. By 2009, the lab around which my story had revolved no longer existed.

When Alain moved from the ENS to the Collège, he reinvented his lab. Aside from himself, I knew no one anymore. Alain Trembleau and Bernadette Allinquant had launched their own labs, which were located elsewhere and centered on questions that had nothing to do with homeoproteins and their nonautonomous transfer. Alain Joliot had also moved to the Collège, but not as member of Alain's lab. He was now director of his own research team. Joliot was still studying homeoproteins, but his research focused on curiosities very different from Alain's. And Michel Volovitch and Brigitte Lesaffre had retired. Of the five seniors who had been responsible for construction work, four were gone.

I felt out of place. The people who now worked for Alain knew little about the history of their research. And perhaps there was no need for them to know about the relational turbulences that had surrounded the idea of a nonautonomous transfer of homeoproteins; about the conceptual provocation that the Bernardian concept of a silent embryogenesis had once been; or about the extensive work of thought on thought that had made possible the experimental system they now relied on and sought to advance. For with the success of the lab, on the level of collaborations and publications, the experimental system that was produced in isolation between 1989 and 2003 had spread. It was now part of a globally circulating technology.[1]

"Did they know about the nocturnal?" I scribbled in my notebook. "Are they aware of the sweeping ethical opening the plastic had been?" At least Alain was still there, still interested in remembering the times we had lived through together.

When I returned for the last time, in 2011, that had changed as well. The once marginal provocateur had become the powerful founding director of the Collège's first ever *département de biologie*. Alain had become one of the big men of Parisian biology in general and of neurobiology in particular. He had become a public intellectual. And he had become tired, I am afraid, of "his" anthropologist. There was hardly any space for me anymore. I knew that Alain had liked the idea of an anthropologist in his lab who would tell the story of his life and work. However, the only story the anthropologist could tell was one that he and his research had long outgrown. What I had to tell, what we could talk about, was a reminiscence. I had become a visitor like many others. He made an hour available; that was all.[2]

For the next year or two I continued to read the papers Alain's lab published, and I still occasionally go online to find out about their most recent publications. I thus learned about the enormous success of his work with Takao Hensch, who has labs at Ricken University in Japan as well as at Harvard. Their laboratories studied the importance of Otx2 nonautonomous transfer for the onset and closure of critical-period plasticity in the visual cortex. By transforming Otx2 into an experimentally controllable plastic force, they had learned to turn the critical period on and off at will.[3] That was, to say the least, spectacular. One could now, with the help of what was once looked at as an experimental artifact, "embryologize" cerebral tissue that was largely immutable, making it plastic in such a way that experience could mold it anew. Their papers were published in the most famous science journals and were accompanied by commentaries that praised the new knowledge they had produced.

But after a while, reading the papers that came out of Alain's lab was like reading simply any other scientific paper written by this or that lab, by a research group that had nothing to do with the one that I studied in the early 2000s.

For a long while I did not know what to do with the distance that had increasingly set apart the unexpected story my fieldwork had given rise to—a story I was still busy putting into words—and the site that Alain's lab was now becoming. Eventually, I concluded that this was one last hint, one final field-based discovery, one final chance to transform contingency into surprise.

I had to let go of what had long let me go.

The Plastic

The word *plastic* first emerged in antiquity. In ancient Greek, *plastikos* means "formable" or "moldable," "good to form or mold," or "susceptible to molding." The verb form, *plássein,* means "to mold" or "to form," as one forms or molds wax or clay. *Plasis* means "the act of forming," and *plasma* is the formed thing—literally, "something that has been formed or molded." Finally, *plástes* (plural *plastikes*) is the one who molds or forms.

To the European Middle Ages the plastic was largely unknown. It emerges in Latin in Pico della Mirandola's (1463–1494) treatise *Oratio de Dignitate Hominis,* where he wrote with Renaissance fervor that man is *plastes et fictus* of himself. The broader context of Pico's *Oratio* was the *paragone,* the debate among the learned about whether architecture and sculpture were superior to painting.

From fourteenth-century Florence, the plastic traveled to seventeenth-century Cambridge, where Ralph Cudworth (1617–1688) coined the phrase *plastic natures* to oppose what he thought of as Descartes' (1596–1650) *morbus mathematicus.* While Descartes had sought to understand nature in terms of mechanical laws, Cudworth, the foremost representative of the Cambridge Platonists, thought nature was plastic.

Pierre Bayle's (1647–1706) *Dictionnaire Historique et Critique* briefly summarized Cudworth's alternative to Descartes and thereby made the concept of plastic natures familiar to the French Enlightenment *philosophes.* Several among them wrote essays about this alternative, making the distinction between the plastic and the mechanical one of the most discussed questions of the eighteenth century. Jean le Rond d'Alambert (1717–1783) later summarized many of these debates in an article, "Des Natures Plastiques," for the *Encyclopédie* and thereby made the plastic relevant to philosophers across Europe.

By the time the *Encyclopédie* was published, several European languages had been referring to sculpture as one of the *plastic arts* for almost two hundred years.

In Britain, meanwhile, the plastic was not opposed to the mechanical but to the particular. The author of this distinction was Anthony Ashley Cooper, the third earl of Shaftesbury. Late in life, Shaftsbury argued, echoing Cudworth's Platonism, that poetry was of a higher order than history, as the former could express *universal* or *plastic truths,* while the latter could attend only to particularities.

Cooper's plastic truths were elegantly linked to questions of sensation by Étienne Bonnot de Condillac's (1714–1780) *Traite sur les Sensation,* which suggested—with reference to William Chesselden's (1688–1752) writings about a young, blind English gentleman—that those who had lost their sight had a more *plastic* (in the sense of haptic) understanding of the world.

In the 1770s, Johann Gottfried Herder (1744–1803) introduced the plastic to Germany. After he read Shaftsbury and Condillac, he visited the garden of Versailles and discovered the plastic beauty of Greek sculptures. Upon his return, Herder wrote *Plastik oder Pygmalions Traum,* which celebrates the plasticity of the human body in partly erotic prose. And Johann Wolfgang von Goethe (1749–1832), who declared "Ich bin ein Plastiker," made the term central to his novels as well as to his studies of nature.

After the plastic had flourished for several decades in nineteenth-century German morphological treatises, and after Darwin published *The Origins of Species*—this one long argument about *plastic variation*—Wilhelm His (1831–1904) discovered that the fundamental plasticity of the human embryo was the key to understanding the wonder of our body form. Subsequently, a generation of embryologists—Roux, Driesch, Spemann, Harrison, Huxley, de Beer, von Dürken—set out to experimentalize the laws of the fundamental plasticity of living things.

Alfred Nobel (1833–1896), in 1875, invented plastic explosives.

H. G. Wells (1866–1946) wrote *The Island of Doctor Moreau* (1896) and *Mankind in the Making* (1903) to express his deep ambivalence about the possibility, opened up by His's successors, to exploit the plasticity of the embryo and to design humans at will.

At the turn of the twentieth century, the word *plastic* arrived in the German *Geisteswissenschaften,* in which scholars from Friedrich Nietzsche (1844–1900) to Georg Simmel (1858–1918) and Max Weber (1864–1920) discussed the plastic forces of history and how they "bred" human types. To many Germans of that period, human plasticity defined the historical potential that set the species apart from nature—and thus the scope of the human sciences.

Only a few years later, Sigmund Freud (1856–1939) distinguished between patients with plastic and those with nonplastic behavior, Pablo Picasso (1881–1973) invented the *peinture plastic,* the deformed faces of World War I boosted plastic surgery—and all the older usages of *the plastic* continued to flourish.

After World War II, synthetic plastic hit the market—and nylons Americanized Europe. In the United States, Jack Cole (1914–1958), cartoonist of *Playboy* magazine, which made its own contribution to plastic surgery, invented the comic strip hero Plastic Man, and Charles Webb (1935–)—just about the time when PVC was first problematized and post-Fordists began to suggest the importance of "flexibility"—advised the graduate that *the future is in plastics.*

And in the late 1990s and early 2000s, after it had been taken for granted for a century that the adult human brain has a strictly fixed cellular structure, just at the time when I arrived in the laboratory of Alain Prochiantz, at the École Normale Supérieure in Paris, neuronal researchers began arguing that they had discovered the fundamental plasticity of the adult human brain—and thereby opened up a whole new, previously unthought-of possibility for thinking about the brain, the human.

A whole new chapter began in the adventures of the plastic.

CODA

PLASTICITY AFTER 2003

When I left Paris in 2003, no one knew yet whether the brain is plastic. No one knew yet what forms cerebral plasticity would assume, or whether only some parts of the brain, perhaps minor, evolutionarily older ones, were plastic. Retrospectively, however, it was just at that time, in 2003, that plasticity was stabilized as a general category of neuronal knowledge production. The aim of this appendix is to provide a schematic sketch of the bits and pieces out of which plasticity is built and to map how they got assembled into a stable form.

THE EARLY 1990s

The idea that some basic embryogenetic processes might continue in adult brains first emerged in the early 1990s, in papers of Alain Prochiantz and Fred Gage (the latter at the Stockholm, now Salk, Institute). While Prochiantz began to wonder whether homeoproteins could be plastic forces, Gage sought to invent a language that would allow thinking the adult brain in terms of its embryogenesis. The background to Gage's conceptual innovation was very different from Prochiantz's. Gage had made a name for himself since the 1970s by grafting fetal brain tissue to mature brains to fight neurodegenerative diseases (mostly Parkinson's). He was interested in reintroducing, through cutting and pasting fetal tissue, the possibility of embryogenetic growth in diseased brains. Then in 1992, Brent Reynolds and Sam Weiss at the University of Calgary published a paper in which they reported that they had isolated neuronal precursor or stem cells in the brain of adult rats.

For Gage, who had been following adult neurogenesis research for years, this was a key moment in his career: if there were stem cells in adult brains, wouldn't this mean that there is an embryogenetic potential in the mature central nervous system?

THE LATE 1990s

In the early 1990s, the works of both Prochiantz and Gage, who know each other well, were empirically informed speculations of rather limited relevance for most of their colleagues. In 1998, when Gage's lab published an article reporting that thousands of new neurons are born in adult human brains, this changed dramatically.

Of course, Gage's discovery was preceded by a long history of experiments that date back to Joseph Altman's electrophysiological studies of the early 1960s. However, it seems that none of the previous reports of the birth of new neurons had actually interpreted the finding in embryogenetic terms, let alone as an opportunity to speculate that embryology could be the science adequate to the adult human brain. The conceptual possibility of understanding the generation, migration, and differentiation of new neurons in adult brains as a silent embryogenesis, and thus as a possibility to think of the central nervous system in terms of its retained embryogenetic potential, marks Prochiantz's and Gage's genuine contribution.

However, Gage's discovery of adult neurogenesis in humans hardly led to a plastic conception of the brain. There is no straight, unbroken line from Gage's 1998 paper to the general category of plasticity as it organizes much of neuronal research today. If there was an immediate effect of Gage's—and Gould's (1997)—article, it was that it produced a powerful uncertainty as to whether the brain is fixed, as had been assumed for so long, or not. Are new neurons born in all parts of the brain, or in only some, perhaps more ancient ones? The significance of the debate that emerged from these question for the emergence of today's concept of plasticity was that it widely circulated the alternative conception of the brain that Gage and Prochiantz had been working on since the early 1990s. More than that, in the course of this debate the term *plasticity* as they had come to define it was quickly cut loose from their names and works and became a general term to indicate the possibility that the adult human brain has retained, in the form of adult neurogenesis, some of its initial, embryogenetic plasticity.

While the debate around whether or not new neurons are born in all parts of the brain continued, two new lines of research emerged that significantly broadened the neuronal understanding of plasticity. The first emanated largely from the lab of Karel Svoboda, then at Cold Spring Harbor (now at Howard Hughes Medical Institute's Janella campus in Virginia).[1] During the 1990s, Svoboda had invented a powerful new technology known as two-photon laser scanning, which allows one to film or to take images of the living brain. When Svoboda then applied this new technique to the neocortex of mice, he found that the dendrites and even more so the dendritic spines have a high degree of motility. Some dendritic spines appear and disappear in the course of a single day, while others become thicker or thinner within just a few hours; and the actual dendrites are mobile too, in the sense that they change their position and form. Follow-up research showed that this motility is experience-dependent and reflects learning and, potentially, memory. When Svoboda and his colleagues began publishing their snapshots of form changes in the neocortex, in 2002–2003, they suggested—and this was an echo, however distant, of the conceptual labor of Prochiantz and Gage—that they indicate the retained embryogenetic plasticity of the adult brain.

The second new line of research emerged from Prochiantz's lab, which began to publish its first articles on the plastic effect of the nonautonomous transfer in parallel to Svoboda' s work (2002–2003).

The effect of these two new lines of research was that they decoupled the term *plasticity* from the (retrospectively) narrow focus on adult neurogenesis and thereby opened up the possibility of using the idea of the plastic in a much broader and general way (much to the delight of Prochiantz, who had consistently argued that adult neurogenesis may be only the most visible form of the adult's embryogenetic potential and that there might be many other, yet unanticipated forms of silent embryogenesis).

It was in the aftermath of Prochiantz's and Svoboda's work (though not necessarily as a consequence of it) that the brain became more and more often described as plastic and that plasticity began to emerge as a general category of neuronal production, as an umbrella term under which one could assemble such heterogeneous things as adult neurogenesis, the emergence of synapses, the continuous sprouting of axons and dendrites, LTP and LTD, form changes, and the thickening and thinning of spines.

Today, all of these neuronal processes are understood as expressions of the retained embryogenetic plasticity of the adult human brain, which most regard as a ceaselessly emerging cellular form—"though perhaps *form,*" as Alain told me with reference to Henri Bergson, "is the wrong term. Because to speak of forms implies some form of stability, while in reality all there is is movement."

NOTES

CHAPTER 1. ENTRY

Epigraph translation: The challenge is to prove that developmental phenomena occur not only in the embryonic but as well in the adult state. Bernard 1956:56.

1. Alain has developed the idea of silent embryogenesis, a term he took from C Bernard 1956, over many years; see Prochiantz 1993, 1995, 1997, 2001. On my use of the term *plasticity,* see the note on technical terms. Regrettably, there is no historical analysis of the use of the term in biology. However, for an excellent analysis of the concept and practice of plasticity made possible by the emergence of tissue culture, see Landecker 2004, 2010. For an effort to articulate a philosophy of plasticity that partly engages the neuronal sciences, see Malabou 2000, 2004, 2005, 2009. For a critical reading of Malabou that seeks to distinguish her history of neuroscience from her philosophy of plasticity, see Rees 2011.

2. Having read about the controversial status that molecular cell biology, classified as an American invention, had in France in the 1960s and 1970s, I was curious to trace how, since the days of geneticists such as Jacques Monod and François Jacob, it had conquered French institutions and research laboratories. To pursue this curiosity, I had prepared to study the belated emergence of French, as compared to American or British, biotechnology. For a history of molecular biology in France, see Gaudellière 2002.

3. Cf. Weber 1958:143.

4. Why did Prochiantz admit me to his lab even though I had no prior knowledge of brain science in general and his work in particular? While I have no clear answer, it seems as if, as a student of Canguilhem, Alain was interested in conceptual conversations and the idea of a historical epistemological study of his lab's work.

5. DEA is short for *diplôme d'étude approfondis,* a kind of master's degree.

6. On homeoproteins, cf. Gehring 1998; Nüsslein-Volhard 2004; Carroll 2005.

7. The third observation was the result of Alain's reading.

8. 'Silent embryogenesis' means that some embryogenetic processes continue in a modest and small scale way in the adult.

9. Until the 1990s, the term *plasticity* was rarely used in the neuronal sciences and, when it was, almost exclusively in one of two ways. Since the late 1950s the term has been used in regeneration studies to refer to the search for which neuronal processes prevent the brain from replacing neurons lost to disease or injury (see especially Raisman 1969; for a comment see Stahnisch and Nitsch 2003). Since the 1970s the term *plasticity* has also been used to refer to the experimental observation that the intensity with which synapses communicate with one another can change (for the prehistory and history of this idea, see chapter 3). Both of these uses have one thing in common: they assumed that the adult human brain has an immutable cellular structure, except on the level of the synapse and of synaptic communication. Most of the available studies of cerebral plasticity tend to confuse these two older uses of the term *plasticity* with the more recent emergence since the late 1990s of an embryogenetic concept of plasticity. See, for example, Mendelzweig 2013 and Abi-Rached and Rose 2013. For a critique of this confusion, see "Histories of Truth" in this volume.

10. In the late 1980s and throughout most of the 1990s Alain had, together with his colleague Jean Didier Vincent, a radio show on the station France Culture.

11. See Gould et al. 1997 for primates, and Erikson et al. 1998 for humans.

12. Alain's idea of continuity in the embryogenetic processes in the adult was informed by a paper on trophic proteins by Fred Gage (1995), with whom Alain had worked in the late 1980s.

13. What I mean by *beauty* is the moment when an established form of knowledge is breaking open and an in-between, irreducibly open state emerges that has not yet been given any directionality and thus defies any teleological effort.

14. Occasionally, the neuronal sciences in general and cerebral plasticity in particular have been associated with neoliberalism. The suggestion here is either that the neuronal sciences contribute to a culture that emanates from neoliberal reforms (Martin 1999, which expands on the extraordinary Martin 1994; Pitts Taylor 2010) or that they contribute forms of self-governance that are congruent with neoliberalism (Abi-Rached and Rose 2013, which partly expands on Rose 2007). Catherine Malabou (2009) has inverted this argument and made plasticity a residue of resistance to neoliberalism.

What makes it difficult for me to relate to these in many ways intriguing studies is that they tend to bypass a thorough historical conceptual analysis of plasticity research in the neuronal sciences. For example, neither for the work of Abi-Rached and Rose nor for that of Malabou is it significant that there is a massive difference between the concept of synaptic plasticity that emerged to dominance in the 1970s (and assumed that the adult brain has an immutable structure) and the embryogenetic plasticity of the late 1990s and early 2000s (which radically overturned the concept of an immutable cellular structure). These works thus miss the event the emergence of plastic reason actually has been. As a consequence, these authors can argue that plasticity emerged in the late 1970s, in parallel with neoliberalism and flourishing alongside it—an argument that is, from the perspective of a careful historical epistemological analysis of the emergence of an embryogenetic conception of the adult human brain since the early 2000s, difficult to maintain. If one takes the emergence of plastic reason into account, the association between—or juxtaposition of—plasticity and neoliberalism loses much of its initial plausibility. (And one could argue, with Collier 2011 and Ferguson 2010, 2013a, 2013b, 2015, that their use of the term *neoliberalism* is almost as undifferentiated as their use of the term *plasticity*.)

15. For example, my understanding of the history of neuronal research grew almost exclusively out of my fieldwork: out of a conversation I by chance overheard, out of an accidental encounter, out of an unexpected event that occurred in the lab. And the same is true for every other aspect of plastic reason. My sense of what is at stake in it, of how it alters the way the brain, its diseases, and its humans are known, is grounded in fieldwork-based discoveries.

16. Different from more classical variants of fieldwork, which aim at the underlying logic that structures a given culture, this was research into the open—first, because I really did not know what my research would be about and, second, because, once I found a theme, it turned out to be about an event that opened up a still emergent way of thinking and knowing. See Rees 2010a, 2010b, 2011.

17. No doubt this is reminiscent of what Lawrence Cohen (1998) has called "thick analysis." I am tremendously grateful to Lawrence for the many discussions— in his office, at Le Cheval, in Café Milano, in the Mission, and in Glen Park—we have had about fieldwork and writing.

18. One important consequence follows. To write a book composed of field-based episodes of surprise—which often provided me with my analytical vocabulary—meant for me to withdraw from theory (the general, the ready-made) on behalf of the singular (the stories and encounters that cannot be reduced to the general, for which no ready-made concepts exist). In vain, therefore, will the reader look for a review of past and present literature. I put such reviews consistently in the footnotes. Not that this literature is unimportant; not that I have not learned from it or that it had not shaped my interest or my questions; but I have opted here for another form.

DIGRESSION: OBSERVATION

1. Yu 1949. See also Le Calvez 1948. A few years later, in 1956, Edward Lewis, Yu's supervisor, identified and located the gene that causes the mutation and called it Anetannapedia (Lewis 1956).

2. The other ones were Aristopedia, Bithorax, and Ultrabithorax. The term *homoeosis* was introduced by William Bateson in his *Materials for the Study of Variation,* published in 1894. At a time when the material basis of inheritance was not known, before even the term *gene* was coined, Bateson collected a large number of oddly disfigured animals and plants in order to see if he could find some logic underlying the seemingly chaotic. To one class of mutants, in which one body part appears

in the place of a structurally similar body part, he gave the name *homeotic,* from the Greek *homoeosis,* meaning "likeness."

Later Bateson was one of the three "rediscoverers" of Mendel's pea studies, the others being Carl Correns and Hugo de Vries. De Vries introduced the term *gene;* Bateson then coined the term *genetics.* Thomas Hunt Morgan began the experimental geneticization of inheritance—much inspired by Bateson—in 1910 at Columbia University. In 1928, with his by then already famous students Briggs and Sturtevant, he moved to Caltech, where they recruited a young PhD student named Edward Lewis—who later became the Thomas Hunt Morgan Professor at Caltech and whose student Sien-chiue Yu first identified and named the Antennapedia mutation.

3. See Lewis 1963, 1964.

4. Walter Gehring (2001:33) suggests that Lewis was the first to use this term. The example that guided Lewis's work in the 1960s and 1970s was the Operan model of Monod and Jacob's repressor gene.

5. Nüsslein-Volhard and Wieschaus 1980. They continued their work throughout the 1980s and 1990s. For a summary of this work, see Nüsslein-Volhard 2006. For a good account of the reasoning behind their experiments of 1979–1980, see Wieschaus 1995.

6. Wieschaus was Gehring's PhD student, and Nüsslein-Volhard his postdoc.

7. Gehring 2001.

CHAPTER 2. RELATIONAL

Epigraph: Malinowski 2014 [1922]. An alternative epigraph would have come from Marilyn Strathern's 1988 *The Gender of The Gift:* "It may sound absurd for an (...) anthropologist to suggest he or she could imagine people having no society." On Strathern's relevance for this chapter, see footnote 11.

1. More specifically, Stéphane had shown that Emx2 doesn't stay in the nucleus but is transported into the axon, where it regulates transcription. This finding was later published as Nédélec et al. 2004.

2. See the biography by her daughter Ève Labouisse (1938).

3. Like Louis Pasteur and, to a lesser extent, Claude Bernard, Marie Curie is celebrated as a heroine of the French people.

4. On Irène Joliot, see Chouchan 1998. On Frédéric Joliot, see Pinault 2000. See also Biquard 1961.

5. On Blum, see Bernstein 2006. On Blum's short-lived political leadership, see Renouvin and Rémond 1967.

6. For Joliot's role in the creation of the CNRS, see Picard 1990:95. For a brief review—and critique—of Joliot's vision, see Gilpin 1968. For a contemporary critique of the postwar organization, see Postel-Vinay 2002. On Frédéric Joliot's role, see Hecht 1986.

7. On the history of atomic energy and weapons in France and for the role the Joliots played in their development, see Hecht 1998.

8. Hélène married Michel Langevin, grandson of the famous physicist Paul Langevin (1872–1946). Paul Langevin was, like Marie Curie, educated at the Institut de Physique Nucléaire. It is said that he had an affair with the widowed Marie Curie, Hélène's grandmother, in 1910. Michel and Hélène have one son, Yves, who became an astrophysicist.

9. Alain, by the way, was deeply upset by such speculations, insisting that Pierre Joliot was actually not one of his allies and had sought to prevent him from getting a lab.

10. A central reference here is Pierre Bourdieu. Bourdieu's work on distinction (2002) and reproduction of the academic milieu (1988) as well as of the French elite is pertinent to the entire chapter.

11. When it comes to understanding the concept of *the relation*, I find two authors unsurpassed. The first is Meyer Fortes, specifically his *Kinship and the Social Order* (1969). I marvel at his understanding of the 'piety of kinship,' lived and in the abstract. Meyer Fortes's effort to capture the forms of relation that human living together has assumed over the course of time, saturated with historical digressions and philosophical curiosity, remains a book that matters.

The second is Marilyn Strathern. Her exploration of the relation as constitutive of self in the context of human living together, which amounts to a powerful rupture with the idea of the individual—or the comprehension of the relation as composed of individual selves—gains contour precisely as what I would describe as a grateful departure from Meyer Fortes (Strathern 1971). With Strathern's explorations of relational thought in Melanesia, it becomes possible to understand humans as constituted by relations, by contexts, by objects, to the degree that they are relationally configured. What self is thus varies—and there is no necessary coherence between the different selves (Strathern 1988, 1992, 1999, 2004). What is particularly striking is the possibility that the individual, this eighteenth-century European concept, is itself a relational configuration (Strathern 2005). Strathern has consistently resisted articulating a philosophy of relations: her work instead is the effort to think through the contemporary by looking at Western phenomena from a Melanesian perspective (Strathern 1995).

12. The relational was not a sense-making category that predated my research. Rather, it became a category for sense making insofar—and only insofar—as my interlocutors provided me with it. It was by listening to my interlocutors—to people like Brigitte, Joliot, and Alain—and by learning from them how to describe almost every aspect of life (and of science) in terms of descent and relation—that I came to understand that one strategy for analyzing (plastic) reason is to think of it as conditioned by relations.

13. The idea for this formulation comes from Eugenides 2002.

14. Prochiantz's career had been straightforward. He entered the École Normale Supérieure in 1969, received his DEA in neurology in 1971, and his PhD in the molecular biology of plants in 1976. Shortly before he earned his degree, he returned to neurology and started working in Glowinski's lab. His excursion into genetics was not a turn away from neurology. At a time when the study of the nervous system

had not yet become molecular, a change of fields was the only way to familiarize oneself with molecular biology. Prochiantz was fascinated by the idea of molecular neurobiology, though at the time he received his degree, such a discipline did not yet exist, at least not in France, where the field was divided between electrophysiology, anatomy, and chemistry. Compelled by the circumstances, he joined Glowinski's lab, where he worked as a neurochemist.

I could go into much detail here about relational lines spun at the ENS and document how they structure academia, in neuroscience as well as in philosophy. However, Alain was always aggressively distancing himself from this club—and, as far as I can tell, he hardly relied on them. He had a certain disgust for the classical ENS story.

15. Glowinski helped invent monoamineoxydase inhibitors, the first commercially available antidepressants.

16. On the history of cell culture biology, see Landecker 2010.

17. Alain had never been a student of Canguilhem in the sense of being supervised by him. However, as a student at the ENS in the early 1970s he frequently attended Canguilhem's seminars.

18. See the excellent account of the debate in Fox-Keller 1995. On experimental embryology, see Kirschner 2003; Maienschain 1991; Mocek 1974; and Querner 1977.

19. There is no need to go into the technical details of the debate here. The difference between a cytoplasmic and genetic theory of inheritance has been reviewed several times. See the brilliant work in Fox-Keller 2002; S. Gilbert 1991, 2000; Haraway 2004; Morange 1998, 2000; Moss 2003; and Sapp (1987).

20. Huxley and de Beer 1934:1–7.

21. Bernhard Dürken, a fellow of Spemann and Driesch, captured the embryologists' conception of life in a poignant formulation when he equated mechanism with "*präformistische Starrheit*" (preformed rigidity) and opposed it to the vitalism of embryologists, which he equated with "*epigenetische Plastizität.*"

22. Huxley and de Beer, 1934:4.

23. Carroll 2005.

24. This dominance is inextricably bound to the Institut Marey, a department for neurophysiology that until the late 1970s was world-class but then missed the emergence of neurobiology, which took place, at least in the United States, in the 1960s, most notably in the lab of Steve Kuffler. See Cowan, Donald, and Kandel 2000 and Albright, Jessel, and Kandel 2000.

25. Prochiantz frequently acknowledged the significance of Gunther Stent (1985) for his own work and his critique of molecular biology.

26. To be clear, the conception of what a gene "is" had changed radically since the time of Morgan's drosophila studies. Genetics had become molecular in the 1940s and 1950s and was no longer exclusively concerned with heredity, but also with cellular events on a molecular level—in development as much as in adulthood. And yet, as far as the theoretical claims are concerned, little seems to have changed since Morgan and his followers had challenged embryological conceptions of development as plastic (cf. Fox-Keller 2000; Morange 1998; Rheinberger 2004).

27. He systematized his view in two publications: Prochiantz 1987, 1989.

28. Joliot was a convenient choice. The year before, he had done an internship in Alain's group, in which he had worked with homeotic genes. In addition, Joliot had just completed a DEA in genetics and hence was familiar with molecular biology— Alain was adamant that he did not know about Joliot's family history at the time.

29. It's is a cliché captured in myriad stories, books, and films that circulate in France and beyond. The film that perhaps best captures the role and place of the *métro* in Parisian life and love affairs is François Truffaut's *Le Dernier Métro* (1980), starring Catherine Deneuve and Gérard Depardieu.

30. Weber 1918.

31. On the gendering of relations, see Strathern 1992. On the gendering of science, see Fox-Keller 1985.

32. Joliot et al. 1991.

33. *PNAS* has a distinctive procedure for reviewing papers for publication, one that makes peer review weigh less heavily. A member of the National Academy of Science may suggest a de facto often controversial or speculative research report for publication, as well as the potential reviewers. In Alain's case, the paper was recommended by Pasko Rakic, longtime president of the American Society of Neuroscience.

34. I quote here just a few—and not even the most critical—reviews.

35. Prochiantz, no doubt in anticipation of a future success, has carefully archived all readers' responses that he and Joliot have received since 1989, and even the faxes, letters, and emails exchanged in order to facilitate publication.

36. Bernard 1957:164.

37. The interview was part of a multimedia play on passions called *Traité de Passion*.

38. *Translation:* If one says, "I aimed to be very good at what I do, but in the end I am not and so it is not worth continuing this whole thing and therefore I kill myself [literally, I shoot myself a bullet in my head]"; then this is not pathetic. It is even good. One would wish it would happen more often. [. . .] It is possible that certain ones of my colleagues think that I am not well and that I am not even aware of it. And so they experience a sentiment of pity or compassion for me. Because they are Christians and so they approve of compassion. Not so for me. But I am sure that some of them have a lot of compassion for me. If I think about this, I feel sick. Last September, one of them told me at the end of a lecture, "If I were you, I would stop this stuff. You are making a fool of yourself. Everyone thinks like me but no one has the audacity to tell you. Stop. You are ruining your career." As I am fragile I wanted to vomit. I felt sick for at least a couple of hours. He further told me, "I am not telling you this because I don't love you but precisely because I love you. I think you could be a good scientist. What you are trying to show is absurd and because none of your friends sufficiently loves you to tell you, I, who have compassion for you, prefer to let you know.

39. On exclusion and outsiders in science, see Harman and Dietrich 2013.

40. Derossi et al. 1994; Derossi et al. 1996.

41. The company that purchased the patent for pAntp wanted to call it Penetrator. Alain and his colleagues intervened and eventually the consensus was Penetratin.

42. For reviews, see Dupont et al. 2002 and Prochiantz 2005.

43. There were a number of indications of his re-entry. Prochiantz, for example, became director of a big CNRS research unit with five subgroups and began to play an increasingly important role in the organization of university courses. In addition, he began occupying important positions within the CNRS, where he increasingly presided over committees on neurobiology. Joliot got his own lab—"Homeoprotein Cell Biology"—that is theoretically separate from Prochiantz's but financially, institutionally, and conceptually part of Prochiantz's CNRS unit. Volovitch, who also got his own small group of researchers in Prochiantz's lab, became professor of molecular biology at Paris VII, and then at the ENS.

44. Research institutions throughout the world quickly showed interest in using the different versions of Penetratin for their work. Perhaps the most important collaborations were with the lab of Michael Shelanski, whom Alain had known since his sabbatical in 1985 and who had moved meanwhile to Columbia University; with Pat Doherty at Guy's Hospital in London, where Derossi later began a postdoc; with Wolfgang Wurst at the Max Planck Institute in Munich; and with Ülo Langel in the Department of Neurochemistry and Neurotoxicology at Stockholm University. The work with Langel was, as far as CPPs are concerned, especially fruitful and led, among other things, to a CPP textbook, which is the main publication on Penetratin and its brothers and sisters.

In addition, Alain's lab was approached by biotech and pharmacology companies. Most notable were the relations with Synthelabo and Fidia, two biotech companies represented by Laura Bossi, a good friend of Prochiantz. What followed, beginning around June 1995, were international collaborations.

45. Alain: "Too many people were against us, you know? [...] Without Penetratin, which was just a step along the way to understanding the in vivo function of homeoproteins exchange, our lab would certainly not have survived."

46. Around 1996 the lab's composition changed. Derossi and Le Roux left, new grad students arrived; several technicians were hired; and with Alain Trembleau, a specialist in axonal guidance and local transcription was recruited.

47. See Joliot et al. 1997; Joliot et al. 1998; Maizel et al. 1999.

48. Maizel et al. 2002.

49. In a 2002 review paper, Prochiantz and Joliot declare programmatically that from now on the question can no longer be whether homeoproteins travel between cells or not. Their work on internalization and secretion, they claim, has firmly established that such a transfer occurs. The main question to be approached now is why, when, and to what ends they transfer: "The physiological significance of [homeoprotein nonautonomous transfer] is unknown. [...] During development, homeoprotein exchange might be necessary for cell-cell recognition. In the adult nervous system, where these proteins still exist, their secretion in the synapse could provide positional information to postsynaptic neurons. Now that molecular and cellular approaches have established the reality of protein transduction, physiological studies can be undertaken that will establish the meaning of this observation" (Prochiantz and Joliot 2003).

50. On the significance of Bernard, D'Arcy Thompson, and Alain Turing, see chapter 4.

51. In 2000, Alain increased his engagement with the media: he was approached by the TV station ARTE and launched a (short-lived) science series.

52. A similar suggestion has been made by Michel Callon, with whom I had the pleasure of discussing my fieldwork. Alain's formulation, though in an unanticipated and inverse way, closely touches on the notion of "boundary objects" as developed in Leigh-Starr 1989 and Leigh-Starr and Bowker 2000.

53. His work, he explained to me, required him to learn how to think of the brain as a continuously emerging form and that is precisely how Jean François, in an interview, defined the work of the artist. "This is for me perhaps the most interesting thing [. . .]. For me the work of theater, but maybe this is true for the work of art in general, is, in the main, the idea of inventing forms."

54. Being with Peyret opened up a space for extensive conversation about what he had been compelled, by the negative reviews and the polemic surrounding his work, to exclude from his official discourse as a scientist—namely, his speculations about an obscure and thus thought-provoking observation, his ideas on the brain's fundamental plasticity.

55. On form/event, see Rabinow 1996a.

56. Goldman and Nottebohm 1983.

57. Rakic 1985:1054.

58. For primates, see Gould et al. 1997; for humans, see Erikson et al. 1998. Rubin (2010) largely follows the arguments of Specter (2001), who had added a bit of sex and crime to Gross 2002. All three seem fairly biased in their value judgments (Specter through Gross, and Rubin through Specter). For the best available overview of the significance of the discoveries by the labs of Gould and Gage (Erikson), see Kempermann 2006, 2012. Cf. Rees forthcoming.

59. That being said, there were certainly fields of neuronal research that were less affected by this controversy.

60. Plasticity research emerged as well in France. In 2001, for example, the Institut Pasteur opened a research center for the study of adult neurogenesis. Only a year later INSERM and CNRS welcomed proposals for plasticity research, with the consequence that several other labs began to work on neurogenesis or aspects of it. And in 2003 the Fondation Ipsen even created the Prix de Plasticité, which was awarded to Arturo Alvarez-Buylla, who had first discovered the birth of new neurons in mice. Prochiantz was centrally involved in all of these events. He was on the advisory board of the Institut Pasteur, had been the driving force at the CNRS, and presented, together with Jean Pierre Changeux, the prize to Alvarez-Buylla.

61. In the 1980s and then again in the late 1990s Prochiantz had collaborated with some of the pioneers of adult neurogenesis, specifically Fred Gage and Anders Björklund. See Gage et al. 2004.

62. On an international scale, one could name, for example, collaborations with labs around the world, invitations to give lectures and attend conferences, articles in

prestigious journals, and the offer he received in fall 2004 from New York's Columbia University (from a group of people he had first worked with in 1985). And on a national scale one could add that Prochiantz became director of the Department of Biology at the ENS, that he received the prestigious Prix Athéna, awarded each year by the Académie de Science and the Assurances Générales de France, that Prochiantz's own biotech company, Elistem Biopharmaceutical, was started based on his ideas about the relevance of homeoprotein exchange for understanding neurodegenerative diseases.

63. Many of my interlocutors characterized Prochiantz's nomination as a final showdown between Prochiantz and his opponents. And his main opponent, as I was frequently told, was Jean Pierre Changeux, professor at the Collège de France, director of research at the Institut Pasteur, a powerful president of several governmental task forces commissioned to modernize French science.

The two stand for fairly different visions of the brain. Changeux, *grand seigneur* of French molecular neuroscience, has spent his academic career illuminating the molecular mechanism of synaptic communication. The conceptual presupposition of this focus has been that synapses are the main active and dynamic element of an otherwise fairly fixed and immutable structure. Understanding the action of neurotransmitters thus could be the key to a brain understood as an information-processing machine (an idea that Changeux strongly advocated in the 1980s and 1990s when he institutionalized cognitive neurobiology in France).

Prochiantz's formulation of an irreducibly plastic brain, according to which not only the synapse but the whole brain is plastic, runs fundamentally counter to Changeux's work. The results are differing ideas concerning the future of neurology and the kind of research one should support.

DIGRESSION: REGIONAL RATIONALITIES

1. For a general account of Bachelard, see Chimisso 2001.

2. As Michel Foucault once noted (1994): "Everyone knows that in France there are few logicians but many historians of science; and that in the 'philosophical establishment'—whether teaching or research oriented—they have occupied a considerable position."

3. On Comte, see the informative works of Juliette Grange (1996, 2000). For the interpretation of Comte as the French Hegel, and for Comte's conception of a history and philosophy of science as corresponding to Hegel's claim that the task of philosophy is to express what is contemporary in terms adequate to the contemporary, see Ritter 1974.

4. For the interpretation of Bachelard's history of science as a *histoire d'esprit humaine,* see Chimisso 2001.

5. Bachelard 1949:103. *Translation:* The trajectories that permit the isotopes to be separated through mass spectrometry don't exist in nature. One has to produce them technically. They are reified theorems.

6. Bachelard 1951:25.

7. For "applied rationalism" and "applied materialism," see Bachelard 1951:5; for the idea that scientific objects have always an emergent—i.e., never actualized—quality, see Bachelard 1951:132–133. The term *realization* is used in Bachelard 1967:61.

8. Bachelard, 1949:119–138.

9. Bachelard, 1949:133.

10. Hans Jörg Rheinberger's concept of experimental system is an explicit continuation of Bachelard's work, and the idea of "epistemic things/objects" is derived from Bachelard's assumption that scientific facts/objects are "reified theorems." See Rheinberger's essay "Wissenschaft des Konkreten," in Rheinberger 2005.

11. Bachelard 1949:133. *Translation:* The challenge to define a general rational language that would make visible what the different regional rationalities have in common, therefore, doesn't pose itself anymore. One would find through this effort nothing but the minimum rationalism used in everyday life. One would erase the structures [that organize the various rationalities] where the actual challenge is to multiply and refine the structures, that is, that which from the point of view of the rationalist has to express itself as a structuration activity, as a determination of the possibility of multiple axioms to cope with the multiplication of the experiences.

12. Bachelard 1949:133 and passim.

13. Bachelard 1949:133.

14. So should one conclude that everything is socially constructed? Certainly not. This is the least one can learn from Bachelard. But certainly it means that what counts as true, for example, about the brain necessarily has a social (or better, relational dimension). This is to say, homeoproteins exist independently of human knowledge and they transferred before Prochiantz observed their transfer. But human knowledge of a homeoprotein n-a-t—or of a continued embryogenesis in the adult—is inseparable from social situations; relations are, so to speak, built into scientific truths.

I would like to thank Ian Hacking for a discussion about his book *The Social Construction of What?*

15. Again thanks are due to Ian Hacking for a discussion about French relational nativism. It is not least because of my emphasis on analytical principles found in the text that the argument presented here diverges from, for example, Berger and Luckmann (1966). Their effort was to present a theory of social construction of reality, a totalizing, all-encompassing theory that explains the world. They presuppose that the social is a human universal, one they never question. And this presupposition structures their analysis. The best Berger and Luckmann can do is to refine their theory. Inquiry is necessary only either to prove that the theory is correct or to refine

it. They leave no space for genuine surprise, for the unanticipated discovery of the possibility that it could be different.

CHAPTER 3. CONCEPTUAL

1. Pasko Rakic has been a major critique of adult neurogenesis. Already in the 1980s when new neurons were first observed in bird brains, he was adamant that in higher vertebrates, neurogenesis is nonexistent (Rakic 1985). He had studied the cellular formation of the cortex for years, in part with Bourgeois, and had not seen new neurons. Eventually, though, when he used a new labeling method (BrmdU labeling), he too detected new neurons in the adult hippocampus and the olfactory bulb, and started publishing papers on his findings. However, he remained an opponent of the effort to use adult neurogenesis to think of the adult human brain in embryogenetic terms.

2. Fixation is a delicate procedure. To avoid the degeneration of the brain's fine structure, one has to cut through the chest to the heart of the living animal in order to inject a fixation.

3. As Jean Pierre Changeux (1985), in whose lab Bourgeois was working, interpreted this phenomenon, "to learn is to eliminate." That is to say, Changeux suggested that this decrease is related to individuation (those possibilities and options we do not use will wither). Gerald Edelman (1987), shortly after Changeux published his work, suggested his theory of "neural Darwinism," which advances, if in a more elaborate way, a similar hypothesis.

4. Rakic et al. 1986; Bourgeois, Jastreboff, and Rakic 1989; Zecevic, Bourgeois, and Rakic 1989; Bourgeois, Rakic, and Goldman-Rakic 1994; Granger et al. 1995; Bourgeois and Rakic 1996; Bourgeois 1997.

5. Chemical because synaptic communication had been known since the early 1950s to be a chemical event. See below.

6. The paper was Bernier et al. 2002. On Hughlings Jackson, see the illuminating work of Allan Young, especially A. Young 1995, 2011.

7. In both cases, the implication seemed to amount to fixity: "it is already wired" translated (for me) as "no more growth," and "a chemical machine" as "a fixed and immutable structure."

8. This was precisely Rakic's argument (1985) against adult neurogenesis. "The brain of primates as well as some other species may be uniquely specialized in lacking the capacity for neuronal production once in the adult stage. One can speculate that a prolonged period of interaction with the environment, as pronounced as it is in all primates, especially in humans, requires a stable set of neurons to retain acquired experiences in the pattern of their synaptic connectivity" (1054). The significance of the relative immutability of the adult cerebral structure goes back to Ramón y Cajal in the early twentieth century (see note 26, this chapter).

9. Purkynĕ 1838; Schwann 1839; Remak 1836, 1837, 1838; Kölliker 1849; Virchow 1846. There are no detailed reliable studies on the enrollment of the brain in Schleiden's cell theory. However, see Clarke and Jacyna 1987; Finger 1994; Shepherd 1991; and van der Loos 1967. On Franz Josef Gall and his significance for the modern conception of the brain as locus of the human, see Hagner 1997.

10. Or one could do so if almost exclusively in German-speaking countries. The analysis of the brain in terms of cell theory was, at first, an almost exclusively German development; it was largely irrelevant for other, cell-independent localization efforts flourishing in, for example, France (in the form of ablation experiments) and England (in the form of phrenology and physiology). This changed only in the twentieth century.

11. Uskoff 1882; His 1883; Bizzozero 1894; Merk 1896.

12. Gerlach's 1873 observation was, as far as I can reconstruct, uncontroversial. Golgi published his observation in 1883 and then again in 1884. He partly departed from Gerlach, but renewed and gave new significance to the reticular theory. The controversy really started only after His 1883, 1886, and Forel 1886.

13. Clarke and Jacyna 1987:58ff.

14. See His 1883, 1885, 1886, 1888, 1889. On His, see Hopwood 1999, 2000, 2002a, 2002b, 2004. On biology in nineteenth-century Germany, see Nyhart 1995.

15. Forel 1887.

16. On Golgi see the helpful biography of his life and work by Mazarello (1999).

17. He later speculated that in the adult brain dendritic spines allow for learning.

18. Ramón y Cajal 1890, 1995 [1897–1904]; see also DeFelipe 2006, 2009.

19. Among the most important supporters were Kölliker and the histologist Wilhelm Waldeyer. Ramón y Cajal describes his 1889 experience in Ramón y Cajal 1991 [1901–1917]:356ff.

20. Of course, the idea of regional specialization is much older. For the history of localization theory, see Clarke and Dewhurst 1974. For the continuity of functional anatomy, see Dumit 2004.

21. As an implicit assumption, fixity had long been a regulatory category. For example, when I read Wolf and von Baer and then later Remak and many others who have established "development" as a distinct category, it seemed as if all of them assumed that once development is over, the brain (or the organism) is "done." But Ramón y Cajal was the first, as far as I can tell, who made fixity, in a conceptually significant way, explicit.

22. I was surprised to find that Ramón y Cajal, who habitually documented the experiments that led him to his conclusions, explained neither how he arrived at the conclusion that the adult brain is essentially fixed nor what he means exactly by "essentially fixed."

In the secondary literature, the *Textura* is often depicted as a kind of architecture book of the brain—as one large blueprint. And indeed, it seems as if for Ramón y Cajal there is a time of construction (large-scale developmental processes) and a time of having been constructed (already developed). The possibility that large-scale construction (developmental) processes occur in the already constructed brain—that neurons continuously die and are replaced by new ones; that they proliferate, differentiate, and migrate; that axons and dendrites appear, disappear, change their directions—appears intrinsically foreign to this architectural logic.

23. Ramón y Cajal 1995 [1897–1904], 2:726. He continues: "Our hypothesis even accounts for greater conservation of older memories—memories of youth in the aged, amnestic, and demented—because association pathways created long ago and repeated for many years obviously acquire even greater strength. In addition, they were formed during a period of life when neuronal plasticity was maximal" (2:726).

24. Ramón y Cajal 1894. The full statement reads: "Mental training cannot better the organization of the brain by adding to the number of cells; we know that nervous elements have lost the property of multiplication past embryonic life; but it is possible to imagine that mental exercise facilitates a greater development of the protoplasmic apparatus [. . .]. In this way, pre-existing connections between groups of cells could be reinforced [. . .]."

25. I am grateful to Javier DeFelipe for several exchanges on Ramón y Cajal's concept of the brain, and for telling me about the histologist's interest in dendritic spines as, in adults, the only remaining locus of growth.

26. In his later work, Ramón y Cajal returned time and again to the question of fixity. In *Regeneration and Degeneration of the Nervous System,* published in 1913–1914, he wrote: "A vast series of anatomic-pathological experiments in animals, and an enormous number of clinical cases that have been methodically followed by autopsy, [have convinced me that it is] an unimpeachable dogma [that] there is no regeneration of the central paths, and [that] there is no restoration of the normal physiology of the interrupted conductors" (Ramón y Cajal 1913–1914:509). "It has been demonstrated, beyond doubt," Cajal concedes, "that there is a production of new fibers and clubs of growth in the spinal cord of tabetics [. . .] and of cones and ramified axons in the scar of spinal wounds of man and animals." However, he goes on, "these investigations, while they have brought out unquestionable signs of repair, which are comparable in principle with those of the central stump of the nerves, have also confirmed the old concept of the essential impossibility of regeneration, showing that [. . .] the restoration is paralyzed giving place to a process of atrophy and definite break-down of the nerve sprouts" (509). At the end of the book, after many hundreds of pages of careful argumentation, Ramón y Cajal then provides a conceptual explanation for the absence of cell generation or cellular outgrowth: "The functional specialization of the brain imposed on the neurones two great lacunae: proliferative inability and irreversibility of intraprotoplasmatic differentiation. It is for this reason that, once the development was ended, the founts of growth and regeneration of the axons and dendrites dried up irrevocably" (750).

27. Goltz wasn't as strict an opponent of the function-specific anatomy conception of the brain as his predecessor Jean Pierre Flourens (1794–1867), who had insisted in the 1810s and 1820s that the localization theory of Franz Josef Gall

(inventor of modern Homo cerebralis) was simply wrong and that the brain had no function-specific organization. By the mid-1850s, the work of Paul Broca (1824–1880), who had taken up arguments by Jean Baptiste Bouillaud (1796–1881), had made Flourens's strict rejection of a function-specific anatomy problematic. Goltz allowed for minimal localization: he held that the posterior cortex was linked to vision, the anterior to movement. For a brief history of how Gall's theory was first anatomized in France and then cellularized in Germany, see Rees 2016b.

28. Langley later became famous for his contribution to the drug receptor concept.

29. Emil du Bois-Reymond, professor of physiology at the University of Berlin, designed the galvanometer, a novel recording instrument for detecting electrical discharges of nerves, and is often described as having almost single-handedly created the field of electrophysiology. The most significant of his publications was his 1848 *Researches on Animal Electricity*. In the same year, while still a professor of physiology in Königsberg, Hermann von Helmholtz (later renowned professor of physiology and anatomy in Berlin) was the first to measure the speed—with a galvanometer he invented for just that purpose—with which electric impulses travel along a nerve path.

30. W. H. Gaskell from Liverpool, where Sherrington moved to as Holt Professor in Physiology, had suggested that he approach the spinal cord from the periphery, rather than from the fairly complex cortex.

31. Much has been written on who introduced the term. The best overview is given in Tansey 1997.

32. Sherrington in Foster 1897:928–929. The two sentences before read thus: "The axon if it leaves the spinal cord ends in one or more end-plates or in other terminal organs. If, as is the case with a large number of cells, the axon continues to run and finally ends in the central nervous system, its mode of termination as well as that of the collaterals to which it may give rise is in the form of an arborescent tuft, which is applied to the body or dendrites of some other cell."

33. Foster 1897:929–930.

34. This modulation of impulses is critical. Interpretation of axons and dendrites as electrical wires along which nervous impulses travel had been offered before, notably by Helmholtz and Exner. Sherrington relies on these authors, but then offers the radically new argument of modulation.

35. Sherrington 1906:21.

36. Sherrington 1899.

37. The two men met twice, once in Spain in 1884, and then again in Cambridge in 1893.

38. Sherrington 1906:389. There is one other instance in which Sherrington uses the terms *plastic* and *plasticity:* in his 1909 article "On Plastic Tonus and Proprioreceptive Reflexes." In this article, however, the terms refer to the plasticity, or elasticity, of the muscle, not to the plasticity of the nervous system.

39. Sherrington 1906:389. The following sentence reads: "The *Bahnung* of a reflex exhibits this faculty in germ." The German word *Bahnung* is borrowed from

Sigmund Exner, who used it to refer to "the overflow of reflex action into the channels belonging primarily to other reflex-arcs than those under stimulation." The terms Sherrington uses alternatively for *Bahnung* are *facilitation,* meaning facilitation of the flow of reflex action, and *reinforcement,* meaning that a repeated stimulus results in a reinforcement of existent pathways. Hence, what Sherrington has in mind when he says that the nervous system is plastic are changes in the effectiveness of a synapsis.

40. Sherrington 1906:17.

41. Nissl 1903. The work of Apáthy, Bethe, Nissl, and Held was widely discussed and, at least in part, taken up and further developed conceptually as well as methodologically. For example, in the 1920s and 1930s, the conception of the brain as an at least partially continuous structure of nerve cells was refined and diversified. Some authors proposed that perhaps not all nerve cells are contiguous, while others (Lorente de Nó 1938) wondered whether a yet "unknown substance" linking axon and dendrite made at least some circuits act as closed, somewhat continuous networks characterized by reveberation. Indeed, reticularism was so alive and well that in the early 1930s, Ramón y Cajal found it necessary to defend his neuron theory against the growing number of reticularists. And even in the 1940s and 1950s some authors claimed that the structure of the nervous system amounted to a syncitium; see Bethe 1952 and Philipp Stöhr 1957, the latter of which received glorious reviews.

There are—and this is a real shortcoming—no studies that attempt to carefully reconstruct the truth possibility—and the conception of the brain/human contained in this truth possibility—that reticularism once was. Somewhat oddly, almost all historical accounts frame reticularism simply as a failure. For a very brief, judgment-neutral history, see Breidbach 1997:189–195.

42. I say neither Langley nor Lucas nor Adrian subscribed to the synapse because they appear never to have made much of Sherrington's functional interpretation of Ramón y Cajal's gap between axon and dendrite. In any case, Langley, who died in 1905, never used the term *synapse* in his work on chemical reception at the neuromuscular junction. And neither in Lucas's 1917 posthumous volume *The Conduction of the Nervous Impulse* nor in Adrian's 1932 *The Mechanism of Nervous Action* is the term ever mentioned. Adrian began using the term *synapse* only after World War II.

Nor could I find a synaptic conception of the brain among the British chemists. Henry Dale and Otto Loewi, who supposedly worked on the chemical makeup of synaptic communication in the 1910s and 1920s, hardly ever uses the term, and for good reason: Loewi and Dale were chemists of the organism rather than of nerve cells. They studied the chemical content of, and the effect of chemicals on, tissue and largely refrained from speculation about the precise mechanisms of chemical diffusion and take-up. For an overview of British neuronal research, see Breidbach 1997.

43. Lucas 1905, 1906, 1907, 1910, 1912; Adrian and Lucas 1912; Adrian 1928, 1932, 1937.

44. For an account of Spanish neuroscience from the 1880s to the 1950s, see DeFelipe 2002, 2009.

45. The work of Emile Du Bois-Reymond and Helmut von Helmholtz unfolded along rather different conceptual lines. Neither the former nor the latter had a neuronal comprehension of the brain, and neither was actually concerned with the brain as a cellular organ.

46. Overviews are provided in Breidbach 1997 and Borck 2005.

47. There were exceptions. Histological studies were offered by Louis-Antoine Ranvier (1835–1922), Mathias Duval (1844–1907), and Aguste Louis César Prenant (1861–1927). Electrophysiological studies were conducted by Louis Lapicque, a French doctor and physiologist (he had a PhD in medicine and another in physiology) who had an extraordinarily wide range of interests. Lapicque was primarily a general physiologist in the tradition of Magendie, but also had an interest, apparently through his wife (who had been his PhD student), in the electrical study of the neuromuscular junction. In 1907 Lapicque published "Recherches quantitatives sur l'excitation électrique des nerfs traitée comme une polarization," in which he introduced the "integrate and fire" theory. Apparently, Lapicque's interest in and research on the electronics of the nervous system were independent of the British school. Jean Gäel Barbara (2005) argues that Lapicque was actually busy shielding French neuronal research from British influences. Only later, with Alfred Fessard and Wilhelm Feldberg, and then again with the creation of the Institut Marey, would this change.

48. A tableaux of French brain research before World War II emerges from Gasser 1991; see also Barbara 2005 and Debru and Barbara 2008, 2009.

Unfortunately, I don't know enough about the Italian tradition of neuroscience in the aftermath of Golgi. The only historically informative publications I could find are Berlucchi 2008 and Mazzarello 1999.

49. The one local tradition for which the synapse, or at least nerve impulse transmission, was the central concept for understanding the brain thus began to spread its web across the Western world just as the two other major lines of research ceased (Germany and Spain).

50. A book-length story is presented in Valenstein 2006. See also Albright, Jessel, and Kandel 2000; Bennett 2001; Changeux 1985; and Cowan, Donald, and Kandel 2000.

51. Dale, Loewi, and Feldberg had a pharmacological conception of the organism and of the nervous system. They had no major stakes in either contiguity or the synapse.

52. Following is a brief description of the technical experiments that established the chemical quality of the nerve cell.

In 1939, independently of the older pharmacological studies of nervous tissue, Alan Hodgkin and Andrew Huxley, who were students of Edgar Adrian at Cambridge and who experimented on the giant axon of the Atlantic squid, succeeded in showing that the release of an electronic impulse changed the electrical charge of the "conducting fluid" outside the axon. When, at the end of World War II, they could return to the bench and continue their work, they documented that the ionic current in a nerve cell during impulse depends on two phases of cell membrane permeability: a rise in impulse needs sodium permeability, and a fall in impulse needs potassium permeability (Hodgkin and Huxley 1945). These observations led them to formulate the ionic theory of transmission, which holds that transmission of impulses involves receptors controlled by ions (Hodgkin and Huxley 1947). They did not use the term *synapse* in their work.

During the war, however, Wilhelm Feldberg, a German refugee who had worked with Henri Dale on acetylcholine, and Alfred Fessard, who had worked with Edgar Adrian at Cambridge, documented that the peripheral nerves of the electric (torpedo) ray released a chemical called eserine (Feldberg and Fessard 1942). Was transmission a chemical event?

John Eccles, Sherrington's last student, did not think so. In part building on the work of Hodgkin and Huxley, Eccles (1948) provided evidence—his focus was on the neuromuscular junction of frogs—for the way synapses integrate and coordinate nervous impulses. Analyzing intercellular recordings with mini-electrodes, he showed that if the arriving impulse is connected to what he called "excitatory synapses of the cell," the excitability of the cell increases, and when the "inhibitory synapses" make the cell respond, the result is a diminution of excitability.

Stephen Kuffler and Bernhard Katz (like Feldberg, they had fled Nazi Germany) disagreed with Eccles. In 1948, Bernard Katz—who had been working under Sherrington, and had collaborated closely with Eccles, sought to establish that nervous communication is not an electrical but a chemical process (he also focused on frogs, as well as on crustacea). In a critique of Hodgkin and Huxley, upholding the work of Feldberg and Fessard, he argued that nervous communication occurs by way of a release of chemicals present in a cell. To be more precise, he showed how acetylcholine causes a large and very brief increase in the ionic permeability of what he called the "synaptic membrane." The consequent ionic influx across the membrane causes the actual electrical potential transmitted "between synapses." This work was refined in Fatt and Katz 1951.

Then, in 1952, Eccles repeated the work of Fatt and Katz and applied it to motor neurons. It was this experiment that convinced him that all transmission is chemical (Brock, Coombs, and Eccles 1952).

53. The synapse as it emerged in the early 1950s had, conceptually speaking, little left to do with Sherrington's "synapsis." To begin with, the referent changed: Sir Charles (he was knighted in 1922) had intended the term to refer to a "special connection"—a "mode of nexus"—but in the 1950s it became customary to associate with the term either a transmitting or a receiving terminal of neurons. What was initially a somewhat immaterial process now referred to a piece of tissue. What had been for Sir Charles an undifferentiated, almost miraculous contact was now stabilized as a linear chemicomechanical process in which one synapse releases a transmitter substance across the synaptic cleft that is in turn taken up by the receiving synapse in such a way that an impulse is triggered along the dendrite to the soma. Lastly, the nature of the brain changed. What had been for Sherrington an electrical event—an event that defined the brain as an electrical entity—was now a chemical process that gave rise to a chemical brain.

54. De Robertis 1954a; Palade and Porter 1954; Palay 1956.

55. One could argue, of course, that most of neuronal research carried out in the 1960s and 1970s was still conducted with the tools of electrophysiology. So why the emphasis on neurochemistry? The answer is that it was generally established that the processes underlying impulse transmission were chemical. This is to say, the tools came from electrophysiology but the actual framework was chemical.

There were actually no tools, before the arrival of molecular biology in the late 1970s, that would have allowed analysis of synaptic communication from a molecular perspective (the first paper was Scheller et al. 1982; see below).

56. Watson 1913; Skinner 1938.

57. Cf. Eccles 1953:216–221.

58. Konorski 1948:79–80.

59. Hebb 1949:xix.

60. Hebb 1949:62. As can be nicely seen in this formulation, Hebb's "dual trace hypothesis" attempted to reconcile structural plasticity à la Ramón y Cajal with functional plasticity à la Lorente de Nó.

61. Konorski suggested that the number of synaptic contacts a single neuron can have has an upper limit. In some neural circuits this limit is reached before birth; these circuits are fixed. In plastic circuits the maximum number of contacts is reached at some point in postnatal development. After that, learning improves the effectiveness of synaptic transmission and potentially leads to the growth of new synaptic contacts.

62. While the works of Konorski and Hebb were provocative to psychologists, they generated positive excitement among neuronal researchers. After the divorce of psychology from brain research in the early twentieth century, neuronal researchers had largely focused their attention on the functional architecture of the nervous system. Whereas their nineteenth-century predecessors moved freely back and forth between brain research and grand speculative statements about human psychology, they had analyzed the brain as an enclosed, autonomous machine and were driven by the effort to discover the intrinsic mechanism that governed the brain. (The heroic ethos of the discipline was, cut the head open, understand how the nervous centers are composed, and withdraw from far-reaching speculative claims about the mind.) As a result, the neuronal organ existed in isolation. Konorski and Hebb's work was exciting in that it provided a concrete, experimentally feasible program to leave this isolation behind.

63. J. Z. Young 1951.

64. Eccles 1953:193.

65. In Eccles's words: "In itself, post-tetanic potentiation has little significance, for it is not effective in increasing the relatively prolonged discharges that are characteristic of natural movements" (Eccles 1953:202).

66. Born in Vienna, Kandel had fled with his brother from the Nazis. For Kandel's life and work, see his biography, Kandel 2006.

I bypass the highly important work of David Hubel and Torsten Wiesel that documented for the first time experience-dependent plasticity. I bypass it because, on the one hand, they showed that there is experience-dependent plasticity and thus linked brain, organism, and environment. On the other hand, they worked on the developing brain and were crystal clear that once adulthood is reached, the brain is a fixed and immutable structure. In 1981, looking back at their work of the 1960s, Wiesel wrote that once adulthood is reached, "plasticity disappears" (Wiesel 1981:69). And Hubel added in 1989: "We have been thinking of the brain as a fully formed, mature machine. We have been asking how it is connected [...]. But that leaves untouched an entirely different and most important question: How did the machine get there in the first place?" (Hubel 1989:191).

67. And in 1954, a nine-hundred-page atlas, *Epilepsy and the Functional Anatomy of the Human Brain* (with Herbert Jaspers).

68. Milner 1954. Penfield had given the 1950 Gordon Wilson Lecture, titled "Mechanisms of Memory."

69. Scoville and Milner 1957; Penfield and Milner 1958; Milner 1954; Milner et al. 1968.

70. That is to say, Tauc used *Aplysia* as a model organism for studying the electric properties of neurons. However, he had not previously attempted to study the neuronal organization of behavior. This was Kandel's distinctive contribution. See Kandel 1979.

71. Tauc and Kandel 1964; Kandel and Tauc 1965a, 1965b.

72. Castellucci et al. 1970.

73. Kandel 1977.

74. The perforant pathway connects areas of the hippocampus to the cortex. Bliss and Lømo 1973:332. See also Lømo 1966; Anderson et al. 1969; Lømo 1971; and Bliss and Lømo 1970.

75. I write "in principle" because there was a caveat to their work. All they showed was that synaptic strength could be increased by artificially applied electrical impulses. Whether synaptic plasticity exists in vivo and is the locus of memory storage remained an open question. Bliss and Lømo concluded their 1973 paper: "Our experiments show that there exists at least one group of synapses in the hippocampus whose efficiency is influenced by activity which may have occurred several hours previously—a time scale long enough to be potentially useful for information storage. Whether or not the intact animal makes use in real life of a property which has been revealed by synchronous repetitive volleys [of impulses] to a population of fibers the normal rate and pattern activity along which are unknown, is another matter."

76. Kandel 1982:35, cited in Gardner1987:280.

77. There is, of course, the work of Joseph Altman (Altman 1962, 1963, 1966, 1967, 1969, 1970; see as well Altman and Das 1965a and 1965b; and Bayer et al. 1973), who reported in the early 1960s on the postnatal emergence of new neurons in the hippocampus of rats, guinea pigs, and mice. But did Altman set out to challenge fixity? In reporting his findings, he suggested that the formation of the brain takes, at least in part, longer than is usually assumed, but did not offer a new, embryogenetic conception of the adult brain. This is to say, Altman did not suggest that the mammalian brain as such is plastic, and he did not suggest, as far as I can tell, that postnatal neurogenesis is a lifelong, functionally significant event. In addition, there

was, in the 1970s, the rediscovery of adult hippocampal neurogenesis by Michael Kaplan. Kaplan attempted to generalize from his observations a conception of the brain as generally plastic. However, a separate oral history project on adult neurogenesis research that I have been conducting suggests that where Altman had offered too little concept work, Kaplan offered too much. He presented claims his work did not support, and thus not even the small community of adult neurogenesis researchers that came into existence in the late 1980s in the aftermath of Nottebohm's work on birds took his claims seriously.

78. Genetic studies of biological signal transduction were of course conducted since the 1960s; see, especially, the work on allosteric proteins in Monod, Wyman, and Changeux 1965. See also Monod, Jacob, and Changeux 1963. A review of this work is provided in Changeux 2012. A synaptic receptor was first isolated and described in Changeux's 1969 analysis of the nicotine receptor of acetylcholine. However, a description and analysis of the genes that regulate synaptic communication was an event of the early 1980s.

79. Scheller et al. 1982.

80. Kandel 2005. On transgenic mice, see Haraway 1997.

81. Such experiments have had ambiguous results. For example, on the one hand, they confirmed the existence of function-specific areas; on the other, they have shown that many cognitive functions previously thought to be site specific in fact engage many, sometimes widely separated areas of the cortex in a seemingly nonhierarchical fashion. For a powerful critique, see Hagner 2006. For a subtle critique, see Dumit 2004.

82. See Squire and Kandel 1999.

83. Nottebohm and Gold first reported on the birth of new neurons in the early 1980s, in the song nuclei of birds. However, the observation was assumed to be restricted to birds. In the 1990s, Arturo Alvarez-Buylla, a postdoc of Nottebohm, and Elizabeth Gould both discovered, independently of each other, the birth of new neurons in rodents, the former in the olfactory system, the latter in the hippocampus. To a degree, they rediscovered what Altman and Kaplan had reported in the 1960s and 1970s. Fred Gage, who entered the field of adult neurogenesis in the mid-1990s, also found new neurons in the hippocampus of rats. These experiments challenged fixity—and thus the exclusive focus on the synapse. There were two problems, however. First, neurogenesis was found only in lower vertebrates but not in human or nonhuman primates. When it then was found—in 1997 and 1998—it did not immediately result in a plastic brain. As Jean Pierre Bourgeois explained, adult neurogenesis was documented only in two small, ancient parts of the brain. Adult neurogenesis thus challenged fixity—but the actual emergence of a genuinely plastic brain, that is, a brain that is no longer essentially fixed and in which functional, synaptic plasticity is not the only dynamic element, occurred only after 2002, as adult neurogenesis research came together with the work of Karel Svoboda on long-term, large-scale structural plasticity and the work conducted in Alain's lab, which documented about then that the n-a-t of homeoproteins has a physiological function. See the coda to this book.

I wish to add another clarifying digression. In popular science literature about the plastic brain (Doidge 2007; Begley 2007, 2009; Schwartz and Begley 2003) one often reads that the work of Michael Merzenich and Jon Kaas in the 1980s marked the advent of plasticity research. Indeed, these authors provided powerful evidence of axonal remodeling in the adult brain (Merzenich et al. 1982)—but (almost) exclusively in response to prolonged (months to years) injury. As Chklovskii et al. (2004:786) put it: "Such pathological subcortical changes might release mechanisms of cortical rewiring that are not normally observed in the brain."

Merzenich did work on cortical representation of the hand digits and showed— with the tools of electrophysiology—that *after he cut the nerve that links a particular digit to a particular area of the cortex*—continuous training or stimulation of surrounding digits results in an expansion of the representation of these surrounding digits in the cortex into the area formerly occupied by the now dysfunctional digit (Merzenich et al. 1984; for a review on how his work developed, see Buonomano and Merzenich 1998). Merzenich called this increase in areal representation "plasticity." What is more, it seems as if, when speculating about the normal, noninjured brain, he explained such area-use increase in purely functional terms. This is to say, it was grounded in the strengthening of existing synaptic connections, pretty much in the way Hebb had predicted (neurons that wire together fire together). It was thus speculative—and in addition it was a chemical, functional plasticity entirely within what one could call the "classical schema": the adult brain is an immutable structure and the only way to account for learning is, as Sherrington put it, the plasticity of "the nervous reaction."

Put differently, Merzenich's was still a synaptic, chemical brain that had very little to do with the emergence of a genuinely plastic brain—in the sense of growth of new, not yet specified, and hence literally plastic tissue. He did not observe how the cortical connections underwent structural changes in response to the functional growth of new synapses, axons, dendrites, and spines (or the disappearance of new synapses).

In sum, Merzenich's maps, spectacular as they were, remained entirely within the fixed brain. For a similar assessment of Merzenich, see Chklovskii et al. 2004.

84. At the time I met Jean Pierre in 2002–2003, plasticity was just beginning to emerge as a general feature of the brain and to powerfully undermine fixity and with it the chemical, synaptic brain.

DIGRESSION: HISTORIES OF TRUTH

1. I refer here to articles published mostly in the *Journal of the History of Neuroscience* (largely run by neuroscientists for neuroscientists); for example, Jones 2000, 2002, 2004; Berlucchi 2002; Stahnisch and Nitsch 2002, 2003; Pascual-Leon et al. 2005; DeFelipe 2002, 2006; Colucci-D'Amato, Bonavita, and Di Porzio 2006; Berlucchi and Buchtel 2009. In addition, a small group of popular-science books

unfold along similar lines: Doidge 2007; Black 2001; Ansermet and Magistretti 2007; Schwartz and Begley 2003; Arden 2010. See also the books by American journalist Sharon Begley (2007, 2009).

2. Note that my historical inquiry in the previous chapter is not focused on the term *plasticity*, which was widely but unsystematically used in morphology from at least as far back as the late eighteenth century, and in biology from the discipline's emergence. Instead, I focus on the idea of anatomical fixity.

3. I learned the phrase "epistemologist of history" from Hans-Jörg Rheinberger's exploration of Canguilhem's work, which he juxtaposes with Gaston Bachelard's historical epistemology. An earlier characterization of Canguilhem as "epistemologist of history" (again juxtaposed with Bachelard as a "historical epistemologist") is offered by Lecourt.

4. In his lecture Canguilhem quotes Bachelard as saying: "Every historian of science is necessarily a historiographer of truth. [...] At various moments in the history of thought, the past of thought and experience can be seen in a new light."

5. On how the brain outgrew its histories, see Rees 2016a.

6. Begley 2007:5; Berlucchi and Buchtel 2009:307.

7. Berlucchi and Buchtel 2009:309. Already in 2002 Berlucchi had offered a similar argument. Then as now he insisted that Ernesto Lugaro (1870–1940), Tanzi's pupil, expanded on Tanzi's "hypothesis by applying the term plasticity to the practice-related synaptic changes envisioned by his teacher" (Berlucchi 2002:305–309). In this account, Ramón y Cajal is said to have known about the work of Lugaro and Tanzi and to have taken the term "plasticity" from them. Berlucchi argued that Cajal simply complemented Tanzi's "hypothesis with his own hypothesis of new connections between cortical neurons." In Berlucchi and Buchtel's 2009 article, essentially a rebuttal of Jones 2004, the authors acknowledge the work of James.

8. Miu 2011:3. See also Jones 2000; Stahnisch and Nitsch 2002; Stahnisch and Nitsch 2003; and Jones 2004.

9. Minea quoted in Jones 2000:37. On the same page, Jones claims: "So far as one can tell, the first use of plasticity in reference to the nervous system came in the thesis of Ioan Minea, written in Romanian and published in Bucharest in 1909."

Jones (2000 and 2004) and, if indirectly, DeFelipe (2006) argue that Ramón y Cajal then took the term from Minea and thus actually followed the French-Romanian rather than the Italian line. And a subset of this third group (DeFelipe 2006) claims that in fact Marinesco learned the term from the Belgian Jean Demoor, who published a paper in 1896 with the title "La plasticité morphologique des neurones cérébraux," or maybe from Mathias Duval, who put forth in 1895 a theory of amoebism.

10. The key author here is Javier DeFelipe (2006). I find DeFelipe's historical knowledge of nineteenth-century neuronal literature unsurpassed. I am grateful to Javier for several exchanges on the topic.

Jones (2004) seems to suggest, taking up DeFelipe's comment that the work of Wiedersheim and Rabl-Rückhard was later explicitly taken up by Lépic and Duval (i.e., two French authors), that either Lépic or Duval may have been the source of Demoor's use of the term *plasticity*, who in turn might have been the source for Marinesco, who actually studied in France. Via Minea, the term would have then reached Ramón y Cajal.

11. Canguilhem 1994:32. On historical epistemology, see Rheinberger 2010.

12. Canguilhem 1994:32, 30.

13. And his concept of psychology was not yet fully differentiated from philosophy.

14. It is true that he frequently speaks about the brain, but this brain is a psychological abstraction, not an anatomical composition.

15. The key passage in James is from chapter IV, "On Habit":

> Plasticity, then, in the wide sense of the word, means the possession of a structure weak enough to yield to an influence, but strong enough not to yield all at once. Each relatively stable phase of equilibrium in such a structure is marked by what we may call a new set of habits. Organic matter, especially nervous tissue, seems endowed with a very extraordinary degree of plasticity of this sort; so that we may without hesitation lay down as our first proposition the following, that the phenomena of habit in living beings are due to the plasticity of the organic materials of which their bodies are composed.

16. In many ways, James is a pre-anatomical, pre-neuronal philosopher reflecting about the brain. Like a Cartesian, he was looking for the seat of the Soul in the brain. James described the mind as fire and the brain as clay, and appears to have assumed that the fire literally burns itself into the clay. He suggested that every single brain cell is endowed with an individual consciousness—and that there is an arch cell that coordinates all the others into a coherent self.

17. The American philosopher's work neither generated a systematic inquiry into neuronal plasticity nor conceptually prefigured today's notion of plasticity. His discourse was not a different regional rationality; it was a different continent.

18. Was Tanzi—in 1893—really suggesting that memory is the product of synaptic, chemical facilitation? How could that have been the case? First, Sherrington invented the term *synapse*—and with it the conception of the brain as an integrative organ that alone allowed for the concept of the synapse—only half a dozen years later (in 1897). Second, Sherrington's synapse was not a chemical but an electrical entity (chemical facilitation was not established until 1952). Tanzi's is conceptually incommensurable with Sherrington's as well as with the neurochemical and today's plastic brain. It was a different organ, differently conceptualized, differently analyzed, differently known.

To complicate things further, how could Ramón y Cajal learn in 1893 from Tanzi about synaptic facilitation (which required a conceptualization of the nervous system that came into existence only several years later)? How could Ramón y Cajal intend his 1894 lecture as a compliment to Sherrington's concept of the synapse, when the synapse was born only three years later? And wasn't Ramón y Cajal, the anatomist of growth, rather critical of Sherrington's functionalization of the nervous system?

19. What is more, in none of these works, as far as I can tell, had the term *plasticity* any programmatic quality: no program was worked out, no new line of research was launched. Plasticity is not a central argument for any one of the cited works. On the contrary, the term is most often mentioned only a few times, usually in the form of a speculative outlook at the end of a longer work. And these researchers' contemporaries either ignored such speculations or denounced them as sheer nonsense.

Put differently, the amateur historians don't recognize—or at least they ignore—that the authors (or at least the passages from the works) they quote were forgotten on purpose: in the eyes of their late-nineteenth-century contemporaries, their reflections on plasticity actually disqualified them. After all, as everybody knew, the brain was essentially fixed. Put differently, plasticity was simply not yet a category of neuronal research for them. James *Principles of Psychology* is well over a thousand pages long, yet the term *plasticity* appears only five times! In Ramón y Cajal's *Textura*—likewise a thousand pages—the term appears even less often. The same applies, as far as I can tell, to Tanzi and Lugaro. And Wiedersheim and Rabl-Rückhard, and Duval, appear not to use the term at all.

20. The only thing they had in common, conceptually speaking, was the belief in adult cerebral fixity.

21. The competing histories of truth order the past in terms of the present—not recognizing that the past did not know our present concepts, problems, and methods.

22. Tanzi is linked explicitly to synaptic facilitation, Minea to sprouting after injury, Wiedersheim to potentiation, and James to synaptic plasticity and LTP.

23. The difference between synaptic plasticity and a more general, embryogenetic plasticity made possible by a silent embryogenesis in adult brains is also missed by Nikolas Rose and Joelle Abi-Rached (2013). They argue: "The belief that up until 1970, the human brain was viewed as immutable after the period of its development in utero and in early childhood has become something of a modern myth" (48) What is more, they suggest that there was always a "general acceptance" of plasticity in the neuronal sciences. In what follows, I critically work through the evidence they assemble to support their argument.

First, they turn to Rita Levi Montalcini, who wrote in 1982: "Is the formation of neuronal circuits in the central nervous system and the establishment of specific connections between nerve fibers and peripheral end organs rigidly programmed and unmodifiable, or are nerve fibers endowed with sufficient plasticity to allow deviation from predetermined routes [...] during neurogenesis?" (48). The quote is surprising, as Levi Montalcini in this passage actually speaks about the process of embryogenesis, as her reference to neurogenesis, which was in 1982 assumed to occur only before birth, clearly shows. The passion with which she wrote these lines were directed toward genetics, as it was claimed at the time that embryogenesis is organized by genes. What is the link to adult cerebral plasticity? It appears that Rose and Abi-Rached miss that Levi-Montalcini speaks about the embryo, not the adult.

Next, they refer to the discovery of critical periods (48/49). As I have sought to show above, however, the discovery of critical periods refers to developmental events: once the critical period is over, the cerebral tissue is immutable. Critical period studies hardly challenged the idea of adult cerebral fixity.

Then, abstracting from the discovery of critical periods, Rose and Abi-Rached suggest that throughout the twentieth century, there was "general acceptance that synaptic connections among neurons were constantly being created and pruned across the life of the organism, as a result of neuronal activity arising from experience" (49). The article that allows them to make this argument is Berlucchi and Buchtel (2009), which projects the discovery of synaptic plasticity by Bliss and Lømo in the 1970s back onto the 1880s and 1890s and then argues that research on synaptic plasticity emerged in the final decades of the nineteenth century. Rose and Abi-Rached, relying on Berlucchi and Buchtel, thus miss the massive conceptual and experimental events the emergence of a synaptic brain in the early 1950s and of synaptic plasticity in the 1970s actually were. Besides, if neuronal researchers always knew that that synapses appear and disappear continuously, why was the discovery of critical periods such an event?

Subsequently, they turn to what they refer to as the "most clearly stated postulate" (49) of plasticity, by Hebb 1949. They quote Hebb as saying: "Any two cells or systems of cells that are repeatedly active at the same time will tend to become associated, so that activity in one facilitates activity in the other." I note that Hebb doesn't use the term *plasticity* in this statement. Instead he speaks about facilitation, which (as shown above, footnote 39, chapter 3), is the English translation of Exner's *Bahnung,* which assumed that the brain is immutable. (Note that when Hebb wrote *The Organization of Behavior* in 1949, the synapse was still an electrical concept, which explains the absence of neurochemical concepts in his work.) As Hebb's big question was how an immutable brain could organize behavior, and as synaptic plasticity was discovered for higher vertebrates only a good twenty-five years after Hebb published *The Organization of Behavior,* it is not surprising that he actually doesn't use the term *plasticity* at all in this book.

I could go on, but think that these examples show that Rose and Abi-Rached consistently focus on the synaptic brain and assume—and this is historically inaccurate—that this synaptic brain has existed since the 1880s. What is more, they consistently miss the sweeping event that the emergence of a general concept of the brain's retained embryogenetic plasticity around the year 2000 actually was. This is shown particularly well by the only reference they make to research concerning adult neurogenesis—which they claim has been shown in "adult rodents [...] and later in primates" (50). They write—thereby repeating the critical voice of the synaptologists—that "there remained many doubts about the functional implications of such newly generated neurons." It is thus as if Rose and Abi-Rached defend the chemical, synaptic brain by belittling the significance that the observation of adult neurogenesis actually had. This is especially curious as their book was published in 2013—that is, long after the significance of adult neurogenesis in the hippocampus was shown to be critical for memory. It is curious also that the only author they reference here is Elizabeth Gould, as if no other researchers contributed to the discovery of adult neurogenesis. How could they miss that Gage, just a year after Gould reported new neurons in the hippocampi of macaque monkeys, discovered adult neurogenesis in humans?

It seems as if Rose and Abi-Rached write the history of the past in terms of the present: they abstract from the contemporary concept of plasticity as it has emerged since roughly 2000, and project it on the past, with the consequence that Levi-Montalcini (1980s), Tanzi (1890s), Hebb (1940s), and Merzenich (1980s) can all be described as plasticity researchers. Hence their argument that plasticity is hardly new.

For the way that led from the discovery of adult neurogenesis to the emergence of a general conception of plasticity in neuronal research, under which synaptic plasticity was then subsumed, see the coda.

CHAPTER 4. NOCTURNAL

Epigraph translation: It is an opportunity to do science differently, to show its nocturnal side, which never appears in the official discourse. […] For this it is necessary that the experience is constructed around an idea.

1. The focus on the technical misses the significance of ideas—and the importance of thinking for technology and the fact that it is constitutive of the possibility for thinking of the brain as plastic, for observing and knowing the brain as plastic.

2. My focus on things experimental was prefigured by the so-called turn to practice, in many ways exemplified by the emergence of laboratory studies. Famously, Michael Lynch (1985:xiv) declared—in part gesturing toward Latour and Woolgar (1979) and Knorr-Cetina (1981), as well as to Shapin and Schaffer (1985)—that science should not be considered "the exclusive property of historians and philosophers." Instead it should be taken up "as matters to be observed and described in the present." Put differently, the challenge was to study what scientists actually do.

As early as the mid-1980s, experimentation had emerged as a major site of science studies. Some authors focused on how scientists socially construct experimental results—through negotiation, judgment, and building social networks (Barnes 1985; Collins, Green, and Drape 1985; Pinch 1986; Pinch, Gooding, and Schaffer 1989; Gooding 1990); others studied the role that context and judgment play in experimentation (Pickering 1992) or how experimental results are realized through the construction of human or nonhuman networks (Latour 1984, 1987; Keating and Cambrosio 2003); yet others sought to understand experimentation as a distinct practice in which thinking and technology come together and constitute epistemic things (Hacking 1983; Galison 1987, 1988; Rheinberger 1992a, 1992b, 1993, 1994, 1996, 1997; Rheinberger, in particular, builds on Fleck 1935 and Bachelard 1949, 1953). It was this third line, the conjuncture of epistemology and experimentation, that I found intriguing.

3. Historical epistemology, just like laboratory studies or even the social construction of truth, does not undermine this assumption, but rather confirms it.

4. It would be easy to extend the critique—reproach—of Alain to the vast majority of historical and sociological studies of experimentation that were to become a key pillar of STS as it emerged over the 1980s and 1990s. In almost none of these works does the nocturnal work with ideas, or the conception of science as an effort to increase the possibilities of truth, have its place.

5. Had I made a discovery? I was aware, if vaguely, that it had been argued before that science has a nocturnal side to it (cf. notably Bachelard 1965; Bernard 1956; Jacob 1997). Although these and the few other publications on the topic I could find differ decisively from the nocturnal work practiced by Alain, almost all of the existing accounts are based on what one could call an ultimately diurnal, experiment-centric understanding of science: scientific practice, for them, is essentially experimentation. They describe nocturnal work as a kind of pre-scientific play. It might be considered as significant play, yet the actual scientific challenge is almost always said to come after one has ideas—to experimentally verify those ideas and thereby to deprive them of their nocturnality, to transform them into diurnal facts (e.g., Jacob 1997).

Some who read an earlier version of this chapter reacted by pointing out that Hans-Jörg Rheinberger, in particular, has explored the nocturnal dimension of scientific practice. Indeed, Rheinberger's work (1997, 2005, 2006) is most significant in this regard, though he has focused exclusively on experimentation. With regard to experiments, he showed that at the core of experimental knowledge production is a calculated form of "imprecision," which he defined as the condition of the possibility of exploring the yet to be known. By modifying a single variable of a given technical arrangement, one ventures into the yet unknown (Rheinberger called this procedure "differential reproduction"). But the work with ideas is absent even from Rheinberger.

Another comment on an earlier version of this chapter pointed to the large body of texts on what Polanyi (1958) called "tacit knowledge." Here too the above applies: the literature on tacit knowledge is overwhelmingly concerned with experimentation, not with nocturnal work.

6. Alain's work here speaks to a growing body of literature focused, on the one hand, on the importance of writing and scribbles (see Campe 1991; Rheinberger 2003, 2008) and, on the other hand, on drawing sketches and visualization—see Latour (1986) and especially the work of German art historians around Horst Bredekamp. The latter have explored the role that drawing and visualization have played in the history of philosophy and science (Bredekamp 2005; Wittman 2009; see also Bredekamp and colleagues' journal *Bildwelten des Wissens*). The key hypothesis of this school, if this is not too scholastic a term, is that drawing images, or pictorialization, provides a nonconceptual orientation central to new scientific discoveries precisely insofar as they are new—and hence beyond logocentric reach.

7. Bernard 1965:1.

8. The phrase "a feeling for the organism" is Alain's. Evelyn Fox-Keller (1984), writing about Barbara McClintock, makes a point similar to the one I aim at with regard to Alain.

9. *Translation:* I have my own idea of texts, my own style of reading. No touch. Pollution of the oeuvre as one pollutes nature.

10. I write "almost" because there were a few other labs, dispersed and unknown to one another, that elaborated the idea of plasticity.

11. Bernard 1957:167.

12. The background to this conceptualization was largely the chemistry of Lavoisier (Holmes 1987).

13. Bernard 1957:163.

14. For the specific French context of cognitive neuroscience, see Chamak. Interestingly, Brigitte Chamak, who is very critical of—and who sets French apart from American—cognitive neuroscience, was a PhD student of Prochiantz.

15. Bernard 1956:56. *Translation:* The challenge is to prove that developmental phenomena not only occur in the embryonic but as well in the adult state. [. . .] To prove, secondly, that developmental phenomena are the cause of all physiological phenomena, of all manifestations of life. Development, its creation [developmental creation], is therefore always the dominant vital phenomenon.

16. Bernard 1956:85. *Translation:* I am happy to admit that if physiology were well advanced, the physiologist could create new animals and plants, just as the chemist can produce minerals that that could exist but that have not yet been realized by nature. [. . .] But in order to achieve such modifications, physiology has to act scientifically and it has to pay attention to what it does [scientifically] because it is going to know the intimate laws of formation of organic bodies, as the chemist knows the laws of formation of mineral bodies. It is thus in the laws of formation of organized bodies that all biological experimental science takes place [can occur].

17. More specifically, Spemann's goal now was to uncover the inductive potency of the different parts of the gastrula, with a particular focus on the so-called medullar plate, an axis out of which the embryo is formed in the course of embryogenesis.

18. Spemann's lab notebook, 1921, quoted in Mangold 1982:170. *Translation:* Such a piece of an organization center could simply be called an organizer. It produces in the indifferent material in which it lies or into which it is grafted an organizational field of a certain direction and expansion.

19. The idea was not new. Spemann, in his 1925 paper with Mangold, had himself speculated that the active force of the organizer could be a chemical substance. However, Spemann soon abandoned this idea and mostly displayed skepticism toward chemical approaches to studying the organizer.

20. Waddington et al., 1935.

21. S. Gilbert 1991:188.

22. Waddington 1952.

23. Waddington 1939:37–44.

24. Cf. S. Gilbert 1991:192, 265.

25. Waddington 1940:88.

26. Turing 1952:37.

27. Turing 1952:37.

28. The idea of infectious entities is taken from Alain's reading of the work of Stanley Prusiner, who has suggested that prions are infectious proteins. Call it another example of nocturnal work with ideas.

29. In addition, one would have to mention, at least, Ovid; Bergson, contemporary of Bernard, philosopher of life as motion and invention; Goethe and Geoffrey, the first, inventor of morphology, the second, his ally, introducer of the concept of homology into comparative anatomy; His and Haeckel, who fought with each other but who both conceived of irreducible forces of formation (e.g., Haeckel's *Plastidulen*); Stephen Gould and Dennis Duboule, to name two contemporary biologists of form and motion; and of course countless scientific papers and articles.

30. Thompson 1942:7.

31. Thompson 1942:1026.

32. Thompson 1942:137

33. Thompson 1942:265.

34. Thompson 1942:155.

35. A transformation brought about not by genetic mutations but by changing the equilibrium among "physical forces" (Thompson 1942:137). "The form of any particle of matter, whether it be living or dead, and the changes in form which are apparent in its movements and in its growth, may in all cases be described as due to the action of force" (155).

36. Thompson 1942:272.

37. Thompson 1942:137.

38. Thompson 1942:137, 155.

39. Thompson 1917:687.

40. Stern 1967:165.

41. The rivalry between Goldschmidt and Morgan reaches back to 1915, the year Morgan published "Theory of the Gene." On how the conflict developed, see Stern 1967.

42. *Translation:* Nature doesn't make jumps.

43. That is why Goldschmidt's genetics is occasionally called "physiological genetics."

44. Goldschmidt's conceptualization of genes changed over the course of his career and is, as Stephen Jay Gould attests, often vague and unclear.

For Morgan, a gene was a discrete, corpuscular substance that could be located on a chromosome. He viewed it as simultaneously a unit of structure, function, mutation, and recombination. Goldschmidt did not deny the possibility of locating genes on chromosomes. However, he rejected the assumption that genes are discrete entities. In place of Morgan's gene (usually called the classical gene), Goldschmidt advocated a dynamic and hierarchically structured interplay of genetic units. This had consequences especially for his understanding of mutation. Whereas Morgan considered mutations to be changes in the chemical constitution of a single, classical gene, Gold-schmidt mutations occur not on the level of a single gene but only insofar as they impact the structure or hierarchy of the interplay between genetic units. It seems at times as if Goldschmidt was ready to discard the gene concept entirely and speak instead of the chemical reorganization of the chromosomes as such.

45. Analyzing these latter results, he found that "an intersex is an individual which has developed as a male (or female) up to a certain time point; from this turning point the development has continued as a female (or male). The increasing degree of intersexuality is an expression of the recession of the turning point, that is, its occurrence at an earlier stage in development" (Goldschmidt 1923:91).

46. Normal expression of a trait, according to Goldschmidt, depends on the corresponding gene's ability to produce enough substance at the right time in the course of development. If this is not the case—for example, if not enough male sex determiners are produced at the right time—an animal that has thus far developed as male will continue to develop as female.

47. In addition, working on caterpillars, he found that large differences in the color patterns of caterpillars resulted from small changes in the timing of development: the effects of a slight delay or enhancement of pigmentation early in growth increased through ontogeny and led to profound differences among fully grown caterpillars.

48. Goldschmidt 1940:297.

49. Goldschmidt 1940:205.

50. Goldschmidt 1940:391. The result, then, is a saltational emergence of a new species: "evolution in a single large step on the basis of embryonic processes produced by one mutation."

51. Quoted from the manuscript "Are Homeoproteins Morphogens?" which Alain sent me in 2003.

52. And, as one will quickly recognize if one searches for further correspondences between Goldschmidt and Thompson, both argue that *natura facit saltum*. Thompson wrote in *On Growth and Form* (1942):

> When we begin to draw comparison between our algebraic curves and attempt to transform one into another, we find ourselves limited by the very nature of the case. [. . .] An algebraic curve has its fundamental formula, which defines the family to which it belongs. [. . .] We never think of "transforming" a helicoid into an ellipsoid, or a circle into a frequency curve. So it is with the forms of animals. We cannot transform an invertebrate into a vertebrate, nor a coelenterate into a worm, by any simple and legitimate deformation [. . .]. Nature proceeds from one type to another [. . .]. To seek for steppingstones across the gaps between is to seek in vain, forever. (1094)

Thompson, like Goldschmidt, argued that macroevolutionary change could occur only in a saltational mode. Abstracting from his analyses of homeotic mutations, Thompson became convinced that the steady continuity of evolutionary change suggested by Darwinism reigns only within a family of species, but that it cannot account for the emergence of different species. Interspecies gaps can be crossed only "per saltum." Such changes could occur, Thompson concluded, only in fundamental rearrangements of developmental growth rates. Thirty years later, Goldschmidt arrived at a similar conclusion.

53. De Beer 1958.

54. He described the claim that ontogeny strictly recapitulates the linear stages of phylogeny as a "mental straight jacket."

55. For this conclusion, de Beer drew especially on the work of Charles Manning Child, Walter Garstang, Edwin Stephen Goodrich, and Julian Huxley.

56. De Beer (1958) wrote: "For instance, teeth were evolved before tongues but in mammals now tongues develop before teeth" (7).

57. De Beer 1958:23.

58. De Beer (1958:8) wrote: "To the alteration and reversal of the sequence of stages the term heterochrony is applied". With the concept of heterochrony, de Beer literally turns Haeckel's biogenetic law upside-down. Whereas the "German Darwin" saw the key for understanding embryology in identifying evolutionary stages, de Beer, who had constructed an index that allowed him to see what Darwin read at any point in his life, saw the study of embryogenetic processes as key to understanding evolution.

59. In a remarkable synthesizing effort, de Beer systematized such heterochronic changes into "eight possible morphological modes." He subsumed these eight modes under the two principles gerontomorphosis and paedomorphosis.

60. De Beer 1958:174.

61. In fact, he depicted evolution as a cyclic back-and-forth of organisms between increases and decreases in plasticity.

62. De Beer 1958:63. The term *neoteny* was first used by the German zoologist Julius Kollmann to refer to amphibians who reached sexual maturity in a larval state.

63. De Beer 1958:68.

64. De Beer 1958:117.

65. De Beer 1958:122, 71.

66. One can see here that Alain, even though his claim of adult cerebral plasticity blurs the classical schema of neuronal research, holds on to the anthropological aspiration constitutive of brain research since the time of Franz Josef Gall.

67. One could further argue that it is the vagueness, the unknownness, of "his artifact" that allows him to correlate passages and to travel from embryology to evolution to anthropology to neuroscience.

68. Spatazza et al. 2013a, 2013b.

69. The effect of my introduction to the nocturnal basis of science was that Alain's laboratory began to appear to me as a factory to explore the spaces of possibility opened up by his nocturnal work. It was still the place of experimentation, of intense discussions about how to conduct, or not to conduct, an experiment; a place of continuous exchange about the technical details of antibodies and anti-antibodies, about temperatures, Western and Northern blots, about confocal micro-

scopes. And yet all of this now had meaning only in relation to nocturnal work, which set it in perspective—which gave this work its perspective.

DIGRESSION: VITAL CONCEPTS

1. This is how Arthur Goldhammer translates Canguilhem:

> Nevertheless, the use of epistemological recursion as a historical method is not universally valid. It best fits the disciplines for the study of which it was originally developed: mathematical physics and nuclear chemistry. Of course there is no reason why one cannot study a particularly advanced specialty and then abstract rules for the production of knowledge that may with caution be extrapolated to other disciplines. In this sense the method can be not so much generalized as broadened. Yet it cannot be extended to other areas of the history of science without a good deal reflection about the specific nature of the area to be studied. Consider, for example, eighteenth-century natural history. Before applying Bachelardian norms and procedures to the study of this subject, one must ask when a conceptual cleavage occurred whose effects were as revolutionary as those of the introduction of relativity and quantum mechanics in to physics.

Goldhammer's attempt is problematic because it loses sight of what Canguilhem actually writes about: whether there are in biology any conceptual fractures that correspond in their effect to the effect quantum mechanics has had in physics. The point here is that Canguilhem actually juxtaposes Bachelard's concept of *déchirures*—which he argues, however indirectly, is specific to physics—with the concept of *fracture*, which he sees more suited to biology.

2. *Translation:* This term "fracture"—so close to [and yet so different from] the terms of "rupture" or "tear," which belong to G. Bachelard—is borrowed from Jean Cavaill's: "[. . .] these fractures of successive interdependence, which each time lift from that which was before the imperious profile of that which comes necessarily after and which exceeds that which was before."

To elaborate: Canguilhem states here with Cavaillès that knowledge is not a linear growth but must be understood as fractures of conceptually independent units of knowledge. Each time new knowledge comes along, it lifts from the previous one the authority it could enjoy only as long as it was unquestionably true, and the new knowledge can necessarily come only after it conceptually exceeds previous knowledge, on which it partly builds (thereby constituting progress). Canguilhem thus himself builds on Bachelard and yet departs from him by replacing the terms *rupture* or *tear* with the terms *fracture* (*fracture*) and *outgrowth* (*dépasser*, "to exceed").

3. *Translation:* We can admit that life unsettles logical reasoning without needing to believe that we'll be better off understanding life by giving up to form concepts and to instead search for some long lost key.

1. Frequently one of my lab mates would stop by, tell me something he or she thought interesting to an anthropologist, smile like an accomplice, and hurry away, often with a frivolous and triumphant laugh. See Marcus 1998.

2. Pax6 is also a paired box gene–protein. For what was known in 2002, see Callaerts et al. 1996 and Gehring 1999. For a more up-to-date overview, see Gehring 2012.

3. Gianfranco later left the lab and became a science and society scholar invested, on the one hand, in the overlap between the arts and science and, on the other hand, in determining the limits of what neuroscience can tell us about our lives. He has published a large body of articles in science journals, as well as a popular science book that seeks to circumscribe what one can and cannot learn from the neuroscience of emotion.

4. A condition of the possibility of creativity is the systematic effort to allow for accidents to derail an experimental setup, as especially Rheinberger 1997 has brilliantly argued. One could argue that the 1989 observation of a non-autonomous transfer of homeoproteins is one such accident—what is the role of the accidental for fieldwork?

5. One consequence of this perspectivism is that experimental knowledge is inevitably partial (Strathern 1991). Experiments are partial connections with and to the real. They can actualize only one among several possible aspects of the thing to be known. The condition for this perspectivism—for this partiality—is grounded in the curious fusion of thinking and technology that allows phenomena to be addressed from various points of view.

6. For an account of the difficulty of the shift from in vitro to in vivo work, see Morange 2002.

7. Which in turn implied the challenge of "seeing" in the available technological knowledge a possibility for conceptualizing the living (the yet to be known) in such a way that one could address the living in technical terms (the already known) without actually reducing it to the technical (that is, while maintaining the possibility of surprise).

8. Not all homeoproteins are relevant for brain formation, and not all of them play an equally significant role in the cellular emergence of the nervous system.

9. Gehring 1995. It was known as a transcription factor (if an unusual one, for Pax6 has two DNA binding sites, a paired domain, coded for by the so-called paired box, and a homeodomain, coded for by the homeobox), and was known to have the three alpha helices necessary for the nonautonomous secretion and internalization, and to be autoregulative, that is, to regulate its own transcription (which was central to the morphogen question).

10. Classical knockout experiments had shown that Pax6 and Pax2 are reciprocal inhibitors. In the absence of Pax2, neuroepithelial pigment cells from the retina are found in the stalk, suggesting a shift in the border. Conversely, in the absence of Pax6, the eyecup is missing and the stalk elongates up to the nonneural ectoderm.

In all of these processes its main role is the regulation of molecules known to affect growth and guidance cues, cell proliferation, migration, adhesion, and signaling.

11. Götz et al. 2002a, 2002b. Today, these claims are clearly established. Pax6 is critical for the transformation of radial glia into neural stem cells or progenitor cells. For the olfactory system (OS) the decisive area is the subependymal zone of the subventricular zone, and for the hippocampus (HP) the decisive area is the amygdala of the dentate gyrus. Furthermore, it seems likely that the progenitors produced in these regions migrate to areas other than OS or HP and that Pax6 is centrally involved in this migration and differentiation of neurons.

Götz's observations led her to suggest that Pax6 is the "master control regulator of modular functions in development as much as in adulthood."

12. Pax2 is genetically determined and cell-autonomous. Pax6, in contrast, is diffusing and nonautonomous. It will expand until it encounters cells already differentiated as Pax2 cells.

13. PCR stands short for "polymerase chain reaction," the term for a method used in amplifying pieces of DNA. For a history of PCR, see Rabinow 1996a.

14. "What is meant by the term 'joking relationship' is a relation between two persons in which one is by custom permitted, and in some instances required, to tease or make fun of the other, who in turn is required to take no offence." Radcliffe-Brown 1952:90.

15. The term *experimental system* here does not, or does only partially, refer to Hans Jörg Rheinberger's work. As Rheinberger himself emphasizes, the phrase is common currency among researchers throughout the world. Prochiantz and his colleagues were no exception to this rule. And, as will be seen below, they had a clear sense of what they meant by the term. Rheinberger took the term from Paul Zamecnik and develops his understanding in a close analysis of Zamecnik's work; see Rheinberger 1997. See footnote 19 for a discusion of Rheinberger's seminal work on experimentation.

16. This discovery has been made several times in the history of the anthropology of science. See, especially, Traweek 1992 and Germer 1997.

17. The relevance of social trust and reliability in experimental work was first emphasized by Shapin (1995), who focuses on the emergence of a gentleman science in seventeenth-century England. For an account of the relevance of trust in the biotech world, see Rabinow 1996a.

18. See, especially, Daston and Galison 1992 and Rheinberger 1997.

Historians of science have argued that the emergence of such mechanical, or machine-based, forms of knowledge production in the late nineteenth century mark the beginning of "objective knowledge." The clue here is that "objectivity" is not a breakthrough to a timeless, universal truth, but a time- and place-specific concept that reflects a particular way of producing knowledge (a clearcut separation of the process of knowledge production from the human senses). It relies on machines, or technological procedures, that force the objects in question to leave traces that form the material basis of experimental knowledge. (In the case of my work with

Gianfranco, these traces were bands on a western blot membrane, fluorescent dots under the Confocal microscope, or stained spots visible on tissue prepared through in situ hybridization.) What interests me here is less a historical provincialization of objectivity, or the powerful ethical effect that the emergence of objectivity, as practice, has actually had for experimenters (how it produces an ascetic self that must efface itself). Rather, I am curious about the epistemological consequences of the recognition that the experimental *Erkenntnisprozess* (process of gaining knowledge) is fundamentally decoupled from human individuals and their faculties.

19. The fact that experiments constitute, rather than discover, things has led some authors to avoid speaking of experimentally known things as if they are discovered "natural" objects or entities. Rather, they suggest, one should speak about "reified theorems," "theoretical entities," or "epistemic things," The term *reified theorems* is taken from Gaston Bachelard (see chapter 3). Undergirding Bachelard's concept of reified theorems is what he called phenomeno-technology. According to Bachelard, the things experiments produce knowledge about do not exist in nature as such; instead, they are technically produced reifications of theories—hence, reified theorems.

Ian Hacking (1983) speaks of "theoretical entities" (e.g., 21). Hacking does not refer to Bachelard. The background of Hacking's argument is his effort to develop, against Kuhn's thesis of the incommensurability of different scientific paradigms, a concept of "scientific realism." "Scientific realism," Hacking writes, "says that the entities, states and processes described by correct theories really do exist." The principle of correctness is that they are technically reified by technical procedures. In Hacking's terms, "So far as I am concerned, if you can spray them [electrons] then they are real" (21).

Rheinberger (1997) introduced the concept of "epistemic things" or "epistemic objects." The context for Rheinberger's concept of epistemic things is his effort to develop Bachelard's initial insight into a broad epistemology of experimental science. At the core of this epistemology is a conception of "experimental systems" as the "smallest integral working units of research" (28). These experimental systems, much along the lines I have developed above, are the material basis of experimental knowledge and produce what is known about experimental objects. As what is known depends on the technical procedures and the epistemological assumptions they stand for, Rheinberger speaks of epistemic things. One can see that Rheinberger draws heavily on Bachelard (and little on Hacking). One could almost say that his epistemic things are a well-elaborated version of Bachelard's conception of reified theorems. Almost, for Rheinberger elegantly adds an important dimension to Bachelard. With multiple references (especially to Derrida, Deleuze, and George Kubler) Rheinberger shows that epistemic things are characterized by their intrinsic potential for producing surprise and the unexpected. Specifically, he makes epistemic things visible as unstable entities that embody a productive vagueness in the form of a not yet exhausted openness, which invites speculation and association. In experimentation, this speculation and association, which according to Rheinberger make visible an intersection point between art and science, comes in the form of a "groping in the dark" or a "differential reproduction" (Rheinberger is citing, as Alain did, Claude Bernard). One constantly repeats experimental procedures, looking for a significant difference that gives contour to the object in question. Once such an object is exhausted, it becomes, so Rheinberger argued, a part of the technical procedures an experimental system consists of. It is evident that in my own understanding of experimental science I owe gratitude especially to Rheinberger. And yet I think that my effort to move beyond a technical description of experimentation—my emphasis on thought, on construction work, on experimental realism, on the poetry of window making—is also an effort to move beyond Rheinberger's (narrow) focus on the technical.

20. Bruno Latour (1987) writes: "The new object, at the time of its inception, is still undefined. At the time of its emergence you cannot do better than explain what the object is by repeating the list of its constitutive actions. The proof is that if you add an item to the list you redefine the object, that is, you give it a new shape" (87–88). It is exaggerated to suggest, as Latour seems to do, that each time a new entry is added to the list, the object becomes something new altogether. However, this does not mean, as Latour seems to imply, that it gains a new shape, as if the whole thing as such changes.

21. The title of this chapter refers to Galison 1987.

22. Although I tried hard several times, I could never find out whether this narrowing of perspective was built into the construction of the Pax6 project, as if Alain and his colleagues expected from the beginning that at one point energy would focus on one of the several issues touched on, or whether it was simply the result of the difficulties encountered in the course of research. Each time I asked Alain, he smiled and then changed topics.

23. In the specific case of Pax6 and eye formation, neurons of the diencephalon express Pax6 and thereby define the "eye anlagen," as Spemann had suggested, if hypothetically, in the 1920s. As the diencephalon evaginates, it comes into contact with the nonneural epithelium. This contact induces the formation of the lens, which also expresses Pax6, but only after the contact and thus, presumably, after Pax6 has been activated by itself.

One can see here the continuity of experimental and nocturnal work. The effort to show that Pax6 is a plastic force is in correspondence with Bernard's, Spemann's, Turing's, and Waddington's ideas that essential plastic forces—organizers, evocators, or morphogens—shape the organism. And if one takes into account that the experiments are meant to shed light on plastic processes in the adult, a second conjuncture of experimental and nocturnal work becomes visible, namely the relevance of the ideas of Thompson, Goldschmidt, Bernard, and de Beer.

24. And besides—Laure's project on Engrailed in the adult substantia nigra had established, in parallel with Brigitte's work, the relevance of the nonautonomous transfer for the survival of dopaminergic neurons in the adult.

25. Nédélec et al. 2004; De Toni et al. 2008; Sugiyama et al. 2008, 2009, Beurdeley et al. 2012; Spatazza et al. 2013.

1. For a brief period in the sixteenth century, wax models were produced as well. However, these earlier models were not known to eighteenth-century sculptors. Anatomical illustrations have been known since at least the fourteenth century, but only in the mid-eighteenth century were sculptors beginning to produce wax models of the anatomical body, and also of plants and of animals.

2. I have relied largely on the following histories of embryology: Hopwood 2000, 2002a, 2002b, 2009, 2015; Maienschein 2003; Oppenheimer 1967; and the essays in S. Gilbert 1991.

3. The formulation "embryos in wax" is taken from Hopwood 2002a. I first learned about His's modeling from Hopwood 1999.

4. Aside from Hopwood—who has focused on the modeling of His and as well on his conflict with Haeckel—surprisingly little has been written about Wilhelm His's plastic anatomies. And even Hopwood, from whom I learned enormously, does not actually write much about His's concept of plasticity. Rather, he discusses His's attempt at three-dimensional thinking. Hopwood (1999) writes:

> Investigating three-dimensional representation devices many not just enrich but also revise our accounts of scientific controversy and change. Innovations [. . .] have been important sources of novelty, but scientists have achieved less consensus on their representational virtues than on those of pictures. Detractors have reluctantly conceded their uses where vividness is at a premium, such as in teaching or communication with laypeople, while advocates have prized them as the ultimate in representational achievement [. . .]. Precisely because they have been so disputed, bringing models in three dimensions into general histories of the sciences may do more than just fill them out. By studying models that some groups promoted or relied on and others ignored or opposed, we can develop new views of what was at stake in struggles over change.(464)

Hence, Hopwood's interest in the role of models in science. Hence, his focus on the conflict between His and Haeckel—a way of studying controversies, so central to STS, from the vantage of models.

His referred to his models as *plastische Anschauung* (plastic views) as early as 1868. In 1880, His began to speak of *plastische Synthese* (plastic synthesis).

5. Haeckel first used the phrase biogenetic law in 1870 (Haeckel 1870:361–362).

6. *Our Body's Form and the Physiological Problem of Its Development,* also published in 1874. He had moved from Basel to Leipzig in 1871, when the University of Leipzig was Germany's most renowned research university, and His directed what was at the time the world's most modern anatomical institute.

7. Daston and Galison 1992; Daston 1999; Hopwood 2006; Daston and Galison 2007:192, 193, 447.

8. A few years before he died, Spemann published *Embryonic Induction,* an overview of his work. Early on in the book he criticized His's modeling as a pre-

experimental embryology (Spemann 1936:8). What Spemann did not recognize, perhaps, was how much his own modeling continued that of His.

1. This was my first time to visit him in his lab, and I was struck by how unfamiliar a space it was. While a cell biology laboratory like Alain's was organized around the cell culture room, an electrophysiology lab seemed to revolve around a set of electronic recording devices. Whereas the former was stuffed with Petri dishes, test tubes, pipettes, and centrifuges, the latter was equipped with electrodes, power cords, and computers. Even the smell was different. Whereas a biology lab's odor came from the ubiquitous calf medium used to culture neurons, the electrophysiology lab smelled of dusty electronics and reminded one a bit of an old radio shop.

2. Fessard, in many ways, was the esteemed founding figure of neuronal electrophysiology in France. Jean Pierre Changeux was a student of Jacques Monod (1910–1976) and François Jacob (1920–2013), two Nobel Prize–winning first-generation molecular biologists. The clashes between the electrophysiologists and molecular biologists marked, in retrospect at least, the beginning of a gradual shift from the predominance of electrophysiological methods to methods of cell biology.

3. Weber (1918) assigns the idea of an unbridgeable gap between life and science to Tolstoy. On Tolstoy's conception of life and science, see Gustafson 1986. On the relationship between Weber and Tolstoy, see Hanke 1993. For a brilliant contextualization of Weber's distinction between life and science in post-Hegelian German intellectual culture, see Schnädelbach 1984. For the relevance of the distinction in Weber's personal life, see Radkau 2005.

To underscore the significance of the belief in an unbridgeable gap in European thought (and also for contemporary American anthropology), I would point to the extraordinary career of this belief among European philosophers. For example, a considerable part of twentieth-century German philosophy was preoccupied with delimiting life from—indeed with philosophically occupying and defending life against—science. Relying on Weber, Karl Jaspers (1919) sought to identify concrete human experiences for which science is irrelevant. Martin Heidegger (1967 [1921]), addressing Jaspers, argued that the task of philosophy is to think of humans precisely from the perspective of those experiences to which science is irrelevant (on the significance for Heidegger of Georg Simmel's distinction between life and science, see Großheim 1991). Hans Georg Gadamer (1960), a prominent student of Heidegger, insisted on the significance of nonscientific truths for things human. What holds true for German intellectual culture is equally true, if in different ways, for France, a country in which (from Claude Bernard and Henri Bergson to Michel Foucault, Gilles Deleuze, and Félix Guattari) the relationship between life and science has been a central concern of philosophers. And via Foucault—be it in the form of biopower, or of the ethical relation between knowledge and subject of knowledge, or of the naïve antimodernism of some quarters of the anthropology of science—the gap between life and science has also become a central topic in American anthropology.

4. For the argument I seek to develop here, the distinction between "morals" in the modern sense and "ethics" in the ancient sense (often referred to as "virtue ethics") is critical. By "morals," one usually refers to a philosophical system that seeks to define what is right or wrong in the abstract. Morality, this is to say, is about rules, about abstract universal rules, independent from concrete situations and lives. In this respect, the idea of a general moral system is inseparably related to European modernity (Jonsen and Toulmin 1990; MacIntyre 1967, 1981). Furthermore, morality is usually concerned exclusively with moral questions. It does not touch on all domains of life—or does so only insofar as they involve moral issues (Striker 1996; Williams 1985). Ethics, at least in the way the ancients understood it, has little to do with what is generally right or wrong. *Ethics,* first and foremost, refers to the effort—the practice—of actively living one's life, the effort of giving a form to one's life always in accordance with reason. Whereas morality requires obeying rules, ethics is an all-encompassing practice: work on the self in which one's very being is at stake. The ideal form of life—and this can be achieved only by continuous exercise—was one that succeeded in making ethos and logos coincide, a life lived in accordance with reason. For a detailed account of the ancient Greek sense of the term *ethics,* see, especially, Rabbow 1954; Hadot 1995; and Foucault 2001. See also Pohlenz 1948 and Nussbaum 1986, 1994.

5. My use of the term *equipment* is reminiscent of Foucault's (2005). See also Rabinow 2003.

6. One could say that I learned from Brigitte that plasticity was a conceptual event only insofar as it also was a relational event; and from Maria-Luz that in the life sciences a conceptual event is always also and perhaps primarily an experimental event. Hence, I not only conducted a conceptual analysis of plastic reason but also a relational and experimental one—and a nocturnal one, for without Alain's nocturnal work, plastic reason would not have been *possible.*

7. The idea to use the ethical as an analytic device for understanding what kind of humans we're in the process of becoming has been prefigured by my reading of Georg Simmel and Max Weber, specifically their conversation about Nietzsche's *Genealogy of Morals* (a conversation first brought to my attention in Hennis 1987:172ff; see also Hennis 1996:101–105). Weber appears to have learned from Simmel's work on Nietzsche—specifically his book *Schopenhauer und Nietzsche* (1995 [1907]) and his essay "Friedrich Nietzsche: Eine moralphilosophische Silhouette" (1896)—to use "the ethical" as a key analytic device to find out "what kind of human beings" (*"welcher Typus Mensch"*) we are in the process of becoming (cf. Hennis 1986:173–174).

I stress this use of "the ethical" as an analytic device in order to avoid misunderstanding. This chapter has nothing to do with the various and often brilliant ways in which anthropologists have touched on ethics (for a general review, see Faubion

2001a:118–138; 2001b). It is guided neither by ethnographies of "their" ethics (of which the ethnographic archive tells us quite a bit; see, e.g., R. B. Brandt 1954 and Geertz 1960, 1973) nor by the (often Foucault-inspired) anthropological inquiries into the ethical self-relations of others (see Mahmood 2005; Hirschkind 2001, 2006). Also, this book is not related to anthropological inquiries into the complex relation between "ethics" and biology or biomedicine (see Cohen 1999; Franklin 1995; Kleinman 1995; Rabinow 2003) or the important reflection of an ethically motivated anthropology (Kleinman and Benson 2006; Farmer 2001, 2004; Das 2006).

8. Waldeyer-Hartz 1891:52–55, 64. As supporters of Ramón y Cajal, Waldeyer-Hartz mentioned Koelliker, His, Lenhossek, and Retzius.

9. Suddenly I had doubts about the whole enterprise. I worried that what awaited me was the tedious labor of deducing ethical ideas from texts not actually written to address ethical questions. But then I made what I came to think of as one of the most important discoveries of my second sojourn in the library: almost every publication I was reading, no matter how narrowly technical it was, spoke directly to questions about life and science—either by making an explicit effort for thinking of things human (from behavior to cognition of reasoning) in neuronal terms or by making implicit recommendations about how one should, from a neuronal perspective, live one's life (from diet to exercise to learning). The longer I stayed in the library and the more I read, the more I found myself intrigued by the idea that the authors of the texts I was reading had all been neurological humans— that they, just like Philippe, Christo, and Alain, had been ethically at stake in their research.

Making explicit the ethical spaces and equipment that different neuronal conceptions of the brain have opened up over time thus hardly meant asking questions external to the texts I was working through. Rather, it meant learning to read them as the ethical reflections their authors intended them to be, at least partly.

10. Ramón y Cajal used the tree and the forest concept widely—and perhaps most famously in his Nobel lecture "Neurons, Structures, and Connections." See the exceptional essay by DeFelipe 2013.

11. Ramón y Cajal 1991 [1901–1917]:155–156.

12. Except, perhaps, on the microscopically small scale of dendritic spines—as he speculated late in his life. Consequently, Ramón y Cajal frequently published articles on the importance of education and public schools.

13. Ramón y Cajal 1913.

14. The term *cytoarchitecture* actually first emerged in Theodor Meynert's *Der Bau der Gross-Hirnrinde und seine örtlichen Verschiedenheiten: Nebst einem patholo-gisch–anatomischen Corollarium* (1872). Meynert (1833–1892) died a year after Waldeyer-Hartz first used the term *neuron*. The neuronalization of cytoarchitecture was left to Meynert's successors.

15. Brodmann (1909), for example, wrote that his task was "eine topographische Analyse der menschlichen Hirnrinde hinsichtlich ihres Zellbaus durchzuführen.

Dieser Aufgabe lag der [...] Gedanke zugrunde, einen von den Hirnanatomen und Pathologen einen längst als Bedürfnis empfundenen histologischen Normalstatus der gesamten Großhirnrindenfläche des Menschen zu schaffen" (The task was to carry out a topographical analysis of the human cortex with respect to its cellular construction. The idea behind this task was to create what anatomists and pathologists long felt was needed: a histological assessment of the normal state of the entire cerebral cortex of humans). The aim was "ein vollständiges Bild des Rindebaus" (a complete picture of the building of the cortex). To be more precise, Brodmann hoped to uncover "die Bildungsgesetze der Großhirnrinde" (the laws of formation of the cerebral cortex) He also speaks of the "Organisationsprinzipien" (organizational principles) that underlay the logic of construction of the entire cortex or of the "Bauplan des Cortex cerebri" (the construction plan of the cerebral cortex).

16. Sherrington 1906 [1904].

17. Lucas 1905, 1906, 1907, 1910, 1912; Adrian and Lucas 1912; Adrian 1928, 1932, 1937.

18. Turing 1937, 1938. What is a Turing machine? Here is an answer from Wikipedia (https://en.wikipedia.org/wiki/Turing_machine): "The Turing machine was invented in 1936. [...] Turing [...] called it an 'a-machine' (automatic machine). The Turing machine is not intended as practical computing technology, but rather as a hypothetical device representing a computing machine. Turing machines help computer scientists understand the limits of mechanical computation. Turing gave a succinct definition of the experiment in his 1948 essay, 'Intelligent Machinery.' Referring to his 1936 publication, Turing wrote that the Turing machine, here called a Logical Computing Machine, consisted of: '[...] an unlimited memory capacity obtained in the form of an infinite tape marked out into squares, on each of which a symbol could be printed. At any moment there is one symbol in the machine; it is called the scanned symbol. The machine can alter the scanned symbol and its behavior is in part determined by that symbol, but the symbols on the tape elsewhere do not affect the behavior of the machine. However, the tape can be moved back and forth through the machine, this being one of the elementary operations of the machine. Any symbol on the tape may therefore eventually have an innings (Turing 1948, p. 3).'"

19. The transfer of the term *computer* from humans who computed to electrical machines occurred in the late 1940s and became more widespread only in the 1950s.

20. Wiener 1948. I did not mention Wiener's *Cybernetics, or Control and Communication in the Animal and the Machine* as significant for cybernetic brain research, because it seems that the significance of Wiener's work was that it provided a general sketch of the possibility of thinking about machines and animals in terms of computation. His chapter "Brain Waves and Self-Organizing Systems" is less the product of research than a review.

21. In 1956 Ashby published *Introduction to Cybernetics,* which was widely read and which popularized the term *cybernetics,* especially in the United Kingdom. On Ashby, see Pickering 2010.

22. Von Neumann 1951.

23. To make explicit the obvious correspondence between cybernetics and behaviorism—both formalizations of the human that revolve around the idea of control—I would add that at a time when the universality of the synapse was proven, computational theory provided a powerful answer to the question of how an immutable brain could allow for memory and learning. Perhaps Donald Hebb was among the first who understood this importance, or so his 1949 *Organization of Behavior* suggests.

24. Eccles's so called Dale principle—one neuron, one transmitter—was largely proven wrong in the 1980s. Many neurons contain more than one neurotransmitter. See Lichtigfeld and Gillman 1991.

25. Schildkraut 1965. For a review of the rise of neurochemistry, see Shepherd 2010 and Rees forthcoming.

26. Rose 2003. For a critique of the neurochemical self-concept, see Rees 2015a.

27. Scheller et al. 1982; Changeux 1985.

28. Of course, the work of Alain was not a turn away from the discoveries and observations made in the aftermath of histology and cytoarchitecture. The extension of embryogenetic processes to the adult human brain was not meant to call into question that neurons have electrical properties, or that they produce neurotransmitters and communicate with one another through synapses, or that genes are critical for synaptic communication. However, with the reconceptualization of neurons as instances of lifelong growth—of ceaseless movement—the release and uptake of chemicals across synaptic clefts as the sole focus of neuronal research was questioned. One could almost argue that the emergence of plastic reason has led to a post-chemical, post-synaptic brain: post-synaptic insofar as the centrality of the synapse had been contingent on the late-nineteenth-century hypothesis that synaptic communication is the only dynamic element of an otherwise immutable cellular structure; and post-chemical because the chemical conception of neurons and the brain had resulted from the discovery of the chemical nature of synaptic communication, understood as key to the brain.

Once it was known that homeoproteins transfer between neurons in adult mammalian brains, that thousands of new neurons are born every day, that axons and dendrites continue to sprout, and that millions of synapses continuously appear and disappear, the once compelling focus on the synapse—on chemistry—became much less obvious. And less compelling. There were now other, more dynamic processes—processes of biological growth—that seemed to better explain behavior, learning, or memory—better than synaptic communication alone.

In a curious twist, the synapse is still considered essential to the plastic brain, though no longer exclusively, perhaps not even primarily, as an instance of chemical communication, but rather as the most prominent instance of plastic growth. To be sure, synapses, even where understood in terms of growth, still release and take up neurotransmitters and thereby trigger electrical signals. But this release and uptake is now assumed to concern the signaling of changes in neuronal form—changes now understood as the actual functional processes of the brain.

29. And I have mentioned here only the most significant, the—retrospectively—dominant ones. Many other half-forgotten moons of neuronal conceptions of the brain existed on the firmament of reason. I think of reticularism, equipotentiality, reverberation.

30. Philippe Ascher and Christo Goridis may well serve as an example for continuity and change in the neurological human. As an electrophysiologist and neurochemist, respectively, they share a single ethical space—for both the brain and hence the organ that makes them human, has to be thought of as a machine organized in fixed structural circuits. But they operate with vastly different ethical repertoires—in Ascher's case, the terminology of electrophysiology (a machine governed by wires), in Goridis's the concepts of neurochemistry (a machine governed by neurotransmitters).

For Ramón y Cajal, this meant the minimal growth of dendritic spines; for Meynert and his successors, I could not find an answer; for Sherrington and Adrian and their many students and postdocs, it mean reverberation and changes in flow; for McCulloch, Walter, and Ashby, it mean that signaling loops could change the dynamics of closed systems; for neurochemists, it meant LTP/LTD.

It was not that there was no space—and yet, in each case the space was minimal at best.

31. From the 1950s to the 1990s, that which is constitutive of the human was made possible by chemical, synaptic communication. That is to say, the substrate of reason, language, behavioral changes, emotions was chemical processes in cells (and each small mutation of what a synapse is or of how synapses communicate had anthropological consequences). With the emergence of plastic reason, the human is no longer the product of the chemical synapse. Instead, the human is made possible by a "silent embryogenesis": the continuous generation of new, yet undifferentiated and hence still plastic cellular tissue that allows for a niche independent existence, that allows for lifelong learning and adaptability. A whole new figure of the neurological human emerged, at home in a novel ethical space, equipped with a whole different—biological and cellular, rather than chemical and synaptic—ethical equipment for (neuronal) sense making.

32. For an account of the rise of anti-romanticism in France, see Friedrich 1935.

33. The emergence of plastic reason in Alain's laboratory had severe consequences for the heroic, for the heroic was heroic only insofar as life had to be lived within the narrow confines of fixity, only insofar as humans had to face the unpleasant but inevitable truth that we are machines. With the rise of what I suggest calling *the plastic*—the ethos of being a continuously emerging cellular form—the heroic becomes a relic, a vestige of a previous epoch in which the brain was misunderstood.

34. Was plasticity a liberation? It was—as far as the relation between life and science is concerned. Plasticity liberated the neurological human from the narrow confines that delimited—that imprisoned—him or her ever since the concept first emerged in 1891. However, it certainly was no liberation if by liberation one means

the release of the human—of life—from knowledge and thought. The central aspect of the relation between life and science—namely, the fact that life is lived within the confines offered by knowledge and thought—is untouched by the plastic. Plasticity is merely a new episode in the effort to think of and know the human.

DIGRESSION: HUMILITY

1. Alain thereby commented, without making it explicit, on a new book by Jean-Pierre Changeux, *L'Homme de Vérité* (2002).

CHAPTER 7. LETTING GO

1. When I say "global," I mean that the plastic brain elaborated in Alain's lab no longer has a center. It has become globally dispersed. The experimental system had itself become a black box, a building block of other experimental systems. The building of this material and global infrastructure brought with it a certain generalization. Plasticity, the n-a-t, was now a general argument about the brain. Groups independent of Alain's lab were working on it.

2. The 1989 discovery, the relational struggles, the nocturnal work, the effort to come up with an experimental in vivo system—all of these were now elements of the past, a mere prelude to the present, a present that revolved around different questions, relations, struggles, and experiments. The present was composed differently— relationally, conceptually, and experimentally.

3. Sugiyama et al. 2008, 2009; Beurdeley et al. 2012; Spatazza et al. 2013a, 2013b.

CODA

1. Trachtenberg et al. 2002; Ottersen and Helm 2002; Harvey and Svoboda 2007; Holtmaat et al. 2009; Holtmaat and Svoboda 2009; Svoboda 2011.

BIBLIOGRAPHY

Abi-Rached, J. M., and N. Rose

2010   "The birth of the neuromolecular gaze." *History of the Human Sciences,* Vol. 23, No. 1, pp. 11–36.

Adrian, E. D.

1928   *The basis of sensation.* New York: W. W. Norton.

1932   *The mechanism of nervous action.* Philadelphia: University of Pennsylvania Press.

1937   "Synchronized reactions in the optic ganglion of Dytiscus." *Journal of Physiology,* Vol. 91, No. 1, pp. 66–89.

Adrian, E. D., and K. Lucas

1912   "On the summation of propagated disturbances in nerve and muscle." *Journal of Physiology,* Vol. 44, pp. 68–125.

Agnihotri, N., R. D., Hawkins, J. C. López Garcia, et al.

1998   "Morphological changes associated with long-term potentiation." Histology and Histopathology, Vol. 13, No. 4, pp. 1155–1162.

Albers, Irene

2002   "Der Photograph der Erscheinungen." In Peter Geimer (ed.). *Ordnungen der Sichtbarkeit: Fotografie in Wissenschaft, Technik und Kunst,* pp. 211–251. Frankfurt am Main: Fischer Verlag.

Albright, D. A., T. M. Jessel, and Eric R. Kandel

2000   "Neural science: A century of progress and the mysteries that remain." *Neuron,* Vol. 25, pp. 1–55.

Altman, J.

1962   "Are new neurons formed in the brains of adult mammals?" *Science,* Vol. 135, No. 3509, pp. 1127–1128.

1963   "Autoradiographic investigation of cell proliferation in the brains of rats and cats." *Anatomical Record,* Vol. 145, No. 4, pp. 573–591.

1966   "Proliferation and migration of undifferentiated precursor cells in the rat during postnatal gliogenesis." *Experimental Neurology,* Vol. 16, No. 3, pp. 263–278.

1967 "Postnatal growth and differentiation of the mammalian brain, with implications for a morphological theory of memory." In G. C. Quarton, T. Mel-
nechuck, and F. O. Schmitt (eds.). *The neurosciences: First program study,*
p. 723. New York: Rockefeller University Press.

1969 "Autoradiographic and histological studies of postnatal neurogenesis. IV.
Cell proliferation and migration in the anterior forebrain, with special
reference to persisting neurogenesis in the olfactory bulb." *Journal of Comparative Neurology,* Vol. 137, pp. 433–458.

1970 "Postnatal neurogenesis and the problem of neural plasticity." In W. A.
Himwich (ed.). *Developmental neurobiology,* pp.197–237. Springfield, IL:
Charles C. Thomas.

Altman, J., and G. D. Das

1965a Autoradiographic and histological evidence of postnatal hippocampal
neurogenesis in rats. In: *Journal of Comparative Neurology,* Vol.
124:319–335.

1965b "Autoradiographic and histological evidence of postnatal hippocampal neurogenesis in rats." *Journal of Comparative Neurology,* Vol. 124, pp. 319–336.

Alvarez-Buylla, A., J. M., García-Verdugo, and A. D. Tramontin

2001 "A unified hypothesis on the lineage of neural stem cells." *Nature Reviews
Neuroscience,* Vol. 2, No. 4, pp. 287–293.

Anderson, P., G. N. Gross, T. Lømo, and O. Sveen

1969 "Participation of inhibitory and excitatory interneurones in the control of
hippocampal cortical output." *UCLA Forum in Medical Sciences,* Vol. 11,
pp. 415–465.

Ansermet, François, and Pierre Magistretti

2007 *Biology of freedom: Neural plasticity, experience, and the unconscious.* London: Karnac Books.

Arden, John B.

2010 *Rewire your brain: Think your way to a better life.* New York: John Wiley
and Sons.

Ashby, Ross

1956 *Introduction to cybernetics.* London: Chapman and Hall.

Bachelard, Gaston

1949 *Le Rationalisme Appliqué.* Paris: PUF.

1951 *L'Activité Rationaliste de la Physique Contemporaine.* Paris: PUF.

1953 *Le matérialisme rationnel.* Paris: PUF.

1965 *Poétique de la Rêverie.* Paris: PUF.

1967 *La Formation de l'Esprit Scientifique.* Paris: Vrin.

Barbara, Jean-Gaëlle

2005 "Les heures sombres de la neurophysiologie à Paris (1909–1939)." *Lettre des
Neurosciences,* Vol. 29, pp. 3–6.

Barbara, Jean-Gaël, and Claude Debru

2009 "Edgar Douglas Adrian et la neurophysiologie en France autour de la Sec-
onde Guerre mondiale." In Robert Fox and Bernard Joly (eds.). *Echanges*

entre savants français et britanniques depuis le XVIIe siècle. Oxford: College Publications.

Barnes, D.M.

1985 "Neurosciences advance in basic and clinical realms." *Science,* Vol. 234, No. 4782, pp. 1324–1326.

Barry, Andrew

2001 *Political machines: Governing a technological society.* London: Athlone Press.

Bateson, William B.

1894 *Materials for the study of variations: Treated with special regards to the discontinuity in the origins of species.* London: Macmillan and Co.

Baxandall, Michael

1988 *Painting and experience in 15th century Italy: A primer in the social history of pictorial style.* Oxford: Oxford University Press.

Bayer S.A., Brunner R.L., Hine R., and Altman J.

1973. "Behavioral effects of interference with the postnatal acquisition of new hippocampal granule cells." In: *Nature: New Biology.* Vol. 18:222–224.

Begley, Sharon

2007 *Train your mind, change your brain.* London: Constable.

2009 *The Plastic Mind.* London: Constable.

Belting, Hans

2004 *Kult und Bild: Eine Geschichte des Bildes vor dem Zeitalter der Kunst.* Munich: C.H. Beck Verlag.

Bennett, Max R.

2001 *A History of the Synapse.* London: Taylor and Francis.

Berger, Peter L., and Thomas Luckmann

1966 *The social construction of reality: A treatise in the sociology of knowledge.* New York: Anchor Books.

Berlucchi, Giovanni

2002 "The origin of the term *plasticity* in the neurosciences: Ernesto Lugaro and chemical synaptic transmission." *Journal for the History of Neurosciences,* Vol. 11, No. 3, pp. 305–309.

Berlucchi, G., and Henry A. Buchtel

2009 "Neuronal plasticity: Historical roots and evolution of meaning." *Experimental Brain Research,* Vol. 192, No. 3, pp. 307–319.

Bernard, Claude

1859 *Leçons sur les propriétés physiologiques et les altérations pathologiques des liquides de l'organisme.* Paris: Editions Baillière et Fils.

1956 *Cahier des Notes.* Paris: PUF.

1957 *An introduction to the study of experimental medicine.* Reprint, New York: Dover.

1965 *Introduction á l'étude de la médecine expérimentale.* Brussels: Culture et Civilisation.

1966 *Leçons sur le Phénomène de la Vie Communs au Animaux et aux Vegetaux.* Paris: Vrin.

1987 *Principes de Médecine Expérimentale.* Paris: PUF.

Bernier, P. J., et al.

2002 "Newly generated neurons in the amygdala and adjoining cortex of adult primates." *Proceedings of the National Academy of Sciences of the United States of America,* Vol. 99, No. 17, pp. 11464–11469.

Bernstein, Serge

2006 *Léon Blum.* Paris: Fayard.

Bethe, Albrecht

1952 *Allgemeine Physiologie.* Heidelberg: Springer.

Beurdeley, Marine, et al.

2012 "Otx2 binding to perineuronal nets persistently regulates plasticity in the mature visual cortex." *Journal of Neuroscience,* Vol. 32, No. 27, pp. 9429–9437.

Biagioli, Mario

1993 *Galileo Courtier: The Practice of Science in the Culture of Absolutism,* Chicago: University of Chicago Press.

Bijker, Wiebke, Thomas P. Hughes, and Trevor Pinch

1989 *The social construction of technological systems.* Cambridge, MA: MIT Press.

Biquard, Pierre

1961 *Frédéric Joliot-Curie et l'Énergie Atomique.* Paris: Harmattan.

Bizzozero, Giulio

1894 "An address on the growth and regeneration of the organism: Delivered before a general meeting on the XIth International Medical Congress, held in Rome, 1894." *British Medical Journal,* Vol. 1, No. 1736, p. 728.

Black, Ira

2001 *The changing brain: Alzheimer's disease and advances in neuroscience.* Oxford: Oxford University Press.

Bliss, T. V. P., and T. Lømo

1970 "Plasticity in a monosynaptic cortical pathway." *Journal of Physiology,* Vol. 207, No. 2, p. 61P.

1973 "Long-lasting potentiation of synaptic transmission in the dentate area of the anaesthetized rabbit following stimulation of the perforant path." *Journal of Physiology,* Vol. 223, pp. 331–356.

Blumenberg Hans

1981 *Die Lesbarkeit der Welt.* Frankfurt am Main: Suhrkamp Verlag.

Borck, Cornelius

2005 "Hirnstrome." In *Eine Kulturgeschichte der Elektroenzephalographie.* Göttingen, Germany: Wallstein.

Bourdieu, Pierre

1988 *Homo Academicus.* Stanford: Stanford University Press.

1996 *The state's nobility: Elite schools in the field of power.* Stanford: Stanford University Press

2000 *Pascalian meditations.* Stanford: Stanford University Press.

2002 *Distinctions: A social critique of the judgment of taste.* Cambridge, MA: Harvard University Press.

Bourgeois, Jean Pierre
  1997 "Synaptogenesis, heterochrony and epigenesis in the mammalian neocortex." *Acta Paediatrica,* Vol. 86, No. S422, pp. 27–33.

Bourgeois, Jean Pierre, P. J. Jastreboff, and Pasko Rakic
  1989 "Synaptogenesis in the visual cortex of normal and preterm monkeys: Evidence for intrinsic regulation of synaptic overproduction." In *Proceedings of the National Academy of Sciences,* Vol. 86, pp. 4297–4301.

Bourgeois, Jean Pierre, and Pasko Rakic
  1996 "Synaptogenesis in the occipital cortex of macaque monkey devoid of retinal input from early embryonic stages." *European Journal of Neuroscience,* Vol. 8,. No. 5, pp. 942–950.

Bourgeois, J. P., P. Rakic, and P. S. Goldman-Rakic
  1994 "Synaptogenesis in the prefrontal cortex of rhesus monkeys." *Cerebral Cortex,* Vol. 4, No. 1, pp. 78–96.

Brandt, Richard B.
  1954 *Hopi ethics: A theoretical analysis.* Chicago: University of Chicago Press.

Brandt, Christina
  2004 *Metapher und Experiment: Von der Virsuforschung zum Genetischen Code.* Göttingen, Germany: Wallstein Verlag.

Bredekamp, Horst
  2005 *Darwins Korallen.* Berlin: Verlag Klaus Wagenbach.

Breidbach, Olaf
  1997 *Die Materialisierung des Ichs: Zur Geschichte der Hirnforschung im 19. und 20. Jahrhundert.* Frankfurt am Main: Suhrkamp Verlag.

Brock, L. G., J. S. Coombs, and J. C. Eccles
  1952 "The recording of potentials from motorneurons with an intracellular electrode." *Journal of Physiology,* Vol. 117, No. 4, pp. 431–460.

Brodmann, K.
  1909 *Vergleichende Lokalisationslehre der Grosshirnrinde in ihren Prinzipien dargestellt auf Grund des Zellenbaues.* Leipzig, Germany: Johann Ambrosius Barth.

Buonomano, D. V, and M. M. Merzenich
  1998 "Cortical plasticity: From synapses to maps." *Annual Review of Neuroscience,* Vol. 21, No. 1, pp. 149–186.

Callaerts, Patrick, et al.
  1996 "Pax-6 and eye development in invertebrates." *Investigative Ophthalmology and Visual Science,* Vol. 37, No. 3, p. 927.
  1997 "Pax-6 in development and evolution." *Annual Review of Neuroscience,* Vol. 20, pp. 483–532.

Callon, Michel
  2004 "Europe wrestling with technology." *Economy and Society,* Vol. 33, No. 1, pp. 121–134.

Callon, Michel, and Koray Caliskon

2005 "Why virtualism paves the way for political impotence: A reply to Danial Miller's critique of the law of the market." *European Electronic Newsletter,* Vol. 6, No. 2, pp. 3–20.

Campe, Rüdiger

1991 "Die Schreibszene: Schreiben." In H. U. Gumbrecht and K. L. Pfeiffer (eds.). *Paradoxien, Dissonanzen, Zusammenbrüche,* pp. 759–772. Frankfurt: Suhrkamp.

Canguilhem, Georges

1955 *La Formation du Concept de Réflexe aus XVIIIe Siècle.* Paris: PUF.

1993 "La Cerveau et la Pensée." In *Philosophe, Historian des Sciences,* pp. 11–37. Paris: Albin Michel.

1994 *Etudes d'Histoire et de Philosophie des Sciences Concernant les Vivants et la Vie.* Paris: Vrin.

2000 *La Connaissance de la Vie.* Paris: Vrin.

Carroll, Sean B.

2005 *Endless forms most beautiful: The new science of evo devo and the making of the animal kingdom,* New York: W. W. Norton.

Castellucci, H., et al.

1970 "Neuronal correlates of habituation and dishabituation of the gill-withdrawal reflex in Aplysia." *Science,* Vol. 167, No. 3926, pp. 1743–1745.

Changeux, Jean-Pierre

1985 *Neuronal man: The biology of mind.* Oxford: Oxford University Press.

2002 *L'Homme de Vérité.* Paris: Odile Jacob.

2012 "Allostery and the Monod-Wyman-Changeux model after 50 years." *Annual Review of Biophysics,* Vol. 41, pp. 103–133.

Changeux, J. P., T. Podleski, and J. C. Meunier

1969 "On some structural analogies between Acetylcholinesterase and the macromolecular receptor of Acetylcholine." *Journal of General Physiology,* Vol. 54, No. 1 (July), pp. 225–244.

Chase, Michael, and Pierre Hadot

2002 *What is ancient philosophy?* Cambridge, MA: Harvard University Press.

Chimisso, Cristina

2001 *Gaston Bachelard: Critique of Science and the Imagination.* London: Routledge.

Chklovskii, D. B., et al.

2004 "Maps in the brain: What can we learn from them?" *Annual Review of Neuroscience,* Vol. 27, pp. 369–392.

Chouchan, Marianne

1998 *Irène Joliot-Curie ou la Science au Coeur.* Paris: Livre de Poche Jeunesse.

Clarke, Edwin, and Kenneth Dewhurst

1974 *An illustrated history of brain function.* Berkeley: University of California Press.

Clarke, Edwin, and L. S. Jacyna

1987   *Nineteenth-century origins of neuroscientific concepts.* Berkeley: University of California Press.

Cohen, Lawrence

1998   *No aging in India: Alzheimer's, the bad family, and other modern things.* Berkeley: University of California Press.

1999   "'Where it hurts': Bioethics and beyond." *Daedalus,* Vol. 128, No. 4, pp. 143–149.

Collier, Stephen J.

2011   *Post-Soviet social: Neoliberalism, social modernity, biopolitics.* Princeton: Princeton University Press.

Collier, Stephen, and Aihwa Ong (eds.)

2004   *Global assemblages: Technology, politics, and ethics as anthropological problems.* London: Blackwell.

Collins, H. M., R. H. Green, and R. C. Draper

1985   "Where's the expertise? Expert systems as a medium of knowledge transfer." In Merry, M. J. (ed.). *Expert Systems 85,* pp. 323–334. Cambridge: Cambridge University Press.

Colucci-D'Amato, L., V. Bonavita, and U. Di Porzio

2006   "The end of the central dogma of neurobiology: Stem cells and neurogenesis in adult CNS." *Neurological Sciences,* Vol. 27, No. 4, pp. 266–270.

Cowan, M. W., H. H. Donald, and Eric R. Kandel

2000   "The emergence of modern neuroscience: Some implications for neurology and psychiatry." *Annual Reviews of Neuroscience,* Vol. 23, pp. 343–391.

Crick, Francis

1966   "On protein synthesis." *Symposium of the Society for Experimental Biology,* Vol. 12, pp. 138–163.

Das, Veena

2006   *Life and words: Violence and the descent into the ordinary.* Berkeley: University of California Press.

Daston, Lorraine

1992   "Objectivity and the escape from perspective." *Social Studies of Science,* Vol. 22, No. 4, pp. 597–618.

1994   "Historical Epistemology." In Arnold Davidson (ed.). *Questions of evidence: Proof, practice, and persuasion across the disciplines,* pp. 282–289. Chicago: University of Chicago Press.

1999   "Introduction: The coming into being of scientific objects." In *Biographies of scientific objects.* Chicago: University of Chicago Press.

2001   *Wunder, Beweise und Tatsachen: Zur Geschichte der Rationalität.* Frankfurt am Main: Fischer Verlag.

2004   "Introduction: Speechless." In Daston, Lorraine (ed.). *Things that talk: Object lessons from art and science.* New York: Zone Books.

Daston, Lorraine, and Katherine Park

2001   *Wonder and the order of nature, 1150–1750.* New York: Zone Books.

Daston, Lorraine, and Peter Galison
  1992 "The image of objectivity." *Representations,* Vol. 40, pp. 81–128.
  2007 *Objectivity.* Cambridge, MA: MIT Press.
Davidson, Arnold I.
  2002 *The emergence of sexuality: Historical epistemology and the formation of concepts.* Cambridge, MA: Harvard University Press.
De Beer, Gavin
  1930 *Embryology and evolution.* Oxford: Clarendon Press.
  1958 *Embryos and ancestors.* Oxford: Clarendon Press.
Debru, C., J. G. Barbara, and C. Cherici (eds.)
  2008 *L'essor des neurosciences: France, 1945–1975.* Paris: Hermann.
DeFelipe, Javier
  2002 "Cortical interneurons: From Cajal to 2001" *Progress in Brain Research,* Vol. 136, pp. 215–238.
  2006 "Brain plasticity and mental processes: Cajal again." *Nature Reviews Neuroscience,* Vol. 7, pp. 811–817.
  2009 *Cajal's butterflies of the soul: Science and art.* Oxford: Oxford University Press.
Deleuzes, Gilles, and Félix Guattarie
  1988 *A thousand plateaus: Capitalism and schizophrenia.* London: Athlone Press.
De Robertis, Eduardo
  1954 "Changes in the 'synaptic vesicles' of the ventral acoustic ganglion after nerve section (an electron microscopic study)." *Anatomical Record,* Vol. 118, pp. 284–285.
De Robertis, Eduardo, and H. Stanley Bennett
  1954 "Submicroscopic vesicular component in the synapse." In *Federation Proceedings,* Vol. 13, No. 35, p. 1954.
Derossi, D., A. Joliot, G. Chassaing, M. Volovitch, and A. Prochiantz
  1994 "The third helix of Antennapedia homeodomain translocates through biological membranes." *Journal of Biological Chemistry,* Vol. 269, pp. 10444–10450.
Derossi, D., S. Calvet, A. Trembleau, A. Joliot, M. Volovitch, and A. Prochiantz
  1996 "Cell internalization of the third helix of the Antennapedia homeodomain is receptor-independent." *Journal of Biological Chemistry,* Vol. 271, pp. 18188–18193.
De Toni, A., et al.
  2008 "Regulation of survival in adult hippocampal and glioblastoma stem cell lineages by the homeodomain-only protein HOP." *Neural Development,* Vol. 3, No. 13, pp. 1–12.
Doidge, Norman
  2007 *The brain that changes itself: Stories of personal triumph from the frontiers of brain science.* New York: Penguin.
Dumit, Joseph
  2004 *Picturing personhood: Brain scans and biomedical identity.* Princeton: Princeton University Press.

Dupont, E., A. Joliot, and A. Prochiantz

2002 "Cell penetrating peptides." In U. Langel U (ed.). *Penetratins*, pp. 23–51. Boca Raton, Florida: CRC Press.

2011 "Penetratin story: An overview." *Cell-Penetrating Peptides Methods in Molecular Biology*, Volume 683, pp. 21–29.

Eccles, John

1948 "Conduction and synaptic transmission in the nervous system." *Annual Review of Physiology*, Vol. 10, No. 1, pp. 93–116.

1953 *The Neurophysiological Basis of Mind: The Principles of Neurophysiology* (Wayneflete Lectures 1952), Oxford: Clarendon Press.

Eccles, John, with M. Ito and J. Szentágothai

1967 *The Cerebellum as a Neuronal Machine*, New York: Springer Verlag.

Economo, Constantin von, and G. N. Koskinas

1925 *Die Cytoarchitektonik der Hirnrinde des erwachsenen Menschen.* Berlin: J. Springer.

Edelmann, Gerald M.

1987 *Neural Darwinism: The theory of neuronal group selection.* New York: Basic Books.

Elias, Norbert

1995 *Über den Prozess der Zivilisation. Soziogenetische und Psychogenetische Untersuchungen* (Two Volumes), Frankfurt am Main: Suhrkamp Verlag.

Erikson, P. S., E. Perefilieva, T. Björk-Eriksson, A. M. Alborn, C. Nordberg, D. A. Peterson, and F. H. Gage

1998 "Neurogenesis in the adult human hippocampus," *Nature Medicine*, Vol. 4, No. 11, pp. 1313–1317.

Eugenides, Jeffrey

2002 *Middlesex: A novel.* New York : Farrar, Straus and Giroux.

Farmer, Paul

2001 *Infections and inequalities: The modern plagues.* Berkeley: University of California Press.

2004 "Rethinking medical ethics: A view from below." *Developing World Bioethics*, Vol. 4, No. 1, pp. 17–41.

Fatt, Paul, and Bernhard Katz

1951a "Conduction of impulses in crustacean muscle fibres." *Journal of Physiology*, Vol. 115, No. 1, p. 45.

1951b "An analysis of the end-plate potential recorded with an intra-cellular electrode." *Journal of Physiology*, Vol. 115, No. 3, pp. 320–370.

Faubion, James D.

2001a "Toward an anthropology of ethics: Foucault and the pedagogies of autopoiesis." *Representations*, Vol. 74, No. 1, pp. 83–104.

2001b *The ethics of kinship: Ethnographic inquiries.* Lanham, MD: Rowman and Littlefield.

Feldberg, Wilhelm, and Alfred Fessard
1942 "The cholinergic nature of the nerves to the electric organ of the Torpedo (*Torpedo marmorata*)." *Journal of Physiology,* Vol. 101, No. 2, pp. 200–216.

Ferguson, James
2010 "The uses of neoliberalism." *Antipode,* Vol. 41, No. 1, pp. 166–184.
2013 "Declarations of dependence: Labour, personhood, and welfare in southern Africa." *Journal of the Royal Anthropological Institute,* Vol. 19, No. 2, pp. 223–242.
2015 *Give a man a fish: Reflections on the new politics of distribution.* Durham, NC: Duke University Press.

Finger, Stanley
1994 *Origins of neuroscience.* Oxford: Oxford University Press.
2000 *Minds behind the brain: A history of the pioneers and their discoveries.* Oxford: Oxford University Press.

Fleck, Ludwig
1929 "Zur Krise der Wirklichkeit" *Die Naturwissenschaften,* Vol. 17, pp. 426–429.
1980 *Entstehung und Entwicklung einer Wissenschaftlichen Tatsache.* 1935. Reprint, Frankfurt am Main: Suhrkamp Verlag.

Fleck, Ludwik, and Lothar Schäfer
1935 *Entstehung und Entwicklung einer wissenschaftlichen Tatsache.* Basel: Schwabe.

Forbes, Alexander
1922 "The interpretation of spinal reflexes in terms of present knowledge of nerve conduction." *Physiological Reviews,* Vol. 2, pp. 361–414.

Forel, Auguste
1887 "Einige hirnanatomische Betrachtungen und Ergebnisse."

Fortes, Meyer
1969 *Kinship and the social order: The legacy of Lewis Henry Morgan.* Chicago: Aldine.

Foster, Michael, and Charles Scott Sherrington
1897 *A textbook of physiology.* London: Macmillan.

Foucault, Michel
1994 "La Vie: L'Expérience et la Science." In Daniel Defert and François Ewald (eds.). *Dits et Écrits IV,* pp. 763–776. Paris: Gallimard.
1997 "On the Geneaology of Ethics." In Paul Rabinow (ed.). *The essential work of Michel Foucault, 1954–1984,* Volume 1: *Ethics: Subjectivity and Truth,* pp. 253–281. New York: New Press.
2001 "Nietzsche, genealogy, history." In John Richardson and Brian Leiter (eds.). *Nietzsche,.* pp. 139–164. Oxford: Oxford University Press.
2005 *The hermeneutics of the subject: Lectures at the Collège de France, 1981–1982.* London: Macmillan.

Fox-Keller, Evelyn
1984 *A Feeling for the organism: The life and work of Barbara McClintock.* New York: Times Books.

1995   *Reconfiguring life: Metaphors of twentieth-century biology.* New York: Columbia University Press.

2000   *The century of the gene.* Cambridge, MA: Harvard University Press.

2002   *Making sense of life; Explaining biological development with metaphors and machines.* Cambridge, MA: Harvard University Press.

Frank, Manfred

1997   *Unendliche Annäherung: Die Anfänge der philosophischen Frühromantik.* Frankfurt am Main: Suhrkamp Verlag.

Franklin, Sarah

1995   "Postmodern procreation: A cultural account of assisted reproduction." In Faye Ginsburg and Rayna Rapp (eds.). *Conceiving the new world order: The global politics of reproduction,* pp. 323–345. Berkeley: University of California Press.

2004   "Stem Cells "R" Us: Emergent life forms and the global biological." In Stephen Collier and Aihwa Ong (eds.). *Global assemblages: Technology, politics, and ethics as anthropological problems,* pp. 59–79. London: Blackwell.

Fried, Michael

1997   "Thoughts on Caravaggio." *Critical Inquiry,* Vol. 24, pp. 13–57.

1998   *Manet's modernism; or, The Face of Painting in the 1860s.* Chicago: University of Chicago Press.

Friedrich, Hugo

1935   *Das antiromantische Denken im modernen Frankreich: Sein System und seine Herkunft.* Munich: Max Hueber Verlag.

Gadamer, Hans Georg

1960   *Wahrheit und Methode: Grundzüge einer philosophischen Hermeneutik.* Tübingen: Mohr.

Gage, F., A. Bjorklund, A. Prochiantz, et al.

2004   *Stem cells in the nervous system: Functional and clinical implications.* Heidelberg: Springer.

Gage, F., G. Kempermann, T. Palmer, D. Peterson, and J. Ray

1998   "Multipotent progenitor cells in the adult dentate gyrus." *Journal of Neurobiology,* Vol. 36, pp. 249–266.

Galison, Peter

1987   *How experiments end.* Chicago: University of Chicago Press.

1988   "Philosophy in the laboratory." *Journal of Philosophy,* Vol. 85, No. 10, pp. 525–527.

Gardner, Howard

1987   *The mind's new science: A history of the cognitive revolution.* New York: Basic Books.

Garland, Allen

1987   "T. H. Morgan and the split between embryology and genetics, 1910–1926." In T. J. Horder, I. A. Witkowski, and C. C. Wylie (eds.). *A history of embryology,* pp. 113–146. Cambridge: Cambridge University Press.

Gasser, Jacques
  1995   *Aux Origines du Cerveau Moderne: Localisation, Langage, et Mémoire dans l'Œuvre de Charcot.* Paris: Fayard.
Gaudillière, Jean-Paul
  2002   *Inventer la biomédecine: la France, l'Amérique et la production des savoirs du vivant, 1945–1965.* Paris: La découverte.
Geertz, Clifford
  1960   *The religion of Java.* Chicago: University of Chicago Press.
  1973   *The interpretation of cultures.* New York: Basic Books.
Gehring, Walter J.
  1995   "New perspectives on eye evolution." *Current Opinion in Genetics and Development,* Vol. 5, No. 5, pp. 602–609.
  1998   *Master control genes in development and evolution. The Homeobox story.* New Haven: Yale University Press, 1998.
  1999   "Lifting the Lid on the Homeobox Discovery." *Nature,* June 10, pp. 521–522.
  2001   "The genetic control of eye development and its implications for the evolution of the various eye-types." *Zoology,* Vol. 104, pp. 171–183.
  2012   "The animal body plan, the prototypic body segment, and eye evolution." *Evolution and Development,* Vol. 14, No. 1, pp. 34–46.
Germer, Soren
  1997   "German experiments in the sciences and politics of evolution." PhD dissertation, Department of Anthropology, University of California, Berkeley.
Gilbert, Charles
  1998   "Adult cortical dynamics." *Physiological Reviews,* Vol. 78, No. 2 (April), pp.467–485.
Gilbert, Scott F.
  1991   "Induction and the origins of developmental genetics." In Scott F. Gilbert (ed.). *A conceptual history of modern embryology,* pp. 181–207. Baltimore: Johns Hopkins University Press.
  2000   "Genes classical and developmental." In Peter J. Beurton, Raphael Falk, and Hans Jörg Rheinberger (eds.). *The concept of the gene in development and evolution: Historical perspectives,* pp. 178–193. Cambridge: Cambridge University Press.
Gilbert, Scott F. (ed.)
  1991   *A conceptual history of modern embryology.* Baltimore: Johns Hopkins University Press
Gilpin, Robert
  1968   *France in the age of the scientific state.* Princeton: Princeton University Press.
Goldman, Steven A., and Fernando Nottebohm
  1983   "Neuronal production, migration, and differentiation in a vocal control nucleus of the adult female canary brain." *Proceedings of the National Academy of Sciences,* Vol. 80, No. 8, pp. 2390–2394.

Goldman-Rakic, P. S.
  1983 "The corticostriatal fiber system in the rhesus monkey: Organization and development." *Progress in Brain Research,* Vol. 58, pp. 405–418.

Goldschmidt, Richard
  1923 *The mechanism and physiology of sex determination.* London: Methuen and Co.
  1933 "Some aspects of evolution." *Science,* Vol. 78, pp. 539–547.
  1940 *The material basis of evolution.* New Haven: Yale University Press.
  1955 *Theoretical genetics.* Berkeley: University of California Press.

Gooding, David Willoughby
  1990 *Experiment and the making of meaning: Human Agency in Scientific Observation and Experiment.* Heidelberg: Springer.

Gould, E., H. A. Cameron, D.C. Daniels, C. S. Wooley, and B. S. McEwen
  1992 "Adrenal hormones suppress cell division in the adult rat dentate gyrus." *Journal of Neuroscience,* Vol. 12, pp. 3642–3650.

Gould, E., B. S. McEwen, P. Tanapat, L. Galea, and E. Fuchs
  1997 "Neurogenesis in the dentate gyrus of the adult shrew is regulated by psychological stress and NMDA recepter activity." *Journal of Neuroscience,* Vol. 17, No. 24, pp. 2492–2498.

Götz, Magdalena, et al.
  2002a "Glial cells generate neurons: The role of the transcription factor Pax6." *New Neuroscience,* Vol. 5, No. 4, pp. 308–315.
  2002b "Radical glial cells as neuronal precursors: A new perspective on the correlation of morphology and lineage restriction in the developing cerebral cortex of mice." *Brain Research Bulletin,* Vol. 57, No. 6, pp. 777–788.

Grange, Juliette
  1996 *La Philosophie d'Auguste Comte: Science, Politique, Religion.* Paris: PUF.
  2000 *Auguste Comte. La Politique et la Science.* Paris: Odile Jacob.

Granger, B., et al.
  1995 "Tempo of neurogenesis and synaptogenesis in the primate cingulate mesocortex: Comparison with the neocortex." *Journal of Comparative Neurology,* Vol. 360, No. 2, pp. 363–376.

Gross, Charles
  2002 "Neurogenesis in the adult brain: Death of a dogma." *Nature Reviews Neuroscience,* Vol. 1, No. 1, pp. 67–73.

Großheim, Michael
  1991 *Von Georg Simmel zu Martin Heidegger: Philosophie zwischen Leben und Existenz..* Bonn: Bouvier Verlag.

Gustafson, Richard
  1986 "Leo Tolstoy: Resident and stranger." *Comparative Literature,* Vol. 4, No. 2, pp. 185–187.

Habermas, Jürgen
  1995 *Theorie des Kommunikativen Handelns.* 2 vols. Frankfurt am Main: Suhrkamp Verlag.

Hacking, Ian

1983   *Representing and intervening.* Cambridge: Cambridge University Press.

1999   "Historical Meta-Epistemology." In Carl, Wolfgang and Lorraine Daston (eds.). *Wahrheit und Geschichte. Ein Kolloquium zu Ehren des 60. Geburtstags von Lorenz Krüger.* Göttingen, Germany: Vandenhoek and Ruprecht.

2000   *The social construction of what?* Cambridge, MA: Harvard University Press.

2002   *Mad travelers.* Cambridge, MA: Harvard University Press.

2004   *Historical ontology.* Cambridge, MA: Harvard University Press.

Hadot, Pierre

1995   *Qu'est-ce que la philosophie antique?* Paris: Gallimard. 2006 *The veil of Isis: An essay on the history of the idea of nature* Cambridge, MA: Harvard University Press.

Haeckel, Ernst

1870   *Natürliche Schöpfungsgeschichte.* 2nd ed. Berlin: Georg Reimer.

1874   *Anthropogenie oder die Entwicklungsgeschichte des Menschen.* Leipzig: W. Englemann.

Hagner, Michael

1997   *Homo Cerebralis: Der Wandel vom Seelenorgan zum Gehirn.* Berlin: Berlin Verlag.

1999   "Moderne Gehirne." In Michael Hagner (ed.). *Ecce Cortex: Beiträge zur Geschichte des Modernen Gehirns.* Göttingen, Germany: Wallstein.

2000   *Homo Cerebralis. Der Wandel vom Seelnorgan zum Gehirn.* 1997. Reprint, Frankfurt am Main: Insel.

2001   "Cultivating the cortex in German neuroanatomy." In Michael Hagner and Cornelius Borck (eds.). "Mindful practices: On the neurosciences in the twentieth century." Special issue, *Science in Context*, Vol. 14, No. 4, pp. 541–565.

2004   *Geniale Gehirne: Zur Geschichte der Elitegehirnforschung.* Göttingen, Germany: Walltsein.

2006   *Der Geist bei der Arbeit: Historische Untersuchungen zur Hirnforschung,* Göttingen, Germany: Wallstein.

Hanke, Edith

1993   "Prophet des Unmodernen: Leo N. Tolstoi als Kulturkritiker." *Der deutschen Diskussion der Jahrhundertwende,* Vol. 38.

Haraway, Donna Jay

1997   *Modest_Witness@Second_Millenium.FemaleMan©_Meets_OncoMouse™: Feminism and Technoscience.* London: Routledge.

2004   *Crystals, fabrics, and fields: Metaphors that shape embryos.* 2nd ed. Berkeley: North Atlantic Books (1st ed., 1976).

Harman, Oren, and Michael R. Dietrich

2013   *Outsider Scientists.* Chicago: University of Chicago Press.

Harrington, Anne

1989   *Medicine, mind, and the double brain.* Princeton: Princeton University Press.

Harvey, Christopher D., and Karel Svoboda

2007 "Locally dynamic synaptic learning rules in pyramidal neuron dendrites." *Nature,* Vol. 450, No. 7173, pp. 1195–1200.

Haubst, Nicole, Jack Favor, and Magdalena Götz

2006 "The role of Pax6 in the nervous system during development and adulthood: Master control regulator or modular function?." In Gerald Thiel (ed.). *Transcription Factors.* Weinheim, Germany: Wiley-VCH Verlag.

Hebb, Donald

1949 *The organization of behavior.* New York: Wiley Press.

Hecht, Gabrielle

1986 "Frederic Joliot-Curie: A man apart." Unpublished thesis, Department of Physics, Massachusetts Institute of Technology, Boston.

1998 *The radiance of France: Nuclear power and national identity after World War II.* Cambridge, MA: MIT Press.

Heidegger, Martin

1967 *Holzwege.* Frankfurt am Main: Vittorio Klostermann.

1972 *Vorträge und Aufsätze.* Frankfurt am Main: Vittorio Klostermann.

Hennis, Wilhelm

1987 *Max Webers Fragestellung.* Tübingen, German: J.C.B. Mohr (Paul Siebeck).

1996 *Max Webers Wissenschaft von Menschen.* Tübingen, Germany: J.C.B. Mohr (Paul Siebeck).

Hirschkind, Charles

2001 "The ethics of listening: Cassette-sermon audition in contemporary Egypt." *American Ethnologist,* Vol. 28, No. 3, pp. 623–649.

2006 *The ethical soundscape: Cassette sermons and Islamic counterpublics.* New York: Columbia University Press.

His, Wilhelm

1868 *Untersuchungen über die erste Anlage des Wirbelthierleibes: Die erste Entwickelung des Hühnchens im Ei.* Leipzig: F.C.W. Vogel.

1870 *Ueber die Bedeutung der Entwickelungsgeschichte für die Auffassung der organischen Natur.* Leipzig: F.C.W. Vogel.

1880 *Anatomie menschlicher Embryonen.* Leipzig: F.C.W. Vogel.

1883 *Ueber das Auftreten der weissen substanz und der Wurzelfasern am Rückenmark menschlicher Embryonen.* Leipzig: F.C.W. Vogel.

1885 *Embryonen bis Ende des zweiten Monats: Atlas, Tafel IX–XIV und Tafel I.* Leipzig: F.C.W. Vogel.

1886 *Zur Geschichte des menschlichen Rückenmarkes und der Nervenwurzeln.* Leipzig: S. Hirzel.

1888 *Zur Geschichte des Gehirns sowie der centralen und peripherischen Nervenbahn beim menschlichen Embryo.* Leipzig: S. Hirzel.

1889 "Die Neuroblasten und deren Entstehung im embryonalen Marke." *Abhandl. Math.-Phys. Class. Königl. Sächs. Gesellsch. Wiss.,* Vol. 15, pp. 313–372.

Hodges, Andrew

1983   *Alan Turing: The enigma,* London Vintage.

Hodgkin, Alan

1994   *Chance and design: Reminiscences of science in peace and war.* Cambridge: Cambridge University Press.

Holmes, Frederic Lawrence

1987   *Lavoisier and the chemistry of life: An exploration of scientific creativity.* Madison: University of Wisconsin Press.

Holtmaat, A., et al.

2009   "Long-term, high-resolution imaging in the mouse neocortex through a chronic cranial window." *Nature Protocols,* Vol. 4, pp. 1128–1144.

Holtmaat, Anthony, and Karel Svoboda

2009   "Experience-dependent structural synaptic plasticity in the mammalian brain." *Nature Reviews Neuroscience,* Vol. 10, pp. 647–658.

Hopwood, Nick

1999   "'Giving bodies' to embryos: Modelling, mechanism, and the microtome in late nineteenth century anatomy." *Isis,* Vol. 90, pp. 426–496.

2000   "Producing development: The anatomy of human embryos and the norms of Wilhelm His." *Bulletin of the History of Medicine,* Vol. 74, pp. 29–79.

2002a   *Embryos in wax: Models from the Ziegler Studio.* Cambridge: Whipple Museum of the History of Science; Bern: Institute of the History of Medicine.

2002b   "Embryonen auf dem Altar der Wissenschaft zu Opfern: Entwicklungsreihen im späten 19. Jahrhundert." In Barbara Duden, Jürgen Schlumbohm, and Patrice Veit (eds.). *Geschichte des Ungeborenen. Zur Erfahrungs- und Wissenschaftsgeschichte, 17.-20. xsJahrhundert,* pp. 237–272. Göttingen: Vandenhoek and Ruprecht.

2004   "Plastic publishing in embryology." In Nick Hopwood and Soraya de Chadarevian. *Models: The Third Dimensions of Science,* pp. 170–207. Stanford: Stanford University Press.

2006   "Pictures of evolution and charges of fraud." *Isis,* Vol. 97, No. 2, pp. 260–301.

2009   "Darwinism's tragic genius: Psychology and reputation." *Isis,* Vol. 100, No. 4, pp. 863–867.

2015   "The cult of amphioxus in German Darwinism; or, our gelatinous ancestors in Naples' blue and balmy bay." *History and Philosophy of the Life Sciences,* Vol. 36, No. 3, pp. 371–393.

Hubel, David

1978   "Vision and the brain." *Bulletin of the American Academy of Arts and Sciences,* Vol. 31, pp. 17–28.

1988   *Eye, brain, and vision.* New York: Freeman.

1989   *Auge und Gehirn: Neurobiologie des Sehens.* Heidelberg: Spektrumder-Wissenschaft-Verlagsgesellschaft.

Huxley, Julian, and Gavin de Beer

1934   *The elements of experimental embryology.* Cambridge: Cambridge University Press.

Jacob, François

1997   *La mouche, la souris, et l'homme.* Paris: Odile Jacob.

James, William

1890   *Principles of psychology.* London: Macmillan.

Jaspers, Karl

1919   *Psychologie der Weltanschauungen.* Berlin: J. Springer.

Jeanerod, Marc

1985   *The brain machine: The development of neurophysiological thought.* Cambridge, MA: Harvard University Press.

Joliot, A., A. Maizel, D. Rosenberg, A. Trembleau, S. Dupas, M. Volovitch, and A. Prochiantz

1998   "Identification of a signal sequence necessary for the unconventional secretion of engrailed homeoprotein." *Current Biology,* Vol. 8, pp. 856–863.

Joliot, A., A. Trembleau, G. Raposo, S. Calvet, M. Volovitch, and A. Prochiantz

1997   "Association of engrailed homeoproteins with vesicles presenting caveolae-like properties." *Development,* Vol. 124, pp. 1865–1875.

Joliot, A. H., A. Triller, M. Volovitch, C. Pernelle, and A. Prochiantz

1991   "a-2,8-Polysialic acid is the neuronal surface receptor of Antennapedia homeobox peptide." *New Biology,* Vol. 3, pp. 1121–1134.

Jones, Edward G.

2000   "NEUROwords 8 plasticity and neuroplasticity." *Journal of the History of the Neurosciences: Basic and Clinical Perspectives,* Vol. 9, No. 1, pp. 37–39.

2002   "Thalamic organization and function after Cajal." *Progress in Brain Research,* Vol. 136, pp. 333–357.

2004   "Plasticity and neuroplasticity." *Journal of the History of the Neurosciences: Basic and Clinical Perspectives,* Vol. 13, No. 3, pp. 293.

Jonsen, Albert R., and Stephen Toulmin

1990   *The abuse of casuistry: A history of moral reasoning.* Berkeley: University of California Press.

Kahn, Fritz

1929   *Das Leben des Menschen.* Stuttgart: Franckh'sche Verlagshandlung.

Kandel, E. R., and L. Tauc

1965   "Mechanism of heterosynaptic facilitation in the giant cell of the abdominal ganglion of *Aplysia depilans.*" *Journal of Physiology,* Vol. 181, No. 1, pp. 28–47.

1965   "Heterosynaptic facilitation in neurones of the abdominal ganglion of Aplysia depilans." *Journal of Physiology,* Vol. 181, No. 1, pp. 1–27.

Kandel, Eric

1963   "Brain and behavior (Vol. I: Proceedings of First Conference 1961)." *Psychosomatic Medicine,* Vol. 25, No. 1, pp. 95–96.

1977   *Cellular basis of behavior.* San Francisco: Freeman.

1979   *Behavioral biology of* Aplysia: *A contribution to the comparative study of opisthobranch molluscs.* San Francisco: Freeman.

1987   "Steps Toward a Molecular Grammar of Learning: Exploration into the Nature of Memory." In *Medicine, Science, and Society, Symposia Celebrating the Harvard Medical School Bicentennial,* New York Wiley, pp. 555ff.

2005   *Psychiatry, psychoanalysis, and the new biology of mind.* Washington, DC: American Psychiatric.

2006   *In search of memory: The emergence of a new science of mind.* New York: W. W. Norton.

Kandel, Eric, James H. Schwartz, and Thomas Jessell
   2000   *Essential of neural science and behavior.* New York: McGraw-Hill Medical.

Katz, Bernhard
   1948   "The electric properties of the muscle fibre membrane." *Proceedings of the Royal Society,* Series B, Vol. 135, pp. 506–534.

Kaufman, Sharon
   2005   … *And a time to die: How American hospitals shape the end of life.* New York: Scribner.

Keating, Peter, and Alberto Cambrosio
   2003   *Biomedical platforms: Realigning the normal and the pathological in late-twentieth-century medicine.* Cambridge, MA: MIT Press.

Kempermann, Gerd
   2006   *Adult neurogenesis.* Oxford: Oxford University Press.
   2012   "New neurons for 'survival of the fittest.'" *Nature Reviews Neuroscience,* Vol. 13, pp. 727–736.

Kilinç, Berna, Gürol Irzik, and Stephen Voss (eds.)
   2007   *Logic and philosophy of science.* Vol 5. of *Proceedings of the Twenty-First World Congress of Philosophy.* Ankara: Philosophical Society of Turkey.

Kirschner, Stefan
   2003   "Wilhelm Roux (1850–1924) und seine Konzeption der Entwicklungsmechanik." *Würzburger medizinhistorische Mitteilungen,* Vol. 22, pp. 67–80.

Kleinman, Arthur
   1995   *Writing at the margin: Discourse between medicine and anthropology.* Berkeley: University of California Press.

Kleinman, Arthur, and Peter Benson
   2006   "Anthropology in the clinic: The problem of cultural competency and how to fix it." *PLoS medicine,* Vol. 3, No. 10, pp. 1673–1676.

Knorr-Cetina, Karin D.
   1981   "Social and scientific method, or What do we make of the distinction between the natural and the social sciences?" *Philosophy of the Social Sciences,* Vol. 11, No. 3, pp. 335–359.

Knott, G., C. Quairiaux, C. Genoud, and E. Welker
   2002   "Formation of dendritic spines with GABAergic synapses induced by whisker stimulation in adult mice." *Neuron,* Vol. 34, pp. 265–273.

Kölliker, Albert

1849   *Berichte von der Königlichen zootomischen Anstalt zu Würzburg zweiter bericht für das Schuljahr 1847–48.* Leipzig: W. Engelmann.

Konorski, Jerzy

1948   *Conditioned reflexes and neuron organization.* Cambridge: Cambridge University Press.

Kupfermann, I., et al.

1970   "Neuronal mechanisms of habituation and dishabituation of the gill-withdrawal reflex in *Aplysia.*" *Science,* Vol. 167, No. 3926, pp. 1745–1748.

Kupfermann, I., and E. R. Kandel

1969   "Neuronal controls of a behavioral response mediated by the abdominal ganglion of *Aplysia.*" *Science,* Vol. 164, No. 3881, pp. 847–850.

Labouisse, Eve

1938   *Madame Curie.* Paris: Gallimard.

Landecker, Hannah

2005   "Living differently in time: Plasticity, temporality and cellular Biotechnologies." In *Culture Machine,* Vol. 7. www.culturemachine .net.

2010   *Culturing life: How cells became technology.* Cambridge, MA: Harvard University Press.

Latour, Bruno

1984   *Les microbes: Guerre et paix; suivi de irréductions.* Paris: LaDecouverte.

1986   "Visualization and cognition." *Knowledge and Society,* Vol. 6, pp. 1–40.

1987   *Science in action: How to follow scientists and engineers through society.* Cambridge, MA: Harvard University Press.

1988   *Science in action: How to follow scientists and engineers through society.* Cambridge, MA: Harvard University Press.

2004   *The politics of nature: How to bring the sciences into democracy.* Cambridge, MA: Harvard University Press.

Latour, Bruno, and Steven Woolgar

1986   *Laboratory life: The construction of scientific facts.* 2nd ed. Princeton: Princeton University Press (1st ed., 1979).

Le Calvez, J.

1948   "'Aristapedia' heterozygote dominante homozygote lethale chez Drosophila melanogaster: Inversion dans le bras droit du chromosome III." *Bulletin Biologique de la France et de la Belgique,* vol. 82, pp. 97–113.

Leigh-Starr, Susan

1989   *Regions of the mind: Brain research and the quest for certainty.* Stanford: Stanford University Press.

Leigh-Starr, Susan, and Geoffrey Bowker

2000   *Sorting things out: Classification and its consequences.* Cambridge, MA: MIT Press.

Le Roux, I., A. Joliot, A. Prochiantz, and M. Volovitch

1995 "Neurotrophic activity of the Antennapedia homeodomain depends on its specific DNA-Binding properties." *Developmental Biology,* Vol. 90, pp. 9120–9124.

Le Roux, I., S. Durharcourt, M. Volovitch, A. Prochiantz, and E. Ronchi

1993 "Promotor specific regulation of gene expression by an exogenously added homeodomain that promotes neurite growth." *FEBS Letters,* Vol. 368, pp. 311–314.

Lesaffre, B., A. Joliot, A. Prochiantz, and M. Volovitch

2007 "Direct non-cell autonomous Pax6 activity regulates eye development in the zebrafish." *Neural Development,* January 17.

Lewis, Edward

1956 "An Unstable Gene in Drosophila Melanogaster." *Genetics,* Vol. 41, No. 5, p. 651.

1963 "Genes and Developmental Pathways." *American Zoologist,* Vol. 3, pp. 33–56.

1964 "Genetic Control and Regulation of Developmental Pathways." In *The role of chromosomes in development,* pp. 231–252. New York: Academic Press.

Leys, Ruth

2011 "The turn to affect: A critique." *Critical Inquiry,* Vol. 37, No. 3, pp. 434–472.

Lichtingfeld, F. J., and M. A. Gilman

1991 "In spite of its validity, has Dale's principle served its purpose? A scientific paradox." *Perspectives in Biological Medicine,* Vol. 34, No. 2, pp. 239–253.

Lømo, Terje

1966 "Frequency potentiation of excitatory synaptic activity in dentate area of hippocampal formation." *Acta Physiologica Scandinavica,* Vol. 68, p. 128.

1971 "Patterns of activation in a monosynaptic cortical pathway: The perforant path input to the dentate area of the hippocampal formation." *Experimental Brain Research,* Vol. 12, No. 1, pp. 18–45.

Lorente de Nó, Rafael

1938 "Analysis of the activity of the chains of internuncial neurons." *Journal of Neurophysiology,* Vol. 1, pp. 207–244.

Lucas, K.

1905 "On the gradation of activity in a skeletal muscle fibre." *Journal of Physiology,* Vol. 33, No. 2, pp. 125–137.

1906 "On the optimal electric stimuli of normal and curarised muscle." *Journal of Physiology,* Vol. 34, Nos. 4–5, pp. 372–390.

1907 "On the rate of variation of the exciting current as a factor in electric excitation." *Journal of Physiology,* Vol. 36, Nos. 4–5, pp. 253–274.

1910 "An analysis of changes and differences in the excitatory process of nerves and muscles based on the physical theory of excitation." *Journal of Physiology,* Vol. 40, No. 3, pp. 225–249.

1912 "Croonian Lecture: The process of excitation in nerve and muscle." *Proceedings of the Royal Society of London: Series B, Containing Papers of a Biological Character,* pp. 495–524.

1917 *The conduction of the nervous impulse.* Vol. 3. London: Longmans, Green and Company.

Lynch, Michael

1985 "Discipline and the material form of images: An analysis of scientific visibility." *Social Studies of Science,* Vol. 15, No. 1, pp. 37–66.

MacIntyre, Alasdair

1967 *Secularization and moral change.* Oxford: Oxford University Press.

1981 *After virtue: A study in moral theory.* Notre Dame, IN: University of Notre Dame Press.

Mahmood, Saba

2005 *Politics of piety: The Islamic revival and the feminist subject.* Princeton: Princeton University Press.

Maienschein, Jane

1991 "The origins of *Entwicklungsmechanik.*" *Developmental Biology,* No. 7, pp. 43–61.

2003 "Ontogeny, anatomy, and the problem of homology: Carl Gegenbaur and the American tradition of cell lineage studies." *Theory in Biosciences,* Vol. 122, Nos. 2–3, pp. 194–203.

Maizel, A., et al.

1999 "A short region of its homeodomain is necessary for engrailed nuclear export and secretion." *Development,* Vol. 126, pp. 3183–3190.

Maizel, A., et al.

2002 "Engrailed homeoprotein secretion is a regulated process." *Development,* Vol. 129, pp. 3545–3553.

Malabou, Catherine

2000 *Plasticité.* Paris: Léo Scheer.

2004 *The future of Hegel: Plasticity, temporality and dialectic.* London: Routledge.

2005 *La plasticité au soir de l'écriture : Dialectique, destruction, deconstruction.* Paris: Broché.

2009 *What should we do with our brain?* New York: Fordham University Press.

Malinowski, Bronislaw

2014 *Argonauts of the western Pacific: An account of native enterprise and adventure in the archipelagoes of Melanesian New Guinea.* 1922. Reprint, London: Routledge.

Mangold, Otto

1982 *Hans Spemann: Ein Meister der Entwicklungsphysiologie.* Stuttgart: Wissenschaftliche Verlagsgesellschaft.

Mao, Tianyi, Deniz Kusefoglu, Bryan M. Hooks, Daniel Huber, Leopoldo Petreanu, and Karel Svoboda

2011 "Long-range neuronal circuits underlying the interaction between sensory and motor cortex." *Neuron,* Vol. 72, No. 1, pp. 111–123.

Marcus, George

1998 "The uses of complicity in the changing mise-en-scène of anthropological fieldwork." In *Ethnography through thick and thin*. Princeton: Princeton University Press.

Marey, Etienne Jules

1878 *La Méthode Graphique dans les Sciences Expérimentales et Particulièrment en Physiologie et Médecine*. Paris: G. Masson.

Markus, Gyorgy

1987 "Why is there no hermeneutics in the natural sciences? Some preliminary theses." *Science in Context*, Vol. 1, pp. 1–12.

Martenson, Robert L.

2004 *The brain takes shape: An Early History*. Oxford: Oxford University Press.

Martin, Emily

2007 *Bipolar expeditions: Mania and depression in American culture*. Princeton: Princeton University Press.

Martin, Emily, and Suzanne R. Kirschner

1994 *Flexible bodies: The role of immunity in American culture from the days of Polio to the age of AIDS*. New York: Beacon Press.

1999 "From flexible bodies to fluid minds: An interview with Emily Martin." *Ethos*, pp. 247–282.

Masters, Maxwell

1869 *Treatise on vegetable teratology an account of the principal deviations from the usual construction of plants*. London: Macmillan Press.

Mazzolini, Renato G.

2004 "Plastic anatomies and artificial dissections." In Nick Hopwood and Soraya de Chadarevian (eds.). *Models: The third dimensions of science*, pp. 19–43. Stanford: Stanford University Press.

McCulloch, Warren S., and Walter Pitts

1943 "A logical calculus of the ideas immanent in nervous activity." *Bulletin Of Mathematical Biophysics*, Vol. 5, No. 4, pp. 115–133.

Mendelzweig, Dros M.

2013 *Performances et défaillances du sujet âgé: Etude anthropologique des recherches sur le vieillissement cérébral*. Genève, Georg, collection Médecine et Société.

Merzenich, M. M., et al.

1982 "Auditory forebrain organization." *Cortical Sensory Organization*, Vol. 3, pp. 43–57.

1984 "Somatosensory cortical map changes following digit amputation in adult monkeys." *Journal of Comparative Neurology*, Vol. 224, No. 4, pp. 591–605.

Merzenich, M. M., and J. H. Kaas

1983 "Reorganization of mammalian somatosensory cortex following peripheral nerve injury." *Trends in Neuroscience*, Vol. 5, pp. 434–436.

Meynert, Theodor

1872   *Der Bau der Gross-Hirnrinde und seine örtlichen Verschiedenheiten: Nebst einem pathologisch-anatomischen Corollarium.* Neuwied, Leipzig: J. H. Heuser.

Milner, Brenda

1954   "Intellectual function of the temporal lobes." *Psychological Bulletin,* Vol. 5, No. 1, pp. 42–62.

Milner, B., et al.

1968   "Further analysis of the hippocampal amnesic syndrome: 14-year follow-up study of HM." *Neuropsychologia,* Vol. 6, No. 3, pp. 215–234.

Mocek, Reinhard

1974   *Wilhelm Roux, Hans Driesch: Zur Geschichte der Entwicklungsphysiologie der Tiere.* Jena, Germany: Fischer.

Monod, J., F. Jacob, J. P. Changeux

1963   "Allosteric proteins and cellular control systems." *Journal of Molecular Biology,* Vol. 6, April, pp. 306–329.

Monod, J., J. Wyman, and J. P. Changeux

1965   "On the nature of allosteric transitions: A plausible model." *Journal of Molecular Biology,* Vol. 12, May, pp. 88–118.

Morange, Michel

1998   *A history of molecular biology.* Cambridge, MA: Harvard University Press.

2000   "The developmental gene concept." In Peter J. Beurton, Raphael Falk, and Hans Jörg Rheinberger (eds.). *The concept of the gene in development and evolution: Historical and epistemological perspectives,* pp. 193–219. Cambridge: Cambridge University Press.

2001   *The misunderstood gene.* Cambridge, MA: Harvard University Press.

2002   "The relations between genetics and epigenetics." *Annals of the New York Academy of Sciences,* Vol. 981, No. 1, pp. 50–60.

Moss, Lenny

2003   *What genes can't do.* Cambridge, MA: MIT Press.

Mountcastle, Vernon B.

1978   "An Organizing Principle for Cerebral Function: The Unit Module and the Distributed System." In Gerald Edelman and Vernon B. Mountcastle (eds.). *The mindful brain.* Cambridge, MA: MIT Press.

Musil, Robert

1994   *Der Mann ohne Eigenschaften.* 2 Vols. 1931. Reprint, Hamburg: Rowolth.

Nédélec, S., et al.

2004   "Emx2 homeodomain transcription factor interacts with eukaryotic translation initiation factor 4E (elF4E) in the axons of olfactory sensory neurons." *Proceedings of the National Academy of Sciences of the United States of America,* Vol. 101, No. 29, pp. 10815–10820.

Nédélec, Stéphane, and Alain Trembleau

2005 "Localisation axonale de Emx2: Quand des facteurs de transcription à homéodomaine interfèrent avec la traduction." *Médecine/Sciences,* Vol. 21, No. 3, pp. 237–239.

Nédélec, S., A. Trembleau, and C. Dubacq

2005 "Morphological and molecular features of the mammalian olfactory sensory neuron axons: What makes these axons so special?" *Journal of Neurocytology,* Vol. 34, pp. 49–64.

Nissl, Franz

1903 *Die Neuronenlehre und ihre Anhänger.* Jena, Germany: Verlag von Gustav Fischer.

Nottebohm, Fernando

1985 "Neuronal replacement in adulthood." In Fernando Nottebohm (ed.). *Hope for a new neurology,* pp 143–161. New York: New York Academy of Sciences.

Nussbaum, Martha

1986 *The fragility of goodness. Luck and ethics in Greek tragedy and philosophy.* Cambridge: Cambridge University Press.

1994 *The therapy of desire: Theory and practice in Hellenistic ethics.* Princeton: Princeton University Press.

Nüsslein-Volhard, Christiane

2004 *Das Werden des Lebens: Wie Gene die Entwicklung Steuern.* München: C. H. Beck.

2006 *Coming to life: How genes drive development.* San Diego: Kales Press.

Nüsslein-Volhard, Christiane, and Eric Wieschaus

1980 "Mutations affecting segment number and polarity in Drosophila." *Nature,* Vol. 287, pp. 795–801.

Nyhart, Lynn

1995 *Biology takes form: Animal morphology and the German universities, 1800–1900.* Chicago: University of Chicago Press.

Oese, Erhard

2002 *Geschichte der Hirnforschung: Von der Antike biz zur Gegenwart.* Frankfurt am Main: Primus Verlag.

Oppenheimer, Jane M

1967 *Essays in the history of embryology and biology.* Cambridge, MA: MIT Press.

Ottersen, O. P., and P. J. Helm

2002 "How hardwired is the brain?" *Nature,* Vol. 420, No. 6917, pp. 751–752.

Palade, G. E., and K. R. Porter

1954 "Studies on the endoplasmic reticulum I. Its identification in cells in situ" in: the Journal of Experimental Medicine, Vol. 100, No. 6, pp. 641–656.

Palay, Sanford

1956 "Synapses in the central nervous system," *Journal of Biophysics, Biochemistry, and Cytology,* Vol. 2., Supp., pp. 193–202.

Paperno, Irina
1997   *Suicide as a cultural institution in Dostoevsky's Russia.* Ithaca, NY: Cornell University Press.
Pascual-Leon, Alvaro, et al.
2005   "The plastic human brain cortex." *Annual Review of Neuroscience,* Vol. 28, pp. 377–401.
Passeron, Jean Claude
2006   *La Raisonnement Sociologique.* Paris: Albin Michel.
Passeron, Jean Claude, and Pierre Bourdieu
1964   *Les Héritiers: Les Étudiants et la Culture.* Paris: Les Editions du Minuit.
1990   *Reproduction in education, society, and culture.* New York: Sage Press.
Penfield, Wilder
1950   "The Gordon Wilson Lecture: The mechanism of memory." *Transactions of the American Clinical and Climatological Association,* Vol. 62, pp. 165–169.
1959   "The interpretive cortex." *Science,* Vol. 129, No. 3365, pp. 1719–1725.
Penfield, Wilder, and Herbert Jaspers
1954   *Epilepsy and the functional anatomy of the human brain.* Oxford: Little, Brown and Co.
Penfield, Wilder, and Brenda Milner
1958   "Memory deficit produced by bilateral lesions in the hippocampal zone." *AMA Archives of Neurology and Psychiatry,* Vol. 79, No. 5, pp. 475–497.
Penfield, Wilder, and Theodor Rasmussen
1950   *The cerebral cortex of man: A clinical study of localization of function.* London: Macmillan.
Peyret, Jean François, and Alain Prochiantz
2002   *La Génisse et le Pythagoricien: Traité de Formes I. D'Après Les Métamorphoses d'Ovide.* Paris: Odile Jacob.
2004   *Les Variations Darwin.* Paris: Odile Jacob.
Picard, Jean François
1990   *La République du Savante.* Paris: Flammarion.
Pickering, Andrew
1992   *Science as practice and culture.* Chicago: University of Chicago Press.
2010   *The cybernetic brain: Sketches of another future.* Chicago: University of Chicago Press.
Pinault, Michel
2000   *Frédéric Joliot-Curie.* Paris: Odile Jacob.
Pinch, Trevor
1986   *Confronting nature: The sociology of solar-neutrino detection.* Doderecht, The Netherlands: Reidel.
Pinch, Trevor J., David Gooding, and Simon Schaffer
1989   *The uses of experiment: Studies in the natural sciences.* Cambridge: Cambridge University Press.

Pinsker, H., et al.

1970a "Habituation and dishabituation of the GM-withdrawal reflex in *Aplysia*." *Science*, Vol. 167, No. 3926, pp. 1740–1742.

1970b "The role of synaptic plasticity in the short-term modification of behaviour." In Gabriel Horn, Robert A. Hinde, and King's College Research Centre (eds.). *Short-term changes in neural activity and behavior*, pp. 281–322. Cambridge: Cambridge University Press.

Pitts Taylor, Victoria

2010 "The plastic brain: Neoliberalism and the neuronal self." *Health*, Vol. 14, No. 6, pp. 635–652.

Pohlenz, Max

1948 *Die Stoa: Geschichte einer geistigen Bewegung.* 2. Vols. Göttingen, Germany: Vandenhoeck and Ruprecht.

Polanyi, Michael

1958 *Personal knowledge: Towards a post-critical epistemology.* Chicago: University of Chicago.

Porter, Theodore

1996 *Trust in numbers.* Princeton: Princeton University Press.

2004 *Karl Pearson: The scientific life in a statistical age.* Princeton: Princeton University Press.

Postel-Vinay, Olivier

2002 *Le grand gâchis: Splendeur et misère de la science française.* Paris: Eyrolles.

Prochiantz, Alain

1987 "In vitro regulation of dopaminergic maturation." In Antonia Vernadakis et al.; Institute of Developmental Neuroscience and Aging (eds.). *Model systems of development and aging of the nervous system,* pp. 193–200. Heidelberg: Springer.

1988 *Les Stratégies de l'Embryon,* Paris: P.U.F.

1989 *La construction du cerveau.* Paris: Hachette.

1990 *Claude Bernard: La Révolution Physiologique.* Paris: PUF.

1993 *La Construction du Cerveau.* Paris: Hachette.

1995 *La Biologie dans le Boudoir.* Paris: Odile Jacob.

1997 *Les Anatomies de la Pensees: A Qoui Pense les Calamars.* Paris: Odile Jacob.

2001 *Machine-Esprit.* Paris: Odile Jacob.

2005 "Protein transduction: From physiology to technology and vice versa." *Advanced Drug Delivery Reviews,* Vol. 57, pp. 491–493.

Prochiantz, Alain, and Alain Joliot

2003 "Are Homeoproteins Morphogen?" Unpublished manuscript.

Purkynĕ, Jan Evangelista

1838 "Bericht über die Versammlung deutscher Naturforscher und Ärzte in Prag im September, 1837." *Anatomisch-physiologische Verhandlungen,* Pt. 3, sec. 5/A, pp. 177–180.

Querner, Hans

1977 "Die Entwicklungsmechanik Wilhelm Roux' und ihre Bedeutung in seiner Zeit." In Gunter Mann and Rolf Winau (eds.). *Medizin, Naturwissenschaft, Technik und das Zweite Kaiserreich*, pp. 189–200. Göttingen, Germany: Vandenhoeck and Ruprecht.

Rabbow, Paul

1954 *Seelenführung: Methodik der Exerzitien in der Antike*. Munich: Kösel.

Rabinow, Paul

1989 *French modern: Norms and forms of the social environment*. Chicago: University of Chicago Press.

1996a *Making PCR: A story of biotechnology*. Chicago: University of Chicago Press.

1996b *Essays in the anthropology of reason*. Princeton: Princeton University Press.

1999 *French DNA: Trouble in purgatory*. Chicago: University of Chicago Press.

2003 *Anthropos today: Reflections on modern equipment*. Princeton: Princeton University Press.

2007 *Marking time: On the anthropology of the contemporary*. Princeton: Princeton University Press.

Radcliffe-Brown, Alfred Reginald

1940 "On social structure." *Journal of the Royal Anthropological Institute*, Vol. 70.

1952 "On joking relationships." In Fred Eggan and Edward E. Evans-Pritchard (eds.). *Structure and function in primitive society*, pp. 90–105. New York: Macmillan.

Radkau, Joachim

2005 *Max Weber: Die Leidenschaft des Denkens*. Munich: Carl Hanser Verlag.

Raisman, George

1969 "Neuronal plasticity in the septal nuclei of the adult rat." *Brain Research*, Vol. 14, No. 1, pp. 25–48.

Rakic, Pasko

1985 "Limits of neurogenesis in primates." *Science*, Vol. 227, pp. 1054–1056.

Rakic, Pasko, J. P. Bourgeois, M. F. Eckenhoof, N. Zecevic, P. S. Goldman-Rakic

1986 "Concurrent overproduction of synapses in diverse regions of the primate cerebral cortex." *Science*, Vol. 232, pp. 232–235.

Ramón y Cajal, Santiago

1890 "A quelle époque apparaisent les expansions des cellules nerveuses de la moëlle épinière du poulet?" *Anatomischer Anzeiger*, Vol. 5, pp. 631–639.

1894 "La Fine Structure des Centres Nerveux." *Proceedings of the Royal Society of London*, No. 55, pp. 444–468.

1913 "Contribucion al conocimiento de la neuroglia del cerebro humano." *Trabajos del Laboratorio de Investigaciones Biologicas*, Vol. 11, pp. 255–315.

1991 *Recollections of my life*. 1st ed., Madrid, 1901–1917; reprint, Cambridge, MA: MIT Press.

1995 *Histology of the nervous system of man and vertebrates*. 2 vols. 1st ed., Madrid, 1897–1904; reprint, Oxford: Oxford University Press.

Rees, Tobias

2006   "Plastic reason: An anthropology of the emergence of adult cerebral plasticity in France." Unpublished PhD thesis, Department of Anthropology, University of California, Berkeley.

2010a Being neurologically human today: Life, science, and adult cerebral plasticity (an ethical analysis)." *American Ethnologist,* Vol. 37, No. 1, pp. 150–166.

2010b "To open up new spaces of thought: Anthropology BSC (beyond society and culture)." *Journal of the Royal Anthropological Institute,* Vol. 16, No. 1, pp. 158–163.

2011a "As if theory is the only form of thinking and social theory the only form of critique." *Dialectical Anthropology,* Vol. 35, No. 3, pp. 341–365.

2011b "So plastic a brain: On philosophy, fieldwork in philosophy, and adult cerebral plasticity." *BioSocieties,* Vol. 6, No. 2, pp. 263–267.

2015   "Developmental diseases: An introduction to the neurological human (in motion)." *American Ethnologist,* Vol. 42, No. 1, pp. 161–174.

2016a "On plasticity—or how the brain outgrew its histories." In Delia Gravus and Stephen Casper (eds.) *Technique, technology, and therapy in the brain and mind sciences.* New Brunswick, NJ: Rutgers University Press.

2016b "Once cell death, now cell life: On plasticity and pathology ca. 1800 to 2014." In David Bates and Nima Bassri (eds.). *Plasticity and pathology.* New York: Fordham University Press.

Remak, Robert

1836   "Vorläufige Mittheilung mikroscopischer Beobachtungen über den inneren Bau der Cerebrospinalnerven und über die Entwicklung ihrer Formelemente." *Archiv für Anatomie, Physiologie und Wissenschaftliche Medicin,* pp. 145–161.

1837   "Weitere mikroscopische Beobachtungen über die Primitivfasern des Nervensystems der Wierbelthiere." *Frorieps Neue Notizen,* Vol. 3, pp. 35–40.

1838   *Obervationes anatomicae et microscopicae de systematis nervosa structura.* Berlin: G. E. Reimer.

Renouvin, Pierre, and René Rémond

1967   *Léon Blum, Chef de Gouvernement.* Paris: Armand Colin.

Rheinberger, Hans Jörg

1992a "Experiment, difference, and writing: I. Tracing protein synthesis." *Studies in History and Philosophy of Science, Part A,* Vol. 23, No. 2, pp. 305–331.

1992b "Experiment, difference, and writing: II. The laboratory production of transfer RNA." *Studies in History and Philosophy of Science, Part A,* Vol. 23, No. 3, pp. 389–422.

1993   "Experiment und Orientierung: Frühe Systeme der in vitro Proteinbiosynthese." *NTM International Journal of History and Ethics of Natural Sciences, Technology & Medicine,* Vol. 1, pp. 237–253.

1994   "Experimentalsysteme, Epistemische Dinge, Experimentalkulturen zu einer Epistemologie des Experiments." *Deutsche Zeitschrift für Philosophie,* Vol. 42, No. 3, pp. 405–418.

1996   *Raeume Des Wissens Repraesentation Codierung Spur.* Berlin: Akademie Verlag.

1997   *Toward a history of epistemic things: Synthesizing proteins in the test tube.* Stanford: Stanford University Press.

2001   "Partikel im Zellsaft." In Hagner, Michael (ed.) *Ansichten der Wissenschaftsgeschichte,* pp. 299–337. Frankfurt am Main: Fischer Verlag.

2003   "Script and scribbles." *MLN,* Vol. 118, No. 3, pp. 622–636.

2004   *From molecular genetics to genomics: The mapping cultures of twentieth-century genetics.* New York: Routledge.

2005   *Iterationen.* Berlin: Merve Verlag.

2006   *Epistemologie des Konkreten: Studien zur Geschichte der modernen Biologie.* Frankfurt am Main: Suhrkamp Verlag.

2008   *Von der Unendlichkeit der Ränder: Liechtenstein-Miszellen.* Berlin: Edition Isele.

2010   *On historicizing epistemology.* Stanford: Stanford University Press.

Rheinberger, Hans Jörg, and Michael Hagner

1997   *Räume des Wissens: Repräsentation, Codierung, Spur.* Berlin: Akademie Verlag.

Richards, Robert J.

2004   *The romantic conception of life: Science and philosophy in the age of Goethe.* Chicago: University of Chicago Press.

Riese, Walther

1959   *A history of neurology.* New York: MD Publications.

Ritter, Joachim

1974   *Subjektivität.* Frankfurt am Main: Suhrkamp Verlag.

Rose, Nikolas

2003   "The neurochemical self and its anomalies." In R. Ericson (ed.). *Risk and morality,* pp. 407–437. Toronto: University of Toronto Press.

2007   *The politics of life itself: Biomedicine, power, and subjectivity in the twenty-first century.* Princeton: Princeton University Press.

Rose, Nikolas, and Abi-Rached, Joelle M.

2013   *Neuro: The new brain sciences and the management of the mind.* Princeton: Princeton University Press.

Rubin, Beatrix

2010   "Changing brains: The emergence of the field of adult neurogenesis." *BioSocieties,* Vol. 4 (December), pp. 407–424.

Sapp, Jan

1987   *Beyond the gene: Cytoplasmic inheritance and the struggle for authority in genetics.* Oxford: Oxford University Press.

Scheller, R., et al.

1982 "A Family of genes that codes for ELH: A neuropeptide eliciting a stereo-typed pattern of behavior in *Aplysia.*" *Cell,* April, pp. 707–719.

Schildkraut, Joseph

1965 "The Catecholamine hypothesis of affective disorders: A review of support-ing evidence." *American Journal of Psychiatry,* November, pp. 509–522.

Schnädelbach, Herbert

1984 *Philosophy in Germany, 1831–1933.* Cambridge: Cambridge University Press.

Schwann, Theodor

1839 *Mikroskopische Untersuchungen über die Übereinstimmung in der Struktur und dem Wachsthum der Thiere und Pflanzen.* Berlin: G. E. Reimer.

Schwartz, J. H., and Sharon Begley

2003 *The Mind and the Brain: Neuroplasticity and the Power of Mental Force,* Harper Perennial.

Scoville, W. B., and B. Milner

1957 "Loss of recent memory after bilateral hippocampal lesions." *Journal of Neurology, Neurosurgery, and Psychiatry,* Vol. 20, No. 1, pp. 11–21.

Shapin, Steven

1995 "Here and everywhere: Sociology of scientific knowledge." *Annual Review of Sociology,* Vol. 21, pp. 289–321.

Shapin, Steven, Simon Schaffer, and Thomas Hobbes

1985 *Leviathan and the air-pump: Hobbes, Boyle, and the experimental life.* Princeton: Princeton University Press.

Shepherd, Gordon

1991 *Foundations of the neuron doctrine.* Oxford: Oxford University Press.

2004 *The synaptic organization of the brain.* 5th ed. Oxford: Oxford University Press.

2010 *Creating modern neuroscience: The revolutionary 1950s.* Oxford: Oxford University Press.

Sherrington, Charles Scott

1899 "Experiments on the value of vascular and visceral factors for the genesis of emotion." *Proceedings of the Royal Society of London,* Vol. 66, No. 424–433, pp. 390–403.

1906 *The integrative action of the nervous system.* Silliman Lectures, 1904. New Haven: Yale University Press.

1909 "On plastic tonus and proprioceptive reflexes." *Quarterly Journal of Experi-mental Physiology,* Vol. 2, No. 2, pp. 109–156.

Simmel, Georg

1896 "Friedrich Nietzsche: Eine moralphilosophische Silhouette," *Zeitschrift für Philosophie und philosophische Kritik,* Vol. 107, pp. 202–215.

1995 *Schopenhauer und Nietzsche.* 1907. Reprint, Champaign: University of Illinois Press.

Skinner, B. F.

1938 *The behavior of organisms as experimental analysis.* New York: D. Apple-ton–Century Co.

Spatazza, J., et al.

2012 "Otx2 binding to perineuronal nets persistently regulates plasticity in the mature visual cortex." *Journal of Neuroscience,* Vol. 32, No. 27, pp. 9429–9437.

2013a "Choroid-plexus-derived Otx2 homeoprotein constrains adult cortical plasticity." *Cell Reports,* Vol. 3, No.6, pp. 1815–1823.

2013b "Homeoprotein signaling in development, health, and disease: A shaking of dogmas offers challenges and promises from bench to bed." *Pharmacological Reviews,* Vol. 65, No. 1, pp. 90–104.

Spemann, Hans

1903 "Entwickelungsphysiologische Studien am Triton-Ei." *Archiv für Entwicklungsmechanik der Organismen,* October 6, pp. 551–631.

1936 *Embryonic development and induction.* New Haven: Yale University Press.

Specter, Michael

2001 "Rethinking the brain: How the songs of canaries upset a fundamental principle of science." *New Yorker,* July 23, pp. 42–53.

Squire, Larry, and Eric Kandel

1999 *Memory: From mind to molecule.* New York: Scientific American Library.

Stahnisch, Frank W., and Robert Nitsch

2002 "Santiago Ramon y Cajal's concept of neuronal plasticity: The ambiguity lives on." *TRENDS in Neurosciences,* Vol. 25, No. 11, pp. 589–591.

2003 "Making the brain plastic: Early neuroanatomical staining techniques and the pursuit of structural plasticity, 1910–1970." *Journal of the History of the Neurosciences,* Vol. 12, No. 4, pp. 413–435.

Stent, Gunther

1985 "Thinking in one dimension: The impact of molecular biology on development." *Cell,* Vol. 40, No. 1, pp. 1–2.

Stepanyants, A., P. R. Hof, and D. B. Chklovskii

2002 "Geometry and structural plasticity of synaptic connectivity." *Neuron,* Vol. 34, pp. 275–288.

Stern, Curt

1967 *Richard Benedict Goldschmidt, 1878–1958: A biographical memoir.* New York: Columbia University Press.

Stöhr, Philipp

1957 *Handbuch der mikroskopischen Anatomie des Menschen.* Heidelberg: Springer.

Strathern, Marilyn

1972. *Women in Between.* London and New York: Seminar Press.

1988 *The gender of the gift: Problems with women and problems with society in Melanesia.* Berkeley: University of California Press.

1992. *After Nature: English Kinship in the Late Twentieth Century.* Cambridge: Cambridge University Press.

1995. *The Relation.* Chicago: Prickly Pear Press.

1999 *Property, substance, and effect: Anthropological essays on persons and things.* London: Athlone Press.

2004　*Commons and Borderlands: Working Papers on Interdisciplinarity, Accountability and the Flow of Knowledge.* Herfordshire: Sean Kingston Publishing.

2005　*Kinship, Law and the Unexpected: Relatives are Always a Surprise.* Cambridge: Cambridge University Press.

2006　"A community of critics? Thoughts on new knowledge." *Journal of the Royal Anthropological Institute,* Vol. 12, No. 1, pp. 191–209.

Striker, Gisela

1996　"Emotions in context: Aristotle's treatment of the passions in the rhetoric and his moral psychology." In Amélie Rorty (ed.). *Essays on Aristotle's rhetoric,* pp. 286–302. Berkeley: University of California Press.

Sugiyama, Sayaka, et al.

2008　"Experience-dependent transfer of Otx2 homeoprotein into the visual cortex activates postnatal plasticity." *Cell,* Vol. 134, No. 3, pp. 508–520.

2009　"Adult neurogenesis modulates the hippocampus-dependent period of associate fear memory." *Cell,* Vol. 139, No. 4, pp. 814–827.

Svoboda, Karel

2011　"The past, present, and future of single neuron reconstruction." *Neuroinformatics,* Vol. 9, No. 2, pp. 97–98.

Tansey, E. M.

1997　"Not committing barbarisms: Sherrington and the synapse, 1897." *Brain Research Bulletin,* Vol. 44, No. 3, pp. 211–212.

Tauc, L., and E. R. Kandel.

1964　"An anomalous form of rectification in a molluscan central neurone." *Nature,* Vol. 202, pp. 1339–1342.

Thompson, D'Arcy Wentworth

1917　*Growth and form.* 1st ed. Cambridge: Cambridge University Press.

1942　*Growth and form.* 2nd, enlarged ed. Cambridge: Cambridge University Press.

Trachtenberg, J. T., et al.

2002　"Long-term *in vivo* imaging of experience-dependent synaptic plasticity in adult cortex." *Nature,* Vol. 420, pp. 788–794.

Traweek, Sharon

1992　*Beamtimes and lifetimes: The world of high energy physics.* Cambridge, MA: Harvard University Press.

Turing, Alan

1936　"On computable numbers, with an application to the Entscheidungsproblem," Proc. London Mathematical Society, ser. 2, 42: 230–265.

1938　"On computable numbers, with an application to the *Entscheidungsproblem:* A correction." *Proceedings of the London Mathematical Society,* Vol. 2, No. 1, pp. 544–546.

1952　"The chemical basis of morphogenesis." *Philosophical Transactions of the Royal Society of London,* Vol. B237, 37–72.

Uskoff, N.

1882   "Zur Bedeutung der Karyokinese." *Archiv für mikroskopische Anatomie,* Vol. 21, pp. 291–295.

Valenstein, Elliot

2006   *The war of the soups and the sparks: The discovery of neurotransmitters and the dispute over how nerves communicate.* New York: Columbia University Press.

Van der Loos

1967   "The History of the Neuron." In H. Hydén (ed.). *The Neuron,* pp. 1–47. Amsterdam: Elsevier.

Virchow, Rudolf von

1846   "Über das granulierte Aussehen der Wandungen des Gehirnvenrtikels." *Zeitschrift für Psychiatrie,* Heft 2, pp. 242ff.

Vogt, Oskar, and Cecile Vogt

1907   *Zur Kenntnis der elektrisch-erregbaren Hinrrinden-Gebiete bei den Säugetieren.* Leipzig, Germany: Johann Ambrosius Barth.

1919a   *Allgemeine Ergebnisse unserer Hirnforschung.* Leipzig, Germany: Johann Ambrosius Barth.

1922   *Erkrankungen der Grosshirnrinde im Lichte der Topistik, Pathoklise und Pathoarchitektonik.* Leipzig, Germany: Johann Ambrosius Barth.

1926   *Die vergeleichend-architektonisce und die vergleichend-reisphysiologische Felderung der Großhirnrinde unter besonderer Berüksichtigung der menschlichen.* Berlin: Julius Springer.

1951   "Importance of neuroanatomy in the field of neuropathology." *Neurology,* Vol. 1, pp. 205–218.

Von Neumann, John

1951   "The general and logical theory of automata." In L. A. Jeffress (ed.). *Cerebral Mechanisms in Behavior: The Hixon Symposium,* pp. 1–31. New York: John Wiley and Sons.

Waddington, Conrad

1939   "Genes as evocators in development." *Growth,* supp. 1, pp. 37–44.

1947   *Organizers and genes.* Cambridge: Cambridge University Press.

Waddington, Conrad, J. Needham, W. Nowinski, and R. Lemberg

1935   "Studies on the nature of amphibian organization centre I: Chemical properties of the evocator." *Proceedings of the Royal Society of London,* Vol. B117, pp. 289–310.

Waldeyer-Hartz, Wilhelm

1891   "Über einige neuere Forschungen im Gebiete der Anatomie des Central-nervensystems." *Deutsche Medizinische Wochenschrift,* Vol. 17, pp. 1213–1218, 1244–1246, 1287–1289, 1331–1332, 1350–1356.

Watson, John B.

1913   "Psychology as the behaviorist views it." *Psychological Review,* Vol. 20, No. 2, pp. 158.

Weber, Max

   1918   "Science as Vocation." Lecture, Munich University.

   1958   *From Max Weber: Essays in Sociology.* Ed. H. H. Gerth & C. Wright Mills. New York: Oxford University Press.

   1968   *Gesammelte Aufsätze zur Wissenschaftslehre,* ed. Johannes Winckelmann. Tübingen. Germany: J. C. B. Mohr Verlag.

Wiener, Norbert

   1948   *Cybernetics or Control and Communication in the Animal and the Machine*

Wieschaus, Eric

   1995   "From molecular patterns to morphogenesis the lessons from drosophila." Nobel Lecture, December 8. Nobelprize.org. http://www.nobelprize.org /nobel_prizes/medicine/laureates/1995/wieschaus-lecture.html. Last accessed August 15, 2015.

Wiesel, Torsten

   1981   "The post-natal development of the visual cortex." Nobel Lecture, December 8. Nobelprize.org. http://nobelprize.org/nobel_prizes/ medicine /laureates/1981/wiesel-lecture.html. Last accessed August 23, 2015.

Williams, Bernard

   1985   *Ethics and the limits of philosophy.* Cambridge, MA: Harvard University Press.

Young, Allan

   1995   *The Harmony of illusions: Inventing Post-Traumatic Stress Disorder.* Princeton: Princeton University Press.

   2011   "Empathy, evolution, and human nature." In J. Decety, D. Zahavi, and S. Overgaard (eds.). *Empathy: From bench to bedside,* pp. 21–37. Cambridge, MA: MIT Press.

Young, J. Z.

   1951   "Growth and plasticity in the nervous system." *Proceedings of the Royal Society of London,* Series B, containing papers of a biological character, Vol. 139, No. 894, pp. 18–37.

Young, Robert

   1970   *Mind, brain, and adaptation in the nineteenth century.* Oxford: Oxford University Press.

Yu, Sien-Chiue

   1949   "A genetic and cytological study of some X-ray induced mutations and reverse mutations in Drosophila melanogaster." PhD dissertation, California Institute of Technology.

Zecevic, N., J. P. Bourgeois, and P. Rakic

   1989   "Changes in synaptic density in motor cortex of rhesus monkey during fetal and postnatal life." *Developmental Brain Research,* Vol. 50, pp. 11–32.

Zito, Karen, and Karel Svoboda

   2002   "Activity-dependent synaptogenesis in the adult mammalian cortex." *Neuron,* Vol. 35, pp. 1015–1017.

INDEX

actualization, 117, 147, 158, 159, 177, 179, 245n7, 268n5
Adrian, Edgar, 73–74, 80, 191, 205–7, 250n42, 251–52n52, 278n30
affiliation, 22, 26, 37, 239n10
algorithm, 208–10
Allinquat, Bernadette, 161–62, 171–72, 224
Altmann, Richard, 64–65, 215
amino acid, xvi, 34, 43–44, 152, 155, 165, 215
anatomy, 59, 61, 63, 66, 68, 74, 77, 86, 88, 92, 93, 110–12, 185, 239n14, 247n20, 249nn27,29; neuroanatomy, 42, 217; plastic, 185–89
animal, 59–61, 65–66, 68, 71–72, 76, 78, 84–85, 87, 109–11, 116, 131, 150, 152, 182, 183, 185, 187, 237n2, 246n2, 248n26, 254n75, 263n16, 265n46, 266n52, 272n1, 277n20
antennapedia, 11–13, 34, 38, 44, 51, 99, 150, 238n2
anthropology, xvii 4, 8–9, 36, 59, 97, 133, 134, 143, 145, 147–148, 191, 195, 225, 245n15, 266nn66,67, 268n1, 273n3, 275n7, 278n31; of knowledge, 7; of reason xiii, 24; relational, 23–24; of science, 269n16, 273n3; of thought, 7
anti-human hemagglutinin (HA), 166, 168, 170
Apáthy, István, 73, 250n41
ape, 133
Aplysia California, 84–85, 87, 254n70
arborization, 70, 93, 199, 201–02, 203
Aristapedia, 117–18

Aristotle, 122
art, 17, 45–48, 51, 53, 58, 106, 149, 243n53, 268n3, 271n19; plastic, 186, 188–89
Ascher, Philippe, 191–97, 207, 213, 218–20, 278n30
Ashby, Ross, 208, 276n21, 278n30
assembly, 71, 79–80, 89

Baer, Karl Ernst von, 27, 247n21
Bayle, Pierre, 227
beauty, 1, 3, 8, 10, 31, 36, 96, 99–100, 155, 228, 236n13
Becquerel, Henri, 16
Bergson, Henri, 34, 140, 234, 264n29, 274n3
Bernard, Claude, 3, 40, 46, 104–5, 108–14, 116, 118, 120–22, 130, 134–35, 140, 188, 224, 235nn1,8, 238n3, 264n29, 271n19, 272n23, 274n3
Bethe, Albrecht, 73, 250n41
Bichat, Xavier, 110
biogenetic law, 131, 187, 266n58, 273n5
biotechnology, 3–4, 8, 87, 192, 196, 235n2
bird, 36, 48, 65, 100, 122, 246n1, 255nn77,83,
blastula, 188–89
Bliss, Tim, 85–86, 93, 254n75, 260n23
Blum, Leon, 18–19, 238n5
bodily enactment, 194–95
Bolk, Louis, 133
boundary object, 243n52
Bourgeois, Jean Pierre, 59, 198, 246nn1,3, 255n83

315

brain: as locus of the human, 8, 63,
function-specific anatomy, 68, 74, 83,
214, 249n27, 255n81; electric, 71, 75,
205–7; neuronal, 88, 93, 207–8, 213,
218; oceanography, 89, 93; plastic,
xii-xiii, 38, 46, 50, ,53, 61, 90, 91–94,
101, 108, 135, 141, 244n63, 255n77,
255–56n83, 259n18, 278n29, 279n1;
regions, 34, 68, 145, 150, 154–56, 183,
202, 221
Bremer, Frédéric, 75
Brodmann, Korbinian, 74, 201–203,
275n15
Buffon, Georges-Louis Leclerc de, 122
Buylla, Arturo Alvarez, 243n60, 255n83

Cahier des Note, 104, 112
Canguilhem, Georges, 26, 55, 91–94,
137–41, 235n4, 240n17, 257nn3,4,
267n1, 267n2
Cartesian subject, 180, 258n16
cat, 65
Cavaillès, Jean, 139, 268n2
cDNA, 164–165, 168
cell-permeable peptides (CPPs), 44–45,
48, 50, 242n44
cell-to-cell sliding, 5–7, 13, 214
Chamak, Brigitte, 263n14
Changeux, Jean Pierre, 32, 45, 53, 59, 192,
213–14, 243n60, 244n63, 246n3, 273n2
Chapeville, François, 42
chemistry, xv, 16, 18, 25–26, 28, 30, 32–33,
37, 43, 109–12, 117, 119, 124, 128–29,
134, 139, 145, 152–53, 172, 215, 239n14,
246n5, 263n12, 267n1, 277–78n28;
immunocyto, 145, 170; neuro, xii, xxii,
8, 24–25, 30, 33, 36–37, 40, 44, 50,
60–62, 74–77, 81–89, 91, 193–95, 197,
199, 209–12, 213, 217, 250n42, 253n55,
258n18, 260n23, 277nn25,26, 278n30
Chesselden, William, 228
chicken, 27, 29, 65, 163–164
Cole, Jack, 228
collaboration, 6, 44, 47, 50, 52–53, 98, 169,
179, 224, 242n44, 243nn61,62, 252n52
Collège de France, 18, 20, 22, 24, 33–34,
40, 52–53, 55, 105, 109, 135, 183, 223,
244n63

computer, 87, 89, 119, 168–69, 195, 207–
211, 217, 273n1, 276nn18,19
concept: epistemological, 140; space, 112;
work, 137, 139–41, 255n77; vital, 137–41
Confocal, 145–146, 170, 172–173, 267n69,
270n18
constriction experiment, 115, 189
contiguity, 65, 69, 73, 76, 90, 91, 251n51
Cooper, Anthony Ashley, 228
CORA, 208
cortex, 50, 59–61, 68–69, 82–83, 86–87,
193, 201, 202, 204, 208, 225, 233, 246n1,
249nn27,29, 254n74, 255n81, 256n83,
276n15
COS cells, 146, 152, 160, 170–74, 176
counterhomeoprotein, 121
creativity, 118, 138, 146, 148, 151, 178
Crick, Francis, 213–14
critique, 32, 51–52, 62, 78, 92, 103, 110, 119,
137, 167, 236n9, 238n6, 240n25, 252n52,
255n81, 277n26, 279n34
Cudworth, Ralph, 227
cultivation, 200, 201, 203, 209
culture, 23, 36, 56, 60, 136, 167–70, 174,
178, 236n14, 237n16, 273–4n3; cell, 1, 5,
25, 34, 36, 38, 48, 96, 105, 144, 145, 160,
170, 172, 214, 235n1, 240n16, 273n1
Curie, Ève, 17–18, 238n2
Curie, Irène, 17–21, 238n4
Curie, Pierre, 16–17, 21
cybernetics, xii, 198, 207–10, 217,
276nn20,21, 277n23
cyclotron, 19, 56
cytoarchitecture, 198, 201–205, 275n14,
277n28
cytoplasm, 6, 43–44, 240n19

d'Alambert, Jean le Rond, 227
Dale, Henri, 75, 250n42, 251n51,
251–252n52
Darwin, Charles, 128, 228, 266n58
de Beer, Gavin, 28–29, 31, 47, 108, 122,
130–34, 187–88, 266nnn55,58,59, 272n23
de Condillac, Étienne Bonnot, 228
De Robertis, Eduardo, 76, 79
dead, 110–111, 195, 264n35
decontextualization, 108, 121
della Mirandola, Pico, 227

form 9–10, 13, 29–30, 47, 122–23, 134, 202,
   215, 233, 256; and growth, 1, 26, 30, 123;
   in motion, 1, 13, 48, 233, 243
form/event, 48, 243n55
Fortes, Meyer, 239n11
Foucault, Michel, 244n2, 273n3, 275n7
France, 3–4, 6–8, 18–21, 23, 24, 32, 37, 42,
   45, 48, 52, 53, 55, 74, 169, 191, 195, 235n2,
   238n7, 239n14, 240n29, 243n60,
   244nnn62,63,2, 247n10, 249n27,
   258n10, 273n2, 274n3, 278n32
Frazzotta, Gianfranco, 145–46, 149–51,
   156–81, 194, 223, 270n18
Frenchness, 170, 178
Freud, Sigmund, 228
function, 29, 34, 74, 202
functional anatomy, 88, 247n20
functional magnetic resonance imagine
   (fMRI), 87–89

Gadamer, Hans-Georg, 274n3
Gage, Fred, 49, 219, 231–33, 236n12,
   243nn58,61, 255n83, 261n23
Gall, Franz Josef, xviii, 247n9, 248n27, 266n66
Gehring, Walter, 12–13, 30–31, 37–38, 238n4
genetics, xvi, 11, 28, 31, 32, 37, 43, 86–88,
   117–18, 123, 127, 129–32, 212–15, 238n2,
   240n26, 260n23, 264n43
Germany, 22, 52, 63, 74, 92, 126–27, 196,
   201, 209, 228, 247n14, 249n27, 251n49,
   273–74n3
global, 74, 77, 178, 211, 224, 279n1
Glowinski, Jacques, 24–25, 30, 33, 36, 44,
   52–53, 239n14, 240n15
Gödel, Kurt, 207
Goldschmidt, Richard, 108, 122, 126–30,
   132, 134, 264nn41,44, 265n46, 266n52,
   272n23
Goltz, Friedrich, 68, 248n27
Goridis, Christo, 193, 278n30
Gould, Elizabeth, 49, 219, 243n58, 255n83,
   262n23
Gould, Stephen Jay, 264n29, 265n44
Grundfest, Harry, 82
gypsy moth, 127, 132

Haller, Albert von, 26–27
Harrison, Ross Granville, 26–27, 114, 188

Hebb, Donald, 77–78, 80–82, 86, 93,
   253nn60,62, 256n83, 260–61n23, 277n23
Heidegger, Martin, 273n3
Held, Hans, 73, 250n41
Hensch,Takao, 225
Herder, Johan Gottfried, 205, 228
heroic, 218–219, 253n62, 278n33
heterochrony, 132–34, 266nn58,59
hippocampus, 50, 61, 82, 83–87, 156, 183,
   193, 246n1, 254nnn74,75,77, 255n83,
   260n23, 269n11
His, Wilhelm, 26–27, 64–65, 185–88, 199,
   228, 247n14, 264n29, 272–73n4,
   273nn6,8, 275n8
histology, 6, 64, 66, 71, 73–74, 77, 86, 93,
   198, 200, 202, 205, 209, 211, 215, 219,
   247nn10,19, 248n25, 251n47, 276n15,
   277n28
history of science, 55, 58, 91, 150, 185, 191,
   244n4, 267n1
history of truth, 91–94, 148
Hitler, Adolf, 127
Hodgkin, Alan, 75, 251–52n52
homeobox, xvi, 12–13, 30–31, 37–39, 118,
   154, 269n9
homeodomain, xvi, 12, 34, 39, 43, 152–153,
   155, 157, 183, 269n9
homeoproteins, xvi-xviii, 5–7, 9, 12–13,
   15–16, 21, 31–52, 60, 62, 90, 98–101,
   106o109, 111, 113, 114, 116, 118, 120,
   124–126, 129–130, 133–135, 141, 145,
   150–160, 171, 176, 183, 193, 198, 217, 219,
   221- 224, 231, 235n6, 239n10, 241n43,
   242nn45,49, 243n52, 244n62, 245n14,
   256n83, 268n4, 268n8, 277n28
Homeostat, 208
homeotic genes, xvi, 5, 11–13, 26, 30–39, 46,
   116, 118, 129, 134, 241n28
human science, 228
humanity, xii-xiii, xvii-xviii, 2, 8, 22,
   59–64, 67, 71, 81, 88–90, 134, 187,
   197–99, 201–20, 229, 277n23, 278n31,
   279n34
Hume, David, 180
humility, 221–22
Husserl, Edumd, 180
Huxley, Andrew, 28–29, 31, 47, 75, 251–
   52n52, 266n55

Morgan, Thomas Hunt, 28, 117, 127–28, 132, 238n2, 240n26, 264n41,44
morphogen, 119–20, 122, 129, 153–54, 156–58, 183, 268n9
morphogenesis, 5, 9, 13, 33–35, 38, 42, 61, 90, 101, 124, 126, 128–29, 135, 154, 160, 176, 217–18, 268n4
morphology, 38, 64–65, 74, 77, 92, 122, 123–24, 130, 201, 203–4, 211, 228, 257n2, 264n29, 266n59
Muller, Herman, 28
mutation, xiii, xvi, 11–13, 118, 123–24, 128–30, 132, 134, 155, 237n1, 238n2 264n35, 265nn44,50, 265n52, 278n31; conceptual, xviii, xix, 53, 89, 140–41, 198, 206, 207, 209, 215, 217; macro, 128–29; of possiblity, 98, 121, 136, 138, 140
Myc, 166–68

native point of view, 15, 23, 245n15
nativism, 55–58, 245n15
Nédélec, Stéphane, 15, 223, 238n1
Needham, Dorothy, 117
Needham, Joseph, 117
neoliberalism, 236–37n14
neotenous. *See* plastic
nerve fibers, 65, 259n23
nervous machine, 192, 194
nervous reaction, 72, 79, 86, 256n83
nervous system, xi-xv, 4–7, 13, 21, 32, 37–38, 46, 49, 52, 59–90, 93, 98–99, 119, 121, 135, 156, 177, 182, 192, 198–199, 205, 208, 219, 232, 239n14, 242n49, 247n14, 248n26, 249n32, 250nnn38,39,41, 251nn47,51, 253n62, 257n9, 259nn18,23, 268n8
neurogenesis, xv-xvi, 7, 48–50, 61, 135, 156, 183, 193, 215, 232–33, 243nn60,61, 246nn1,8, 255nn77,83, 260–61n23
neurological human, 196–220, 275n9, 278nn30,31, 279n34
neuronal network, 88
neuron, xv-xviii, 2fig,60–61, 66–70, 76; circuit, xii, 80, 83, 193, 259n23; culture, 25, 36, 96, 105, 145, 170; doctrine, 66, 73; tree, xii, 65, 67, 200–201
neuropharmacology. *See* pharmacology

neurotransmitter, xii, xv, 76, 82, 87, 211, 213–15, 218, 244n63, 277n24, 277–78n28, 278n30
newt, 114, 116–17, 188
Nietzsche, Friedrich, 228, 275n7
Nissl staining, 73, 202
Nissl, Franz, 73, 202, 250n41
Nobel Prize, 16, 18, 24, 66, 273n2
Nobel, Alfred, 228
nocturnal 96–135, 140, 153–54, 197, 224, 262nn4,5, 274n6; grounds, 96–97, 103, 267
nonautonomous transfer (n-a-t), 37–40, 42, 45, 47–48, 50–52, 60, 62, 90, 101, 106, 108, 111, 114, 120–21, 126, 129–30, 133–34, 141, 144–45, 152–6, 158, 163, 168, 172, 176, 182–83, 198, 217, 223–25, 233, 245n14, 256n83, 279n1
Nottebohm, Fernando, 48–49, 219, 255n83
nucleus, 5–6, 34, 38, 43–45, 70, 95, 99, 238n1

olfactory bulb, 156, 193, 246n1
On Growth and Form, 122–24
ontogeny, 131, 265n47, 266n54
ontology, 148, 245n15
openness, 8, 59, 196, 217, 271n19
organizer, 116–18, 120, 122, 154, 264nn18,19, 272n23
Otx2, 183, 225

paedomorphosis, 132–33, 266n59
Palade, George, 76
Palay, Sanford, 76, 79
Pander, Christian Heinrich, 27
pAntp, 34–36, 38–39, 43, 45, 241n41
Pax2, 156–58, 182, 269nn10,12,
Pax6, 52, 145–46, 150–51, 156–83, 268nnn2,9,10 269n12, 271nn22,23
pellet. *See* western blot
Penetratin, 44, 51, 173, 175, 241n41, 242nn44,45
Penfield, Wilder, 75, 82–83, 254n68
peptide, 34, 38–39, 44, 145, 152, 154–55, 157, 161, 163–66; mini, 155–56, 158, 165, 183
perspectivism, 148, 151, 158, 175, 177, 268n5
Petri dish, 1, 30–31, 34, 99, 152, 154, 170, 273n1

Waddington, Conrad Hal, 108, 117–22, 134

Waldeyer, Wilhelm, 66, 198, 247n19

Walter, W. Grey, 208, 278n30

Watson, John, 78

wax, 185–89, 227, 272nn1,3

Webb, Charles, 228

Weber, Max, 191, 228, 273–74n3, 275n7

Weiss, Sam, 231

Wells, Herbert George, 228

western blot, 160–68

Wiedersheim, Robert, 92–93, 257n10, 259nn19,22

Wiener, Norbert, 208, 276n20

window making, 144–51, 271n19

window. *See* window making

Wolff, Caspar Friedrich, 26–28

work: bench, 25, 145, 147–148, 150–51, 158; construction, 150–51, 158–59, 175–76, 224, 271n19; field, xi-xiii, 1, 3–5, 8–10, 237nnn15,16,17; nocturnal, 97–98, 102–8, 118, 120–22, 126, 135–41, 148, 180, 197, 262n5, 263n6, 264n28, 267n69, 272n23, 275n6, 279n2; technical, 105, 147, 151, 174, 178

writing, 103–07, 121, 221, 237n17, 263n6

Yu, Sien-chiue, 11, 238n2

Zamecnik, Paul, 269n15

zebra fish, 182–85, 189,

Ziegler, Adolf, 186–88